# Prostate Cancer

Diagnosis and clinical management

# Prostate Cancer

Diagnosis and clinical management

EDITED BY

## Ashutosh K. Tewari M.D., M.Ch.

Ronald P. Lynch Professor of Urologic-Oncology
Director
Center for Prostate Cancer
Weill Cornell Medical College and New York Presbyterian Hospital
Director
LeFrak Center of Robotic Surgery, NYPH
Weill Cornell Medical College
New York Presbyterian Hospital
New York, USA

## Peter Whelan MS, FRCS

Community Urologist, Leeds, UK
Emeritus Consultant Urological Surgeon
Pyrah Department of Urology
St. James's University Hospital
Leeds, UK

## John D. Graham FRCP, FRCR

Consultant in Clinical Oncology
Beacon Centre
Musgrove Park Hospital
Taunton
Somerset, UK
Director, National Collaborating Centre for Cancer
Cardiff, UK

WILEY Blackwell

This edition first published 2014 © 2014 by John Wiley & Sons, Ltd.

*Registered office:* John Wiley & Sons, Ltd, The Atrium, Southern Gate, Chichester,
West Sussex, PO19 8SQ, UK

*Editorial offices:* 9600 Garsington Road, Oxford, OX4 2DQ, UK
The Atrium, Southern Gate, Chichester, West Sussex, PO19 8SQ, UK
111 River Street, Hoboken, NJ 07030-5774, USA

For details of our global editorial offices, for customer services and for information about how to apply for permission to reuse the copyright material in this book please see our website at
www.wiley.com/wiley-blackwell

The right of the author to be identified as the author of this work has been asserted in accordance with the UK Copyright, Designs and Patents Act 1988.

*Library of Congress Cataloging-in-Publication Data*

Prostate cancer (Tewari)
    Prostate cancer : diagnosis and clinical management / edited by Ashutosh K. Tewari,
Peter Whelan, John Graham.
        p.  ;  cm.
    Includes bibliographical references and index.
    ISBN 978-1-118-34735-5 (pbk.)
    I. Tewari, Ashutosh, editor of compilation.   II. Whelan, Peter, 1947– editor of compilation.
III. Graham, John, 1955– editor of compilation.   IV. Title.
    [DNLM: 1. Prostatic Neoplasms–diagnosis.   2. Prostatic Neoplasms–therapy.
3. Patient Care Management.   4. Prostate–pathology.   5. Prostate–surgery. WJ 762]
    RC280.P7
    616.99′463–dc23                                                    2013034289

A catalogue record for this book is available from the British Library.

Wiley also publishes its books in a variety of electronic formats. Some content that appears in print may not be available in electronic books.

Cover image: back drop © author Ch 03; inserts © author Ch 05
Cover design by Meaden Creative

Set in 9.5/13pt Meridien by Aptara Inc., New Delhi, India
Printed and bound in Singapore by Markono Print Media Pte Ltd

1   2014

# Contents

*Color plate section can be found facing page 148*

# Contributors

**Hashim U. Ahmed, FRCS(Urol.), BM, BCh, BA(Hons.)**
MRC Clinician Scientist and Clinical Lecturer in Urology
Division of Surgery and Interventional Science, University College London, London, UK; *and*
Department of Urology,
University College London Hospitals NHS Foundation Trust, London, UK

**Adnan Ali, MBBS**
Clinical Research Fellow
Center for Prostate Cancer,
Weill Cornell Medical College,
New York Presbyterian Hospital,
New York, NY, USA

**Anastasios Anastasiadis, MD, FEBU**
Fellow in Endourology and Laparoscopy
Clinical Research Fellow
EAU Section of Uro-Technology (ESUT),
Academic Medical Center
Amsterdam, The Netherlands

**Manit Arya, MBChB, MD(Res), FRCS(Glas), FRCS(Urol)**
Consultant Urological Surgeon
Department of Urology,
University College London Hospitals NHS Foundation Trust,
London, UK; *and*
Barts Cancer Institute,
Queen Mary University London,
London, UK

**Diletta Bianchini, MD**
Specialist Oncologist
Prostate Cancer Targeted Therapy Group and Drug Development Unit,
The Royal Marsden NHS Foundation Trust and The Institute of Cancer Research,
Surrey, UK

**L. Boccon-Gibod, MD**
Former Chairman and former head of surgery
Department of Urology,
CHU Bichat,
Paris, France

**Philippa J. Cheetham, MD**
Attending Urologist
Department of Urology,
Winthrop University Hospital,
New York, NY, USA

**J. Conibear, MBBCh, BSc, MSc, MRCP, FRCR**
Clinical Oncology Specialist Registrar
Mount Vernon Cancer Center,
Middlesex, UK

**Ernesto R. Cordeiro, MD, FEBU**
Fellow in Endourology and Laparoscopy
Clinical Research Fellow
Endourological Society,
Academic Medical Center,
Amsterdam, The Netherlands

**William Richard Cross, BMedSci, BMBS, FRCS(Urol.), PhD**
Consultant Urological Surgeon
Department of Urology,
St. James's University Hospital,
Leeds Teaching Hospitals NHS Trust,
Leeds, UK

**Annie Darves**
Medical Student
Stony Brook University and Winthrop University Hospital, New York

**Johann de Bono, MD, FRCP, MSc, PhD, FMedSci**
Professor of Experimental Cancer Medicine
Prostate Cancer Targeted Therapy Group and
Drug Development Unit,
The Royal Marsden NHS Foundation Trust and
The Institute of Cancer Research,
Surrey, UK

**Jean J.M.C.H. de la Rosette, MD, PhD**
Chairman Department of Urology
Chairman Clinical Research Office
Endourology Society
Executive Board Member Société
Internationale d'Urologie
Academic Medical Center,
Amsterdam, The Netherlands

**Theo M. de Reijke, MD, PhD, FEBU**
Senior Staff Urology Department
Academic Medical Center,
Amsterdam, The Netherlands

**Harveer Dev MA, MB BChir, MRCS**
NIHR Academic Clinical Fellow in Urology
Cambridge
University Hospitals NHS Foundation Trust
Cancer, Research UK Cambridge,
Institute Cambridge Biomedical Campus
Cambridge, UK

**Mark Emberton, FRCS(Urol.), FRCS(Eng.), MD, MBBS, BSc**
Professor of Urology and Director, Honorary
Consultant Urologist
Division of Surgery and Interventional Science,
University College London, London, UK; *and*
Department of Urology,
University College London Hospitals NHS
Foundation Trust,
London, UK

**John D. Graham, FRCP, FRCR**
Consultant in Clinical Oncology
Beacon Centre,
Musgrove Park Hospital,
Taunton,
Somerset, UK; *and*
Director, National Collaborating Centre for
Cancer,
Cardiff, UK

**P. J. Hoskin, MD, FRCP, FRCR**
Consultant in Clinical Oncology
Mount Vernon Cancer Centre
Northwood UK; *and*
Professor in Clinical Oncology
University College London

**Aaron Katz, M.D.**
Chairman of Department of Urology
Winthrop University Hospital, New York

**Frederic Lecouvet, MD, PhD**
Division of Radiology,
Cliniques universitaires Saint Luc,
Institut de Recherche Clinique,
Université catholique de Louvain,
Brussels, Belgium

**Norman Maitland, PhD**
YCR Professor of Molecular Biology and
Director
Department of Biology,
YCR Cancer Research Unit,
University of York,
York, UK

**Aurelius Omlin, MD**
Clinical Research Fellow
Prostate Cancer Targeted Therapy Group and
Drug Development Unit,
The Royal Marsden NHS Foundation Trust and
The Institute of Cancer Research,
Surrey, UK

**Jon Oxley, BSc, MD, FRCPath**
Consultant in Cellular Pathology
Southmead Hospital,
North Bristol NHS Trust,
Bristol, UK

**Joe Park**
Medical Student
Stony Brook University and Winthrop
University Hospital, New York

**Carmel Pezaro, MBChB, FRACP, DMedSc**
Clinical Research Fellow
Prostate Cancer Targeted Therapy Group and
Drug Development Unit,
The Royal Marsden NHS Foundation Trust and
The Institute of Cancer Research,
Sutton, UK

**Yiannis Philippou MA(Cantab), MBBChir**
Foundation Year 2
Department of Surgery,
The Royal Marsden NHS Foundation Trust,
Sutton, UK

**Jonathan Richenberg, BM, BcH, MA, MRCP, FRCR (Hon. Sen. Lect.), BSMS**
Consultant Radiologist
Department of Imaging,
Royal Sussex County Hospital,
Brighton, UK

**Nicholas James Smith, MBChB, FRCS(Urol.), PhD**
Specialist Registrar
Department of Urology,
St. James's University Hospital,
Leeds Teaching Hospitals NHS Trust,
Leeds, UK

**Prasanna Sooriakumaran, MD, PhD, FRCSUrol, FEBU**
Senior Fellow in Robotics and Urology
Honorary Consultant Urological Surgeon
Nuffield Department of Surgical Sciences,
University of Oxford,
Oxford, UK; *and*
Visiting Assistant Professor
Department of Molecular Medicine and
Surgery,
Karolinska Institute,
Stockholm, Sweden

**Martin Spahn, MD**
Associate Professor
Senior Consultant
Department of Urology,
University Hospital Bern, Inselspital Anna
Seiler-Haus,
Bern, Switzerland

**Ashutosh Tewari, MD, MCh**
Ronald P. Lynch Professor of
Urologic-Oncology
Director
Center for Prostate Cancer,

Weill Cornell Medical College, New York
Presbyterian Hospital;
New York, NY, USA; *and*
Director
LeFrak Center of Robotic Surgery, Weill
Cornell Medical College,
New York Presbyterian Hospital,
New York, NY, USA

**George Thalmann, MD**
Professor of Urology
Director and Chairman
Department of Urology,
University Hospital Bern, Inselspital Anna
Seiler-Haus,
Bern, Switzerland

**Bertrand Tombal, MD, PhD**
Professor of Urology
Division of Urology,
Cliniques universitaires Saint Luc,
Institut de Recherche clinique,
Université catholique de Louvain,
Brussels, Belgium

**Massimo Valerio, MD, FEBU**
Clinical Research Fellow, PhD candidate
Division of Surgery and Interventional Science,
University College London, London, UK; *and*
Department of Urology
University College London Hospitals NHS
Foundation Trust,
London, UK; *and*
Centre Hospitalier Universitaire Vaudoi,
Lausanne, Switzerland

**Peter Whelan, MS, FRCS,**
Community Urologist, Leeds, UK
Emeritus Consultant Urological Surgeon,
Pyrah Department of Urology,
St. James's University Hospital,
Leeds, UK

**Matias Westendarp, MD**
Fellow in Endourology and Laparoscopy
Clinical Research Fellow
Academic Medical Center,
Amsterdam, The Netherlands

# Preface

With the advent of new drugs and innovative technologies with which to treat prostate cancer in the last few years, and the realization that over-diagnosis and hence overtreatment have been a feature of the recent past; it was felt timely to produce a short, comprehensive book on all aspects of prostate cancer, leaving the details for the expert to the many excellent contemporary monographs.

We are privileged to have had an internationally known team of contributors ranging across the field. Aaron Katz and colleagues set the scene with the all important review of the epidemiology and natural history of the disease. Jon Oxley sets the contemporary context of histopathology; Philippa J. Cheetham gives us an exhaustive review of the current state of markers in this disease, whereas Jonathan Richenberg brings us up to date with imaging of the disease both locally and distantly. In an innovatory chapter, William Richard Cross reviews what informed consent means and the evidence we have, stage by stage, with which to advise our patients.

The management of localized disease is discussed from all aspects of possible therapies, starting with a discussion on active monitoring, a counterintuitive concept when dealing with cancer in not offering treatment immediately, and why it is valid in prostate cancer, by L. Boccon-Gibod. Ashutosh Tewari gives an authoritive description of surgical treatment, whereas P.J. Hoskin examines both external beam radiotherapy and brachytherapy to help us understand why, numerically, these are the most frequent treatments utilized. Hashim U. Ahmed and Mark Emberton review the role of emerging therapies to which they have contributed so much.

In linked chapters, Theo M. de Reijke, George Thalmann, and Bertrand Tombal, together with their colleagues, explore what options there are when definitive therapies appear to have failed. It is hoped that these, taken together with William Richard Cross's chapter, will allow all readers to reflect on the two important components of prostate cancer treatment:

evidence and timescale. Johann de Bono brings his immense experience and expertise to discuss the exciting developments of new therapies in this disease. Peter Whelan looks at the progress and lack of it, from the beginning of anatomical radical prostatectomy through the PSA era to the current day, whereas John D. Graham reminds us that this is a malignant disease with which we are dealing and some patients progress and some die from it. In a sensitive account, he sets out how our patients may be supported to have a "good death."

Finally, we thought it appropriate to ask a scientist, Norman Maitland, who has spent more than 30 years in this field, to give a scientific rather than a clinical take on future prospects.

We hope this book will prove useful to the experts to enable them to understand where other experts are "coming from," what their therapies have to offer, and what are these therapies' inevitable limitations to the generalist who can use this book to help guide patients through the bewildering options available, and sincerely to include the lay reader, both patient and their relatives. We hope that it will provide a comprehensive summary, an accessible narrative, and a starting point for discussions patients will have with their treating physicians.

Andrew von Eschenbach, a urologist and ex-director of the US National Institute of Cancer, stated that the hope was to turn prostate cancer into a chronic disease. This has largely been achieved in the current era with many men living a quarter or even a third of their lives after the diagnosis. We hope this book shows how this came about and how men can and must be persuaded to live out their lives as fully as possible, and that there are always options, and one will probably fit an individual's needs.

We are grateful to all at Wiley especially Oliver Walter who commissioned this volume, and to Kate Newell and Claire Brewer.

# CHAPTER 1

# Prostate Cancer Epidemiology

*Annie Darves-Bornoz[1], Joe Park[1], and Aaron Katz[2]*

[1] Stony Brook University and Winthrop University Hospital, New York
[2] Department of Urology, Winthrop University Hospital, New York

## United States—recent trends in incidence and mortality

### Incidence

Prostate cancer is the most common non-skin cancer diagnosed among American males, affecting roughly one in six men (16.15%) over the course of their lifetime. Prostate cancer is also the second leading cause of cancer-related deaths in American men. According to the most recent data from the Surveillance Epidemiology and End Results (SEER) database, an estimated 241 740 men were diagnosed with prostate cancer and over 28 000 died of it in the United States in 2012 [1]. The incidence of prostate cancer spiked in the United States in the early 1990s because of the advent of more aggressive prostate-specific antigen (PSA) screening [2]. This was followed by a sharp decline from 1992 to 1995 during which incidence rates returned to a new baseline which remained approximately two and a half times the pre-PSA era rate, likely due to the fact that increased screening in prior years had successfully diagnosed much of the previously undetected prostate cancer patients in the population.

### Mortality and survival

Most recent data show that mortality rates due to prostate cancer have been declining, with a 3.5% decrease between 2000 and 2009 [3]. In addition, 5-year survival rates have also been increasing, jumping from 76% between 1983 and 1985 to 98% between 1992 and 1998 [4]. While this staggering rise in survival and decline in mortality can in part be attributed

*Prostate Cancer: Diagnosis and Clinical Management*, First Edition.
Edited by Ashutosh K. Tewari, Peter Whelan and John D. Graham.
© 2014 John Wiley & Sons, Ltd. Published 2014 by John Wiley & Sons, Ltd.

to the recent trend in earlier detection and more aggressive treatment [5], screening overdiagnosis of preclinical prostate cancers which may never progress clinically is likely a major contributor as well. Overall, 5-year relative survival is nearly 100%, relative 10-year survival is 98%, and relative 15-year survival is 93%.

The stage of the prostate cancer is a major contributor to survival, as patients with local and regional disease had relative 5-year survival rates nearing 100%, while patients with distant metastasis had a relative 5-year survival of only 28% [6]. As screening is advancing, there has been an increase in incidence of organ-confined and regional diseases and a decrease in incidence of metastatic diseases [7].

### International trends

Prostate cancer is the second most common cancer among men in the United States and fifth most common cancer worldwide [8]. However, incidence and mortality of this disease differ greatly depending on the geographical area. Incidence is highest in Scandinavia and North America (especially among African-Americans, with an annual rate of 236.0 per 100 000 men) and lowest in Asia (1.9 cases per 100 000 annually) [1, 8]. With respect to mortality rates, the highest rates are found in the Caribbean (at 26.3 deaths per 100 000 annually) and the lowest rates are found in Asia (<3 deaths per 100 000 annually). There are numerous explanations for these drastically different mortality rates among countries. Two major factors are differences in treatment and misattribution of cause of death. Environment is likely to play a role as well. One study comparing Japanese men living in the United States with Japanese men living abroad found that Japanese men living in the United States had more similar rates of prostate cancer to persons of similar ancestry living in the United States than to the Japanese men living in Japan [9].

## Advancing age

Advancing age is the principal risk factor for acquiring prostate cancer. From 2005 to 2009, the median age of diagnosis was 67 years, with approximately 90% of diagnoses occurring at the age of 55 years and above. In addition, older men are more likely to be diagnosed with high-risk prostate cancer leading to lower overall and cancer-specific survival [1].

## Race/ethnicity

Race is a major risk factor for prostate cancer, both with respect to incidence and mortality; however, the reasons as to why are less clear. African-Americans have the highest incidence of prostate cancer than any other race or ethnicity in the United States (between 2005 and 2009, 236.0 per 100 000 men annually). This is in contrast to other groups living in the United States, including white American males (146.9 per 100 000 men annually), Asian/Pacific Islanders (85.4 per 100 000 men annually), American Indian/Alaska Natives (78.4 per 100 000 men annually), and Hispanics (125.9 per 100 000 men annually). African-Americans also have the highest mortality rate (between 2005 and 2009, 53.1 per 100 000 men annually) once diagnosed with prostate cancer. Again, white American males (21.7 per 100 000 men annually), Asian/Pacific Islanders (10.0 per 100 000 men annually), American Indian/Alaska Natives (19.7 per 100 000 men annually), and Hispanics (17.8 per 100 000 men annually) all had significantly lower mortality rates in comparison [1].

There are numerous explanations for this disparity in outcomes among races. Higher mortality in African-Americans has been attributed to lower socioeconomic status [10–12], less frequent PSA screening [13], less aggressive treatment [14], and a lack of access to advanced treatment facilities [15]. However, even in studies which seemingly control for economic status, PSA screening, diagnostic approaches, and treatment barriers worse outcomes are still found in African-American males [16, 17]. Further research is warranted to elucidate both biologic and societal causes of such disparate outcomes among races.

## Family history

Family history is one of the strongest risk factors when considering who will develop prostate cancer. Having an affected relative, the number of affected relatives, and the age of onset of prostate cancer in the affected relative are all risk factors for developing prostate cancer. Risk of prostate cancer doubles for a male who has one affected first-degree relative [18–22]. For males with more than one affected relatives, the risk is further increased [20]. Age of onset in affected first-degree relatives is also important, as younger age of onset correlates with increased risk as well [20, 23]. Another study from Sweden found prognostic correlation in families where both the father and son had prostate cancer. When comparing fathers who survived for 5 or more years versus fathers who survived less than 2 years, sons of fathers who survived for 5 or more years had a hazard ratio of 0.62 (95% CI) [24].

These familial factors point to a possible hereditary component in the development of prostate cancer. This notion is corroborated by a study of 45 000 twin pairs from Sweden, Denmark, and Finland which found that there was a higher concordance for prostate cancer diagnosis in monozygotic twins (18%) versus dizygotic twins (3%). This study estimated that potentially 42% of the risk of developing prostate cancer could be due to heritable causes [25]. Inheritance patterns of prostate cancer are not yet well understood, although segregation analyses of prostate cancer families point to an autosomal dominant [26], X-linked, or recessive inheritance [27].

## Hormonal factors

### Androgens

Androgens are important for the normal development of the prostate gland and are likely important in the carcinogenesis of the prostate as well. The results of the Prostate Cancer Prevention Trial demonstrated that inhibition of the conversion of testosterone to dihydrotestosterone by finasteride, a 5α-reductase inhibitor, significantly decreased incidence of prostate cancer, thus confirming the role of androgens in the development of prostate cancer [28]. However, a meta-analysis of 18 studies showed that normal variations in serum androgen levels were not correlated with an increased risk of developing prostate cancer [29].

### Insulin-like growth factor-1

Higher concentrations of insulin-like growth factor-1 (IGF-1), which normally promotes proliferation and apoptotic inhibition of normal prostate cells [30], have been associated with an increased risk of prostate cancer [31]. A pooled analysis of 12 studies also found that IGF binding protein 3 was weakly associated with increased risk of prostate cancer as well [31]. IGF-1 levels are both genetically and nutritionally dependent, which may be a reason why certain countries and populations have higher or lower rates of prostate cancer.

## Lifestyle decisions

### Smoking cigarettes

A meta-analysis determined that smoking was not associated with increased risk of developing prostate cancer, but was associated with fatal prostate cancer [32]. Smokers had a 24–30% increased risk of death due to prostate cancer compared with nonsmokers. A large study also found that smokers actually had an 18% decreased risk of developing prostate cancer, but a 67% increased risk of mortality due to prostate cancer [33].

### Alcohol

Most studies have shown that there is no effect of alcohol consumption on the incidence or mortality of prostate cancer [34–36]. Additionally, red wine has not been shown to have any protective effect on prostate cancer [35]. These studies suggest that alcohol consumption does not play a major role in the development of prostate cancer.

## Diet

### Obesity

The role of obesity, as defined by high body mass index (BMI), in the pathogenesis of prostate cancer is not well defined. Many studies show that excess body weight does not lead to increased cases of prostate cancer [37–39], although some have shown a positive association [40, 41]. What studies have shown more conclusively is that obesity is associated with cases of higher-grade and fatal prostate cancer [42, 43].

### Fats

Early studies found a positive correlation between fat consumption and prostate cancer incidence and mortality [44]. Subsequent case–control studies, including one comparing various races [20], also found a positive association between increased fat consumption and risk of developing prostate cancer [45]. In addition to increased incidence, a handful of prospective studies have shown that fat intake correlated with the higher-stage disease [20, 46]. The causes of these findings are likely multifactorial, including increased oxidative stress due to increased adipose tissue, increased difficulty of prostate detection in obese men, and increased production of IGF-1. However, the European Prospective Investigation into

Cancer and Nutrition (EPIC) study, a meta-analysis of seven prospective studies, failed to demonstrate any association between fat consumption and incidence of disease or stage of disease [47]. Currently, it is unclear if fat consumption does indeed raise the risk of developing prostate cancer.

### Lycopene

Lycopene, a carotenoid with potent antioxidant properties found primarily in tomatoes, has been hypothesized to reduce the risk of prostate cancer, but the results have been inconclusive. A meta-analysis found that when comparing the group with the lowest consumption of raw tomato products with the highest-consumption group, there was an 11% reduction in the risk of prostate cancer. This reduction was increased to 19% when cooked tomato products were considered [48]. However, a recent nested case–control study examining the effect of lycopene on various cancers found no reduction in prostate cancer risk [49].

### Soy

Soy is high in phytoestrogens, compounds which may reduce $5\alpha$-reductase activity, induce differentiation of prostate cells, and modulate estrogen receptors which inhibit androgen activity [50]. A meta-analysis of six case–control and two cohort studies [51], as well as the US Multiethnic Cohort Study [52], showed a reduction in the risk of prostate cancer in males with high soy consumption. The latter study also found a 30% reduction in the risk of being diagnosed with advanced disease. Thus, Asian soy-based diets may be contributing to lower rates of prostate cancer in this population. However, active surveillance studies have failed to produce the same results [53]. Although promising, the benefit of soy in reducing prostate cancer risk has not been substantiated.

## Vitamins/minerals/trace elements

### Vitamin D/calcium

No association between vitamin D intake and prostate cancer has been found in studies which have examined this relationship [54–56]. Conversely, numerous studies, including the Cancer Prevention Study II Nutrition Cohort, have reported positive associations between high calcium intake and increased incidence of as well as increased mortality from prostate cancer [55, 57, 58]. With the abundance of calcium supplementation in the United States, more studies are needed to evaluate these potentially increased risks.

## Vitamin E

Results of the Selenium and Vitamin E Cancer Prevention Trial (SELECT) as well as the Physicians' Health Study II were equivocal when examining the effect of vitamin E on the risk of prostate cancer [59, 60]. However, α-tocopherol, the most potent form of naturally occurring vitamin E, has shown to decrease the risk of prostate cancer in smokers [61]. Interestingly though, subsequent follow-up of this same cohort showed no association of vitamin E with incidence of prostate cancer [62], blurring the validity of this association.

## Selenium

The Nutritional Prevention of Cancer Study showed that selenium supplementation reduced the risk of prostate cancer by 65% compared with placebo [63]; these results have been corroborated by subsequent studies [64, 65]. However, these findings conflict with the results of the SELECT trial [59]. Further research is needed before any steadfast conclusions can be made regarding selenium's protective role in prostate cancer.

## Genetics

### Single-nucleotide polymorphisms (8q24 region)

Genome-wide association studies have demonstrated that certain genetic variations called single-nucleotide polymorphisms (SNPs) when found in aggregate in a male are associated with an increased risk of developing prostate cancer [66]. Allelic foci have been found in the 8q24 [67, 68] and 17q regions [66].

### BRCA1/BRCA2 mutations

Risk of developing prostate cancer is increased if a BRCA1 (17q21) or BRCA2 (13q12) mutation is present. BRCA1 mutations roughly double the risk of prostate cancer [69, 70]. BRCA2 mutation carriers have a five- to sevenfold increase in risk [71], an early onset of disease [72], a worse prognosis [72, 73], and a higher Gleason score [74].

## Natural history of prostate cancer

The natural history of a disease is the course a disease takes if left untreated. In other words, it is the prognosis of the disease and the incidence of parameters of interest over time. It is of great interest that physicians are aware of the natural history of diseases, and particularly that of prostate cancer, as many prostate cancers grow slowly and the treatment is not without any side effects. A cost–benefit analysis must be done to determine whether treatment at all and what treatment is appropriate on an individual basis.

The incidence of prostate cancer is high. Autopsy studies have demonstrated that 60–70% of older men have some area showing cancer within the prostate [75, 76]. It is estimated that a 50-year-old man has a lifetime risk of 42% of developing prostate cancer, but only a 9.5% risk of developing the disease clinically and being diagnosed and a 2.9% risk of dying from prostate cancer [77]. This shows the highly protracted course and natural history of prostate cancer. However, our understanding of prostate cancer's natural history is incomplete and an individual's prognosis proves difficult to predict. With the advent of PSA screening, prostate cancer is being detected at earlier stages. The clinical behavior can vastly differ in different men with prostate cancer of similar staging, PSA levels, and histological appearance. Of the 234 460 men diagnosed with prostate cancer yearly, 91% present with localized disease [78]. Clinicians are faced with the challenge of predicting more aggressive forms of localized disease and "clinically insignificant" forms of disease (organ-confined cancer <0.5 mL, no Gleason grade 4 or 5).

A majority of prostate cancers turn out to be small, low grade, and non-invasive with doubling times of 2–4 years. It has been shown that up to 20% of cancers found on pathology after prostatectomy fit in this category and pose no immediate risk to the patient's health [79], suggesting possible overtreatment of prostate cancer. Making the diagnosis of prostate cancer more complicated is the fact that it can be a multifocal disease. Studies have shown the presence of multiple carcinomas in at least 50% of radical prostatectomy specimens, typically having different grades [80]. This can lead to sampling errors and difficulty predicting the true grade of a patient's prostate from a standard biopsy. Standard TRUS biopsy may underestimate the grade and extent of disease, thus many physicians recommend curative treatment for even low-risk cancers found on biopsy.

It is unknown whether low-risk tumors over time acquire the necessary mutations to progress or if they undergo a dedifferentiation process. In one study of patients undergoing active surveillance for the prostate cancer, 17% were found to have higher-grade cancers (poorer differentiation) on repeat biopsies within 6 years [81]. However, it is difficult to conclude whether this is due to dedifferentiation of the initial cancer biopsied or reflect prostate heterogeneity and a sampling error in the initial diagnosis.

## Watchful waiting

Watchful waiting is an approach to conservative management of prostate cancer where treatment is not begun until the man develops clinical signs of progression, at which time androgen-deprivation therapy is started. This modality of treatment is sometimes used for older men with shorter life expectancies or with comorbidities. In these cases, curative treatment may not prolong the man's life and may instead pose a risk to his health. Clinical studies following men designated to a watchful waiting protocol allows us to look at the natural history of prostate cancer.

Outcomes of 828 men with prostate cancer who were conservatively managed with watchful waiting were assessed in a pooled analysis. In this study, they measured disease-specific survival 10 years after the diagnosis, which was found to be 87% for low-grade cancers, and 34% for those with high-grade cancers. About 81% of those with low-grade cancers at diagnosis remained metastasis-free, whereas only 26% of those with high-grade cancers were metastasis-free [82].

In a prospective cohort study done in Sweden [83–85], 223 men were followed for over three decades. A total of 223 subjects were diagnosed with localized prostate cancer and initial treatment was deferred. It was initially found that these men had good disease-specific survival after 15 years [83], demonstrating an indolent course at first; however, mortality rates increased with further follow-up between 15 and 20 years after diagnosis. Survival without metastases decreased from 76.9% at 15 years to 51.2% at 20 years, and disease-specific survival decreased from 78.7% to 54.4%. At 15 years, the prostate cancer mortality rate was 15 per 1000 person-years and increased to 44 per 1000 person-years at 20 years post-diagnosis. The authors concluded from this prospective study that watchful waiting may be appropriate for men who have less than 15 years of life expectancy, as prostate cancer seemed to rapidly progress after 15 years. As of June 2011, this cohort had been followed for 32 years at which point only 3 of the 223 original patients were alive. As per the initial protocol of the study, men who developed symptomatic progression or metastasis of prostate cancer were treated with hormone therapy. About 142 of the 223 men (64%) remained untreated over the course of the trial. They remained metastasis-free and did not die of prostate cancer, indicating that a majority of the men had a cancer that never became clinically significant. In contrast to this good prognosis, 38 of the 79 men (almost 50%) who were hormonally treated died of prostate cancer [85]. In contrast to their prior study, no increase in the rate of progression and mortality was found when follow-up was extended beyond 20 years. It is likely that the increase in progression after 15 years was likely due to the small size of the surviving subjects. Supporting this is another watchful waiting study, a retrospective cohort review of 767 men diagnosed with localized prostate cancer followed up with a mean observation of 24 years. No significant difference in the rate of progression or mortality after 15 years was found [86]. In this cohort, men with high-grade cancer (Gleason score 8–10) at the time of diagnosis had a much higher probability of dying from prostate cancer (121 deaths per 1000 person-years) compared with those with low-grade cancer (Gleason score 2–4, 6 deaths per 1000 person-years) [86].

The diagnoses of the subjects in these studies were made prior to the use of PSA screening, which makes it difficult to correlate it to today's patients. Tumors detected by PSA screening have a lead time between 5 and 7 years [87] and may progress differently than those found clinically as in the studies above. The first watchful waiting study done in the PSA era found the highest predictive parameters for progression of localized disease were PSA level at time of diagnosis and Gleason score of the initial biopsy [88]. In a prospective cohort study done during the contemporary PSA era, disease-specific survival rates were found to be more favorable, reflecting the lead time discussed above and the indolent course of prostate cancer. The 10-year prostate-cancer-specific mortality was 8.3% for men with well-differentiated tumors, 9.1% for those with moderately differentiated tumors, and 25.6% for those with poorly differentiated tumors [89].

The natural history of prostate cancer still leaves much to the unknown. Although localized cancer often remains clinically insignificant, progression and metastasis may still develop after several years. Factors including PSA level, Gleason score, patient's age, and overall health should be assessed when determining appropriate treatment. However, it is important to consider that these are not concrete risk factors, as some men who possess the high-risk factors do not progress to a clinically significant cancer and, similarly, the low-risk men do not always maintain an indolent course.

# References

1 Howlader N, Noone AM, Krapcho M, *et al.* (eds). SEER Cancer Statistics Review, 1975–2009 (Vintage 2009 Populations). SEER Fact Sheets: Prostate. Available at http://seer.cancer.gov/statfacts/html/prost.html.. 2012–2013. Last accessed January 2, 2013.

2 Potosky AL, Miller BA, Albertsen PC, Kramer BS. The role of increasing detection in the rising incidence of prostate cancer. *J Am Med Assoc* 1995;273(7):548–552.

3 Jemal A, Simard EP, Dorell C, *et al.* Annual Report to the Nation on the Status of Cancer, 1975–2009. Featuring the burden and trends in human papillomavirus (HPV)-associated cancers and HPV vaccination coverage levels. *J Natl Cancer Inst* 2013;105(3):175–201.

4 Siegel R, Naishadham D, Jemal A. Cancer statistics, 2012. *CA Cancer J Clin* 2012;62(1):10–29.

5 Walsh PC. Cancer surveillance series: interpreting trends in prostate cancer–part I: evidence of the effects of screening in recent prostate cancer incidence, mortality, and survival rates. *J Urol* 2000;163(1):364–365.

6 Survival rates for prostate cancer. http://www.cancer.org/cancer/prostatecancer/ detailedguide/prostate-cancer-survival-rates: American Cancer Society; 2013 [cited 2013 February 24].

7 Derweesh IH, Kupelian PA, Zippe C, *et al.* Continuing trends in pathological stage migration in radical prostatectomy specimens. *Urol Oncol* 2004;22(4):300–306.

8 Parkin DM, Bray F, Ferlay J, Pisani P. Global cancer statistics, 2002. *CA Cancer J Clin* 2005;55(2):74–108.

9 Shimizu H, Ross RK, Bernstein L, *et al.* Cancers of the prostate and breast among Japanese and white immigrants in Los Angeles County. *Br J Cancer* 1991;63(6):963–966.

10 Albano JD, Ward E, Jemal A, *et al.* Cancer mortality in the United States by education level and race. *J Natl Cancer Inst* 2007;99(18):1384–1394.

11 Mordukhovich I, Reiter PL, Backes DM, *et al.* A review of African American–white differences in risk factors for cancer: prostate cancer. *Cancer Causes Control* 2011;22(3):341–357.

12 Tewari AK, Gold HT, Demers RY, *et al.* Effect of socioeconomic factors on long-term mortality in men with clinically localized prostate cancer. *Urology* 2009;73(3):624–630.

13 Carpenter WR, Howard DL, Taylor YJ, *et al.* Racial differences in PSA screening interval and stage at diagnosis. *Cancer Causes Control* 2010;21(7):1071–1080.

14 Schwartz K, Powell IJ, Underwood W, *et al.* Interplay of race, socioeconomic status, and treatment on survival of patients with prostate cancer. *Urology* 2009;74(6):1296–1302.

15 Onega T, Duell EJ, Shi X, *et al.* Race versus place of service in mortality among medicare beneficiaries with cancer. *Cancer* 2010;116(11):2698–2706.

16 Hoffman RM, Gilliland FD, Eley JW, *et al.* Racial and ethnic differences in advanced-stage prostate cancer: the Prostate Cancer Outcomes Study. *J Natl Cancer Inst* 2001;93(5):388–395.

17 Platz EA, Rimm EB, Willett WC, *et al*. Racial variation in prostate cancer incidence and in hormonal system markers among male health professionals. *J Natl Cancer Inst* 2000;92(24):2009–2017.

18 Bruner DW, Moore D, Parlanti A, *et al*. Relative risk of prostate cancer for men with affected relatives: systematic review and meta-analysis. *Int J Cancer* 2003;107(5):797–803.

19 Hemminki K, Czene K. Age specific and attributable risks of familial prostate carcinoma from the family-cancer database. *Cancer* 2002;95(6):1346–1353.

20 Whittemore AS, Wu AH, Kolonel LN, *et al*. Family history and prostate cancer risk in black, white, and Asian men in the United States and Canada. *Am J Epidemiol* 1995;141(8):732–740.

21 Zeegers MP, Jellema A, Ostrer H. Empiric risk of prostate carcinoma for relatives of patients with prostate carcinoma: a meta-analysis. *Cancer* 2003;97(8):1894–1903.

22 Johns LE, Houlston RS. A systematic review and meta-analysis of familial prostate cancer risk. *BJU Int* 2003;91(9):789–794.

23 Gronberg H, Damber L, Damber JE. Familial prostate cancer in Sweden. A nation-wide register cohort study. *Cancer* 1996;77(1):138–143.

24 Hemminki K, Ji J, Forsti A, *et al*. Concordance of survival in family members with prostate cancer. *J Clin Oncol*. 2008;26(10):1705–1709.

25 Lichtenstein P, Holm NV, Verkasalo PK, *et al*. Environmental and heritable factors in the causation of cancer–analyses of cohorts of twins from Sweden, Denmark, and Finland. *N Engl J Med* 2000;343(2):78–85.

26 Gong G, Oakley-Girvan I, Wu AH, *et al*. Segregation analysis of prostate cancer in 1,719 white, African-American and Asian-American families in the United States and Canada. *Cancer Causes Control* 2002;13(5):471–482.

27 Monroe KR, Yu MC, Kolonel LN, *et al*. Evidence of an X-linked or recessive genetic component to prostate cancer risk. *Nat Med* 1995;1(8):827–829.

28 Thompson IM, Goodman PJ, Tangen CM, *et al*. The influence of finasteride on the development of prostate cancer. *N Engl J Med* 2003;349(3):215–224.

29 Endogenous Hormones and Prostate Cancer Collaborative Group, Roddam AW. Allen NE, *et al*. Endogenous sex hormones and prostate cancer: a collaborative analysis of 18 prospective studies. *J Natl Cancer Inst* 2008;100(3):170–183.

30 Cohen P, Peehl DM, Rosenfeld RG. The IGF axis in the prostate. *Horm Metab Res* 1994;26(2):81–84.

31 Roddam AW, Allen NE, Appleby P, *et al*. Insulin-like growth factors, their binding proteins, and prostate cancer risk: analysis of individual patient data from 12 prospective studies. *Ann Intern Med* 2008;149(7):461–471.

32 Huncharek M, Haddock KS, Reid R, Kupelnick B. Smoking as a risk factor for prostate cancer: a meta-analysis of 24 prospective cohort studies. *Am J Public Health* 2010;100(4):693–701.

33 Watters JL, Park Y, Hollenbeck A, *et al*. Cigarette smoking and prostate cancer in a prospective US cohort study. *Cancer Epidemiol Biomarkers Prev* 2009;18(9):2427–2435.

34 Gong Z, Kristal AR, Schenk JM, *et al*. Alcohol consumption, finasteride, and prostate cancer risk: results from the Prostate Cancer Prevention Trial. *Cancer* 2009;115(16):3661–3669.

35 Sutcliffe S, Giovannucci E, Leitzmann MF, *et al*. A prospective cohort study of red wine consumption and risk of prostate cancer. *Int J Cancer* 2007;120(7):1529–1535.

36  Chao C, Haque R, Van Den Eeden SK, *et al.* Red wine consumption and risk of prostate cancer: the California men's health study. *Int J Cancer* 2010;126(1):171–179.

37  Nilsen TI, Vatten LJ. Anthropometry and prostate cancer risk: a prospective study of 22,248 Norwegian men. *Cancer Causes Control* 1999;10(4):269–275.

38  Habel LA, Van Den Eeden SK, Friedman GD. Body size, age at shaving initiation, and prostate cancer in a large, multiracial cohort. *Prostate* 2000;43(2):136–143.

39  Giovannucci E, Rimm EB, Stampfer MJ, *et al.* Height, body weight, and risk of prostate cancer. *Cancer Epidemiol Biomarkers Prev* 1997;6(8):557–563.

40  Calle EE, Rodriguez C, Walker-Thurmond K, Thun MJ. Overweight, obesity, and mortality from cancer in a prospectively studied cohort of U.S. adults. *N Engl J Med* 2003;348(17):1625–1638.

41  Veierod MB, Laake P, Thelle DS. Dietary fat intake and risk of prostate cancer: a prospective study of 25,708 Norwegian men. *Int J Cancer* 1997;73(5):634–638.

42  Gong Z, Neuhouser ML, Goodman PJ, *et al.* Obesity, diabetes, and risk of prostate cancer: results from the prostate cancer prevention trial. *Cancer Epidemiol Biomarkers Prev* 2006;15(10):1977–1983.

43  MacInnis RJ, English DR. Body size and composition and prostate cancer risk: systematic review and meta-regression analysis. *Cancer Causes Control* 2006;17(8):989–1003.

44  Rose DP, Boyar AP, Wynder EL. International comparisons of mortality rates for cancer of the breast, ovary, prostate, and colon, and per capita food consumption. *Cancer* 1986;58(11):2363–2371.

45  Kushi L, Giovannucci E. Dietary fat and cancer. *Am J Med* 2002;113(Suppl. 9B):63S–70S.

46  Giovannucci E, Rimm EB, Colditz GA, *et al.* A prospective study of dietary fat and risk of prostate cancer. *J Natl Cancer Inst* 1993;85(19):1571–1579.

47  Crowe FL, Allen NE, Appleby PN, *et al.* Fatty acid composition of plasma phospholipids and risk of prostate cancer in a case–control analysis nested within the European Prospective Investigation into Cancer and Nutrition. *Am J Clin Nutr* 2008;88(5):1353–1363.

48  Etminan M, Takkouche B, Caamano-Isorna F. The role of tomato products and lycopene in the prevention of prostate cancer: a meta-analysis of observational studies. *Cancer Epidemiol Biomarkers Prev* 2004;13(3):340–345.

49  Peters U, Leitzmann MF, Chatterjee N, *et al.* Serum lycopene, other carotenoids, and prostate cancer risk: a nested case–control study in the prostate, lung, colorectal, and ovarian cancer screening trial. *Cancer Epidemiol Biomarkers Prev* 2007;16(5):962–968.

50  Setlur SR, Mertz KD, Hoshida Y, *et al.* Estrogen-dependent signaling in a molecularly distinct subclass of aggressive prostate cancer. *J Natl Cancer Inst* 2008;100(11):815–825.

51  Yan L, Spitznagel EL. Meta-analysis of soy food and risk of prostate cancer in men. *Int J Cancer* 2005;117(4):667–669.

52  Park SY, Murphy SP, Wilkens LR, *et al.* Legume and isoflavone intake and prostate cancer risk: the Multiethnic Cohort Study. *Int J Cancer* 2008;123(4):927–932.

53  Kumar NB, Cantor A, Allen K, *et al.* The specific role of isoflavones in reducing prostate cancer risk. *Prostate* 2004;59(2):141–147.

54  Chan JM, Giovannucci EL. Dairy products, calcium, and vitamin D and risk of prostate cancer. *Epidemiol Rev* 2001;23(1):87–92.

55  Kristal AR, Cohen JH, Qu P, Stanford JL. Associations of energy, fat, calcium, and vitamin D with prostate cancer risk. *Cancer Epidemiol Biomarkers Prev* 2002;11(8):719–725.

56  Giovannucci E, Rimm EB, Wolk A, *et al.* Calcium and fructose intake in relation to risk of prostate cancer. *Cancer Res* 1998;58(3):442–447.

57  Skinner HG, Schwartz GG. Serum calcium and incident and fatal prostate cancer in the National Health and Nutrition Examination Survey. *Cancer Epidemiol Biomarkers Prev* 2008;17(9):2302–2305.

58  Rodriguez C, McCullough ML, Mondul AM, *et al.* Calcium, dairy products, and risk of prostate cancer in a prospective cohort of United States men. *Cancer Epidemiol Biomarkers Prev* 2003;12(7):597–603.

59  Lippman SM, Klein EA, Goodman PJ, *et al.* Effect of selenium and vitamin E on risk of prostate cancer and other cancers: the Selenium and Vitamin E Cancer Prevention Trial (SELECT). *J Am Med Assoc* 2009;301(1):39–51.

60  Gaziano JM, Glynn RJ, Christen WG, *et al.* Vitamins E and C in the prevention of prostate and total cancer in men: the Physicians' Health Study II randomized controlled trial. *J Am Med Assoc* 2009;301(1):52–62.

61  Heinonen OP, Albanes D, Virtamo J, *et al.* Prostate cancer and supplementation with alpha-tocopherol and beta-carotene: incidence and mortality in a controlled trial. *J Natl Cancer Inst* 1998;90(6):440–446.

62  Virtamo J, Pietinen P, Huttunen JK, *et al.* Incidence of cancer and mortality following alpha-tocopherol and beta-carotene supplementation: a postintervention follow-up. *J Am Med Assoc* 2003;290(4):476–485.

63  Clark LC, Combs GF, Jr., Turnbull  BW, *et al.* Effects of selenium supplementation for cancer prevention in patients with carcinoma of the skin. A randomized controlled trial. Nutritional Prevention of Cancer Study Group. *J Am Med Assoc* 1996;276(24):1957–1963.

64  Brooks JD, Metter EJ, Chan DW, *et al.* Plasma selenium level before diagnosis and the risk of prostate cancer development. *J Urol* 2001;166(6):2034–2038.

65  Li H, Stampfer MJ, Giovannucci EL, *et al.* A prospective study of plasma selenium levels and prostate cancer risk. *J Natl Cancer Inst* 2004;96(9):696–703.

66  Zheng SL, Sun J, Wiklund F, *et al.* Cumulative association of five genetic variants with prostate cancer. *N Engl J Med* 2008;358(9):910–919.

67  Eeles RA, Kote-Jarai Z, Giles GG, *et al.* Multiple newly identified loci associated with prostate cancer susceptibility. *Nat Genet* 2008;40(3):316–321.

68  Haiman CA, Patterson N, Freedman ML, *et al.* Multiple regions within 8q24 independently affect risk for prostate cancer. *Nat Genet* 2007;39(5):638–644.

69  Struewing JP, Hartge P, Wacholder S, *et al.* The risk of cancer associated with specific mutations of BRCA1 and BRCA2 among Ashkenazi Jews. *N Engl J Med* 1997;336(20):1401–1408.

70  Warner E, Foulkes W, Goodwin P, *et al.* Prevalence and penetrance of BRCA1 and BRCA2 gene mutations in unselected Ashkenazi Jewish women with breast cancer. *J Natl Cancer Inst* 1999;91(14):1241–1247.

71  Cancer risks in BRCA2 mutation carriers. The Breast Cancer Linkage Consortium. *J Natl Cancer Inst* 1999;91(15):1310–1316.

72  Tryggvadottir L, Vidarsdottir L, Thorgeirsson T, *et al.* Prostate cancer progression and survival in BRCA2 mutation carriers. *J Natl Cancer Inst* 2007;99(12):929–935.

73  Narod SA, Neuhausen S, Vichodez G, *et al.* Rapid progression of prostate cancer in men with a BRCA2 mutation. *Br J Cancer* 2008;99(2):371–374.

74  Mitra A, Fisher C, Foster CS, *et al.* Prostate cancer in male BRCA1 and BRCA2 mutation carriers has a more aggressive phenotype. *Br J Cancer* 2008;98(2):502–507.

75  Rullis I, Shaeffer JA, Lilien OM. Incidence of prostatic carcinoma in the elderly. *Urology* 1975;6(3):295–297.

76  Sakr WA, Grignon DJ, Crissman JD, *et al.* High grade prostatic intraepithelial neoplasia (HGPIN) and prostatic adenocarcinoma between the ages of 20–69: an autopsy study of 249 cases. *In Vivo* 1994;8(3):439–443.

77  Scardino PT. Early detection of prostate cancer. *Urol Clin North Am* 1989;16(4):635–655.

78  Jemal A, Siegel R, Ward E, *et al.* Cancer statistics, 2006. *CA Cancer J Clin* 2006;56(2):106–130.

79  Epstein JI, Walsh PC, Brendler CB. Radical prostatectomy for impalpable prostate cancer: the Johns Hopkins experience with tumors found on transurethral resection (stages T1A and T1B) and on needle biopsy (stage T1C). *J Urol* 1994;152(5 Pt 2):1721–1729.

80  Miller GJ, Cygan JM. Morphology of prostate cancer: the effects of multifocality on histological grade, tumor volume and capsule penetration. *J Urol* 1994;152(5 Pt 2):1709–1713.

81  Porten SP, Whitson JM, Cowan JE, *et al.* Changes in prostate cancer grade on serial biopsy in men undergoing active surveillance. *J Clin Oncol* 2011;29(20):2795–2800.

82  Chodak GW, Thisted RA, Gerber GS, *et al.* Results of conservative management of clinically localized prostate cancer. *N Engl J Med* 1994;330(4):242–248.

83  Johansson JE, Holmberg L, Johansson S, *et al.* Fifteen-year survival in prostate cancer. A prospective, population-based study in Sweden. *J Am Med Assoc* 1997;277(6):467–471.

84  Johansson JE, Andren O, Andersson SO, *et al.* Natural history of early, localized prostate cancer. *J Am Med Assoc* 2004;291(22):2713–2719.

85  Popiolek M, Rider JR, Andren O, *et al.* Natural history of early, localized prostate cancer: a final report from three decades of follow-up. *Eur Urol* 2013;63(3):428–435.

86  Albertsen PC, Hanley JA, Fine J. 20-year outcomes following conservative management of clinically localized prostate cancer. *J Am Med Assoc* 2005;293(17):2095–2101.

87  Draisma G, Etzioni R, Tsodikov A, *et al.* Lead time and overdiagnosis in prostate-specific antigen screening: importance of methods and context. *J Natl Cancer Inst* 2009;101(6):374–383.

88  Kattan MW, Cuzick J, Fisher G, *et al.* Nomogram incorporating PSA level to predict cancer-specific survival for men with clinically localized prostate cancer managed without curative intent. *Cancer* 2008;112(1):69–74.

89  Lu-Yao GL, Albertsen PC, Moore DF, *et al.* Outcomes of localized prostate cancer following conservative management. *J Am Med Assoc* 2009;302(11):1202–1209.

# CHAPTER 2

# Diagnosis and Screening

*Yiannis Philippou[1], Harveer Dev[2], and Prasanna Sooriakumaran[3]*

[1]Department of Urology, East Surrey Hospital, Redhill, UK
[2]Department of Surgery, Cambridge University Hospital, Cambridge, UK
[3]Surgical Intervention Trials Unit, Nuffield Department of Surgical Sciences, University of Oxford, Oxford, UK

Prostate cancer is a significant burden to men's health. It represents the most frequently diagnosed nondermatological malignancy and the second leading cause of death due to cancer in men [1]. In 2009, just over 40 000 patients were diagnosed with prostate cancer in the United Kingdom, with approximately 10 000 deaths occurring each year. Global rates for prostate cancer generally mirror those found in the United Kingdom, with the highest primarily in the developed countries of Europe, North and South America, and the Oceanic nations.

The natural progression of prostate cancer in most men is relatively slow. Most tumors remain organ confined and will never surface clinically during the patient's lifetime, either because they are indolent or because death occurs from competing causes before clinical manifestation of the malignancy.

The causes of prostate cancer most likely reflect a complex interplay between environmental and hereditary genetic factors, most of which remain to be identified, that interact and lead to a critical acquisition of DNA mutations in prostate cancer cells. As the growth of prostatic cancer cells initially relies on circulating testosterone metabolites, hormonal factors are likely to have an important role in the natural history of the disease. A slight increase in incidence of prostate cancer has been predicted with high consumption of meat, dairy products, and fats [2]. Although the evidence reveals at best, weak associations are incredibly difficult to interpret in the face of multiple confounding factors.

*Prostate Cancer: Diagnosis and Clinical Management*, First Edition.
Edited by Ashutosh K. Tewari, Peter Whelan and John D. Graham.
© 2014 John Wiley & Sons, Ltd. Published 2014 by John Wiley & Sons, Ltd.

Hitherto, major environmental risk factors that are amenable to primary prevention measures have not been identified [3]. The Selenium and Vitamin E Cancer Prevention Trial (SELECT), the largest ever cancer prevention trial, countered evidence from previous epidemiological studies that suggested that daily selenium and vitamin E taken alone or in combination could decrease the risk of prostate cancer. In fact, the trial reported that taking vitamin E or selenium supplement alone or in combination might increase the risk of developing prostate cancer [4]. Dutasteride, a 5-alpha-reductase inhibitor (used in the treatment of benign prostatic hyperplasia, BPH), can reduce serum prostate-specific antigen (PSA) levels by approximately 50% at 6 months and total prostatic volume by 25% after 2 years. The Reduction by Dutasteride of Prostate Cancer Events (REDUCE) trial suggested that dutasteride might potentially play a role as a chemoprevention agent in individuals at high risk of developing prostate cancer [5].

## Symptoms

The diagnosis of prostate cancer can be made in a number of stages. Symptoms due to prostate cancer are rarely the cause for patient presentation and investigation. If symptomatic, localized prostate cancer can result in urinary symptoms including hematospermia, although the presence of voiding lower urinary tract symptoms (LUTS), hematuria, and/or perineal/voiding discomfort is likely to result from coexisting BPH/prostatitis. Advanced disease may present with rectal obstruction, bone pain, and more systemic features of malignancy [6].

## First line investigations

First line tests include completion of the physical examination with a digital rectal examination (DRE), and measurement of serum PSA; suspicious findings on either of these tests is followed by more sophisticated diagnostic techniques, beginning with transrectal ultrasound (TRUS) and guided systematic biopsy. Until as recently as the early 1990s, prostate cancer was typically diagnosed as a result of symptomatic metastases or when found during DRE in a patient presenting with urinary complaints. In addition, the biomarker "prostatic acid phosphatase" would often be elevated with the presence of bone metastases. However, the advent of the PSA blood test assay, developed by Kurlyama *et al.* in the 1980s, transformed the diagnostic landscape for prostate cancer, as the antigen became one of the most commonly used tumor markers in modern medicine.

## Prostate-specific antigen

Prostate-specific antigen (PSA) is a glycoprotein consisting of 240 amino acids. It is a serine protease secreted by prostate into semen where it causes lysis of seminal coagulum, although its function in the serum is less well understood. PSA in blood occurs in three forms: free PSA, PSA complexed with alpha-1 antichymotrypsin, and PSA complexed with β1-antichymotrypsin [7]. In conjunction with DRE, PSA has since become a widely used clinical tool to help identify men with prostate cancer [8], as well as its subsequent staging and monitoring post-diagnosis. PSA levels may be elevated in men with prostate cancer because PSA production is increased within the cancerous tissue and in addition tissue barriers between the prostate gland lumen and the capillary are disrupted, releasing more PSA into the serum. Studies have estimated that PSA elevations can precede clinical disease by 5–10 years [9].

Although PSA was originally introduced as a tumor marker to detect cancer recurrence or disease progression following treatment, it was widely adopted for cancer screening by the early 1990s [10]. Subsequently, various professional organizations issued guidelines condoning the routine use of PSA in the detection of prostate cancer [11]. The routine use of the PSA blood test as a diagnostic/screening tool has resulted in a substantial increase in the incidence of prostate cancer recorded worldwide. Although the PSA test allows for earlier detection of prostate cancer, critics state that such numbers represent overdetection of subclinical disease, with the potential for widespread use of relatively aggressive curative treatments by radical surgical, chemotherapeutic, and radiation strategies [12].

The traditional cutoff for an abnormal PSA level has been 4.0 ng/mL [11, 13]. The American Cancer Society systematically reviewed the literature to assess the PSA test performance [14]. When reviewing the performance of a diagnostic test, several parameters need to be assessed. These include sensitivity (probability of identifying true positives with the disease), specificity (probability of identifying the true negatives), and positive/negative predictive values (probability that a test positive/negative individual actually has/does not have the disease). According to the American Cancer Society, the estimated sensitivity of a PSA cutoff of 4.0 ng/mL is 21% for detecting any prostate cancer and 51% for detecting high-grade cancers (Gleason ≥8). Using a cutoff of 3.0 ng/mL increased the sensitivities to 32% and 68%, respectively. The estimated specificity was 91% for a PSA cutoff of 4.0 ng/mL and 85% for a cutoff of 3.0 ng/mL. PSA testing however has poorer discriminating ability in men with symptomatic BPH [15]. Overall, the positive predictive value for a PSA level >4.0 ng/mL is approximately 30%, meaning that slightly less than one in three men with an elevated PSA will have prostate cancer detected on biopsy [16]. For PSA levels between 4.0 and 10.0 ng/mL, the positive predictive value is about 25% and this increases to 42–64% for PSA levels >10 ng/mg [17]. Several factors have been reported to affect the measured level of serum PSA thus affecting the specificity of the PSA blood test. These include BPH, diagnostic examinations such as DRE, physical exercise, ejaculation, and prostatitis. PSA levels have also been shown to correlate with prostate volume and the age of the patient.

Many studies have used DRE and PSA to screen for the presence of prostate cancer. [17–19]. The results of these studies are twofold. First of all, the studies suggest that DRE alone can detect some tumors not detectable by PSA testing, but overall its levels of sensitivity and specificity are inferior to PSA. These results suggest that the PSA test is a more accurate screening tool in detecting prostate cancer compared with DRE, with significantly greater sensitivity, specificity, and positive predictive values. As expected, these studies highlight that on combining DRE and PSA, the testing results in better prostate cancer detection rates. A multicenter screening study by Catalona *et al.* of 6630 men reported a detection rate of 3.2% for DRE, 4.6% for PSA, and 5.8% for the two methods combined. PSA detected significantly more of the cancers than DRE (82% vs. 55%) [17]. Overall, 45% of the cancers were detected only by PSA, whereas just 18% were detected solely by DRE. In a separate study of 1000 men by Galić *et al.*, the positive predictive value for prostate cancer was 48.7% for abnormal finding of DRE, 47% for PSA > 4 ng/mL, and 80% for the combination of both [20]. Further manipulations of PSA, based on density (PSA/unit volume of prostate), kinetics (change in PSA/unit time), and free:bound ratios have all been used to attempt to further improve the predictive value of PSA, although no one measure has been established as superior. In general, large trials looking at the efficacy of screening for prostate cancer have relied on the level of PSA alone.

## Transrectal ultrasound

Transrectal ultrasound (TRUS) is the most commonly used imaging technique for evaluating prostate cancer. In addition to its role in diagnosing prostate cancer, it also allows estimation of prostate size, guides needle biopsies, provides local staging information, and monitors disease prior to and after treatment. TRUS is not normally used as a primary screening measure but to confirm the diagnosis of prostate cancer in combination with prostate biopsy for those with raised PSA or lesions suspicious on DRE. Technical advances, selection biases, observer differences in TRUS scanning, and the lack of UK studies mean that the evidence concerning the accuracy and effectiveness of TRUS for the detection and diagnosis of prostate cancer remains variable. It is however generally accepted that when used in conjunction with DRE and PSA measurement, TRUS can add to the detection rate of localized prostate cancer.

## Transrectal ultrasound-guided biopsy

Needle biopsy is used to confirm the diagnosis of prostate cancer and to provide histological grading information. In the context of the increasing use of the PSA assay, the number of biopsies undertaken in urological practice has increased considerably in recent years. Core biopsy involves the use of a spring-loaded automatic biopsy gun, equipped with an 18-gauge needle. The needle is reliably placed into suspicious lesions in the gland using TRUS which helps to ensure accurate targeting [21]. Foci of cancerous cells within the prostate can appear as hypo- (or even hyper-) echoic lesions on TRUS, although are frequently isoechoic, warranting a standard protocol biopsy (e.g., 12-core). Biopsy does not have a role in first line screening, although it is considered the gold standard diagnostic investigation for histological confirmation of prostate cancer.

The ability to grade and stage prostate cancer accurately is of vital importance for prognosis and the choice of suitable treatment options. Biopsy specimens are graded histologically based on the architectural differentiation of the tumor cells [22]. The predominant histological system is the Gleason grading system in which sections of tumor are graded from 1 (least aggressive) to 5 (most aggressive). The two highest grades from each tumor are added to give a score ranging from 2 to 10. In addition to using the Gleason score as a predictor of the biological aggressiveness of prostate cancer, other parameters can also be combined with the

Gleason score to estimate disease severity. D'Amico *et al.* suggested a stratification of patients into low, intermediate, and high-risk groups by combining the Gleason score, the PSA measurement, and the clinical stage [23]. The TNM system is the major method used for the staging of prostate cancer. Although physical examination and the DRE provide the basis for clinical staging, imaging in the form of TRUS, MRI, CT, radionuclide bone scans, and pelvic lymph node evaluation are used to further evaluate the stage of prostate cancer.

## Evaluating population screening for prostate cancer

A number of criteria are commonly used to determine the suitability of a condition for population screening for disease as outlined by Wilson and Jungner in 1968 [24]. We can consider each of these criteria together with the available evidence from randomized control trials (RCTs) and observation trials in order to evaluate a prostate cancer screening program.

- Epidemiology: It is of no doubt that prostate cancer is indeed a major health problem and a public health concern, as the second most common cause of cancer death among men. With an increasing life expectancy, improvements in diagnostic techniques, and a rise in public knowledge and demand for testing, the incidence and prevalence of disease will continue to rise.
- Natural history: In contrast to breast and cervical cancer (where national screening programs are established), the natural history of prostate cancer remains poorly understood. The severity of prostate cancer ranges from nonfatal slow-growing tumors, which remain asymptomatic and probably require no treatment, to aggressive fast-growing tumors that metastasize quickly, often before symptoms become evident. In between are those cancers that are confined to the prostate in the early stages and in these a screening program would seek to target.
- Diagnostic tests: Diagnostic screening tests need to be simple to perform, relatively inexpensive, and provide accurate information about the presence or absence of the disease. The front-line screening tests for prostate cancer include DRE and PSA (see above), both of which are relatively inexpensive and easy to perform but show wide variations in specificity and sensitivity between studies. In addition, the interval between screening tests also proves problematic to define, due to our limited understanding of the natural history of the disease, and requires further careful evaluation.

- Acceptability of test: The initial diagnostic tests need to be acceptable to both the population to be tested and the clinicians performing the tests. In the first stage of screening for prostate cancer, these tests would involve taking a blood sample and a DRE. It is generally assumed that these are acceptable to most patients and clinicians, although little work has been published to confirm this. Further evaluation is required relating to quality of life in screened and nonscreened men with prostate cancer to assess the social and psychological effects of the screening investigations, as well the impact of additional year(s) of knowledge of a diagnosis during active surveillance or watchful waiting.
- Case selection: There should be an agreed policy on whom to treat as patients.
- Treatment: Broadly, there are three main treatments for localized prostate cancer each with its own risk–benefit profile: radical prostatectomy, radiotherapy, and conservative management where surveillance is preferred with active treatment if symptoms then develop. Although there is evidence that all of the above treatment modalities can be effective in the treatment of localized prostate cancer, the question still remains as to whether early detection and active treatment of prostate tumors can significantly enhance life expectancy and the quality of life [25].
- Resources and services: Currently, there is no national screening service for prostate cancer in the United Kingdom, although *ad hoc* screening by general physicians has increased due to patient-led demand for PSA testing. This has resulted in increasing referrals to hospital urology clinics, which may not currently have the facilities to accommodate population screening. If screening were to be introduced, further substantial investment in diagnostic and treatment facilities would be necessary.
- Costs: Cost analyses for establishing and maintaining a prostate cancer screening service has yet to be performed; however, estimates suggest that the funding of such a service would be considerable. A recent study by Benoit *et al.* estimated that the cost per year life saved by prostate cancer screening with PSA and DRE results in a cost per year life saved of $2339–$3005 for men aged 50–59 years, $3905–$5070 for men aged 60–69 years, and $3574–$4627 overall for men aged 50–69 years [26]. It is also likely that costs of following up false positives in a prostate screening program would also be considerable in addition to the cost incurred on managing the complications associated with treatment of localized prostate cancer.

## Screening studies

A number of observational trials and RCTs have been performed to assess the effectiveness of screening, mainly in North America and Europe. Over the last few years, several large multicenter RCTs have been undertaken to assess whether screening for prostate cancer using PSA and DRE has had any impact on prostate cancer mortality. One of the first was a Canadian trial called the Quebec Prospective Randomized Controlled Trial, which was originally reported in 1999 [27]. The Prostate, Lung, Colorectal and Ovarian (PLCO) Cancer Screening Trial and the European Randomized Study of Screening for Prostate Cancer (ERSPC) were both larger multicenter trials published in 2009 [28, 29]. The results from these latter two trials have been the most quoted by health organizations, both in Europe and the United States when making recommendations for national prostate cancer screening programs.

The Quebec Prostate Cancer Trial involved 46 193 men aged 45–80 years who were randomized to no screening, or screening with PSA and DRE at their initial visit (and with PSA alone thereafter); a PSA level of 3 ng/mL prompted further workup with TRUS and biopsy. The end point was prostate cancer mortality and the patients were followed up for 7 years. The study reported 137 deaths due to prostate among 38 056 nonscreened men and only 5 deaths among 8137 screened individuals. An odds ratio of 3.25 ($p$-value <.01) in support of prostate screening was found. The analysis of data as an observational study instead of a RCT invited criticism by the introduction of several biases that were felt to ultimately overestimate the effects of screening and as a result this study has fallen out of favor [30].

The PLCO Screening Trial was a US-based multi-institutional RCT of 76 693 men between the ages of 55 and 74 years who were randomly assigned to annual screening with PSA and DRE or their usual care [28]. A PSA level above 4.0 ng/mL or an abnormal DRE were indications for biopsy. A total of 7 years of follow-up was provided. The PCLO trial reported information on prostate cancer incidence, cancer-specific mortality, all-cause mortality, and cancer staging and is one of few studies with high compliance rates and total patient accrual. The reported incidence of prostate cancer per 10 000 person-years in the screening group was 116 compared with 95 in the control group (rate ratio, RR = 1.22; 95%CI = 1.16–1.29). The cancer-specific mortality per 10 000 person-years was 2.0 in the screened group and 1.7 in the unscreened population (RR = 1.13; 95%CI = 0.75–1.70). The percentage of those diagnosed with low stage

I or II cancers was also similar regardless of the group. Based on these results, neither prostate cancer incidence nor cancer-specific mortality demonstrated significant differences due to screening. Although the PLCO Trial has several methodological strengths, mainly the high number of participants and high compliance rates, there are some weaknesses. While the trial appears to be equally randomized between the study groups, approximately 44% of patients had received a PSA test prior to randomization in the control group and in addition by the sixth year of the study 52% of the control population had been screened. The fact that a significant proportion of the control population had already received screening prior to randomization suggests that men who are less likely to have prostate cancer and in addition less likely to have higher-stage or life-threatening disease may have been introduced into the control arm of the RCT, hence contributing to the lack of a significant difference in cancer incidence and mortality due to screening. A further weakness of the PLCO Trial was the short follow-up period of 7 years, which was addressed with the publication of 13-year follow-up data (92% follow-up through 10 years; 57% through 13 years); this found a 12% higher incidence of prostate cancer in the intervention arm (RR = 1.12; 95%CI = 1.07–1.17) with no significant difference in prostate cancer mortality compared with the control group (RR = 1.09; 95%CI = 0.87–1.36) [31]. Furthermore, the PLCO Trial used a PSA level of 4 ng/mL to trigger further workup, although it is generally accepted that lower cutoff PSA values may lead to detection of more cancers.

The ERSPC Trial was an European multi-institutional RCT initiated in the 1990s with participation of 182 160 men aged 50–74 years who were randomly assigned to PSA screening every 4 years or a control group that was offered no screening; median follow-up was 9 years [29]. This study used different recruiting and randomization procedures across seven centers in Europe and used a PSA cutoff of 2.5–4.0 ng/mL (with most centers using cutoff of 3.0 ng/mL) as indication for referral for TRUS and biopsy. After a median follow-up of 11 years, for the 162 243 men aged 55–69 years, the primary outcome of prostate cancer mortality was 21% lower in the group offered screening (RR = 0.79; 95%CI = 0.68–0.91). To prevent one death from prostate cancer at 11 years follow-up, 1055 men would need to be invited for screening and 37 cancers would need to be detected [32]. Furthermore, there was a 41% reduction of metastatic cancers detected in the screening group in addition to the identification of a higher percentage of patients with low-risk disease (Gleason scores 6 and 7 of 72.2% and 27.8%, respectively, in the screened group vs. 54.8%

and 45.2% in the control group). All-cause mortality was not reduced with screening (18.2 vs. 18.5 deaths per 1000 person-years; RR = 0.99; 95%CI = 0.97–1.01). In 2012, Schroder *et al.* consolidated their previous finding about ERSPC Trial published in 2009 that PSA-based screening significantly reduced mortality from prostate cancer but did not affect all-cause mortality.

Several factors could have contributed to this finding of no effect in all-cause mortality. About 24% of subjects invited for screening did not undergo PSA testing [29] and in addition a substantial proportion of the control group received PSA testing as 31% of cancers in the control group were in fact detected through PSA screening. Furthermore, additional analysis of the ERSPC data may further improve the mortality reduction and screening benefit found in the study. A subsequent analysis of the Rotterdam site data estimated that after adjustment for noncompliance in the screening population and contamination in the control arm, the mortality benefit found in the ERSPC population might be as high as 30% [33]. Furthermore, similar to the PLCO Trial, the 5–10-year lead time associated with PSA testing may mean the follow-up duration was insufficient to accurately estimate the survival benefit. A modeling study using data from all ERSPC sites concluded that the screening benefit could increase over time, with numbers needed to screen (NNS) of 837 at year 10 and 503 at year 12 [34].

Like all screening trials, the results of the ERSPC should be examined with certain caveats. First, several biases could have favored the screening group. A higher proportion of cancers diagnosed in the screening group was aggressively treated in a tertiary setting with radical prostatectomy compared with the control group where aggressive cancers were mostly treated with radiotherapy, expectant management, or hormonal therapy, so some of the survival outcome differences could be related more to improved treatment than screening [35]. While demonstrating a mortality benefit associated with screening, the ERSPC Trial also revealed a high likelihood of overdiagnosis and overtreatment with risk of overdiagnosis estimated to reach about 50%. It is of vital importance to note that any survival benefit from screening would not be realized for many years, while the burdens of screening and treatment, including harms from overdiagnosis and overtreatment, would occur immediately and potentially have lifelong consequences. Finally, of the seven individual centers included in the mortality analysis, two (Sweden and the Netherlands) demonstrated statistically significant reductions in prostate cancer deaths with PSA screening. The magnitude of effect was considerably greater in these two centers than in other countries.

The Göteborg Sweden Trial was a screening study involving 20 000 men aged 50–64 years who were randomized to screening with PSA every 2 years versus no screening. The primary end point was cancer-specific mortality, which was determined after a 14-year follow-up period [36]. The ERSPC site from Göteborg, Sweden, subsequently reported a cumulative mortality reduction of 44% for the PSA screening group after a median 14 years of follow-up (RR for death of 0.56 in those screened vs. nonscreened). Additionally, compared with the results reported by the ERSPC study, the NNS and numbers needed to treat (NNT) were 293 and 12, respectively, in the Göteborg Trial.

The Göteborg study demonstrated better outcomes with screening compared with both the larger ERSPC and PLCO trials. Different parameters in the Göteborg Trial design included a younger patient population (median 56 years of age compared with >60 years in ERSPC/PLCO trials), shorter interval of screening (every 2 years compared with 4 years in the ERSPC Trial), a lower rate of PSA testing prior to entry (approximately 3% compared with 44% in the PLCO Trial), a lower rate of contamination in the control group, and a longer duration of follow-up from randomization (median 14 years); these may contribute to the finding of a benefit for prostate cancer screening. The 44% relative risk reduction in deaths as demonstrated from this study may be the strongest evidence that screening for prostate cancer with PSA can be effective in lowering cancer-specific mortality.

Despite the publication of the results of several long-awaited RCTs, the controversy surrounding prostate cancer continues because the interpretation of this level-one evidence is varied. Although the ERSPC and the Göteborg Sweden trials suggest that screening with PSA can be effective in lowering cancer-specific mortality rates, there are still concerns over statistical analyses issues, contamination of control groups, insufficient follow-up time, differing levels of PSA triggering further workup, and inappropriate screening intervals.

In addition to the recent publication of RCTs to determine whether screening for prostate cancer will reduce prostate cancer mortality, certain RCTs have compared active treatments for localized prostate cancer with watchful waiting. These studies endeavored to determine whether aggressive treatment of localized prostate cancers detected by PSA will reduce morbidity and mortality when compared with watchful waiting. The PIVOT study, conducted in the United States, included men with prostate cancer detected after the initiation of widespread PSA testing. The trial randomly assigned 731 men aged 75 years or younger (mean age, 67 years) with a mean PSA level of <10 ng/mL and clinically localized prostate cancer to radical prostatectomy versus watchful waiting. On the basis of PSA level, Gleason score, and tumor stage, approximately 43% had low-risk tumors, 36% had intermediate-risk tumors, and 21% had high-risk tumors. After a median follow-up of 10 years, prostate cancer-specific or all-cause mortality did not statistically significantly differed between men treated with surgery versus observation (absolute risk reduction, 2.6% [95%CI = −1.1–6.5] and 2.9% [95%CI = −4.1–10.3], respectively) [25]. Subgroup analysis found that the effect of radical prostatectomy compared with observation for both overall and prostate cancer-specific mortality did not vary by patient characteristics (including age, race, health status, Charlson comorbidity index score, or Gleason score), but there was variation by PSA level and possibly tumor risk category. In men in the radical prostatectomy group with a PSA level >10 μg/L at diagnosis, there was an absolute risk reduction of 7.2% (95%CI = 0.0–14.8%) and 13.2% (95%CI = 0.9–24.9%) for prostate cancer-specific and all-cause mortality, respectively, compared with men in the watchful waiting group. However, prostate cancer-specific or all-cause mortality was not reduced among men in the radical prostatectomy group with PSA levels of 10 μg/L or less or those with low-risk tumors [25, 37]. This study suggests that although a PSA blood test may detect low-grade localized prostate cancers, their aggressive treatment with surgery has no survival benefit when compared with watchful waiting.

## Screening recommendations from international health organizations

### USA screening guidelines

The current prostate cancer screening recommendations from several US national health organizations are not in agreement. The American Cancer Society (ACS), National Comprehensive Cancer Network (NCCN), United States Preventive Services Task Force (USPSTF), and American Urological Association (AUA) all differ regarding their recommended approach to screening of prostate cancer using the PSA blood test. A commonality of these studies is the emphasis on informed decision-making between physician and patient. Given the important trade-offs between potential benefits and harms involved with either screening or not screening for prostate cancer, and the lack of definitive data on screening outcomes, it is particularly important that patients make informed decisions about undergoing testing [38].

The AUA guidelines suggest that a baseline DRE and PSA at 40 years of age should be taken. Men who wish to be screened should make an individualized decision after discussion of the risks and benefits of screening with a healthcare provider. Those who wish to be screened will receive both a DRE and PSA test. Screening should normally be stopped at age of 75 years, but may be continued if the patient has a life expectancy of 10 years or more [39].

In October 2011, the USPSTF issued a draft report on PSA-based screening for prostate cancer, giving it a grade D recommendation, that is, "the USPSTF recommends against the service" because it has concluded that "there is moderate or high certainty that the service has no net benefit or that the harms outweigh the benefits." This recommendation, which contradicts the view that PSA-based screening saves lives by reducing the risk of death from prostate cancer, was met with considerable controversy [40]. The recommendations are based predominantly on analysis of data from the PLCO and ERSPC trials. The strength of their argument lies in the fact that these two RCTs reported conflicting results. The PLCO Trial did not demonstrate any reduction of prostate cancer mortality. The ERSPC Trial found a reduction in prostate cancer deaths of approximately 1 death per 1000 men screened, but the USPSTF argues that this result was heavily influenced by the results from two countries; five of the seven countries reporting results did not find a statistically significant reduction. In addition, the report states that the reduction in prostate cancer mortality after 10–14 years is at most very small and stresses that all-cause mortality in the European trial was nearly identical in the screened and nonscreened groups [41]. The USPSTF underlines the harms that can be associated with screening and treatment of screen-detected cancer. They describe false-positive PSA results that can result in negative psychological effects, including persistent worry about prostate cancer. Men who have a false-positive test result are then likely to proceed to TRUS and biopsy. New evidence from a RCT of treatment of screen-detected cancer indicates that roughly one in three men who have prostate biopsy experience pain, fever, bleeding, infection, and transient urinary difficulties and approximately 1% of men require hospitalization [42]. It is well established that surgery and radiotherapy are associated with serious risks, including perioperative death, cardiovascular complications, urinary incontinence, and erectile dysfunction. The USPSTF argue that the high likelihood of false-positive results from PSA testing coupled with its inability to distinguish indolent from aggressive tumors means that a substantial number of men undergo biopsy and are overdiagnosed with and overtreated for prostate cancer. They highlight the rate of overdiagnosis, as found in the ERSPC Trial, of up to 50%.

The conclusions drawn by the USPSTF have been criticized from many sources, including the coordinator of the ERSPC Trial who pointed out a number of weaknesses in the USPSTF report [43]. First, it relied heavily on a meta-analysis that combined higher- and lower-quality evidence which were all given equal weight. This seems unjustified given that certain RCT such as the PLCO Trial had an excessive contamination rate in the control group as more than 40% of subjects had undergone PSA testing before randomization. The USPSTF did not take into account data from the Göteborg study which showed that after 14 years of follow-up the NNS and NNT reported in the ERSPC Trial are likely to improve with long-term follow-up. Further, they did not consider the strong evidence that suggests that the concurrent use of PSA testing with DRE and TRUS has a higher sensitivity, specificity, and positive predictive values in the detection of localized prostate cancer compared with PSA testing alone. Schroder suggested that overtreatment can be at least temporarily avoided by offering active surveillance to men who have a low risk of prostate cancer; however, these men would be taking a small risk of having progressive disease that goes unnoticed.

## European and international screening guidelines

The variation in international prostate cancer screening guidelines reflects the different clinical environments found in different healthcare systems. The European Association of Urology (EAU), United Kingdom National Health Services (UK NHS), New Zealand National Health Committee (NHC), and Japanese Urological Association (JUA) differ in opinion regarding the role of PSA and DRE for national screening of prostate cancer. The EAU position statement published in May 2009 states that the current available evidence argues against national screening for prostate cancer because of significant risk of overtreatment [44]. The UK NHS and the NHC present a similar guideline statement as the EAU that there is currently insufficient evidence at this time to recommend national screening protocols for prostate cancer [45, 46]. In contrast, the JUA makes a firm recommendation in favor of prostate cancer screening and suggests that men should obtain a PSA with or without DRE starting at 50 years of age and those with a positive family history should have a PSA test at 40 years of age [47].

The differing position between health organizations, and particularly the USPSTF with its recent controversial recommendations, provides a mixed message to the general patient population and healthcare-provider alike. This controversy in the literature means that no "standard of care" exists for prostate cancer screening at the present time. For two decades, primary care physicians have been expected to present a screening test to patients through an elaborate ritual of informed decision-making. Almost all guidelines uphold and stress the importance of informed decision-making and patient-centered care. However, it remains challenging to initiate truly informed discussion with a patient with regards to PSA testing with so many probability estimates and uncertainties. What PSA cut-off is best? What level should trigger repeat PSA testing or biopsy? How often should we repeat the PSA test? What is the patient's pretest probability of cancer? What is the chance that a PSA test plus a biopsy will find cancer and if cancer is found will it be clinically important? It seems unlikely that such uncertainties can be addressed by today's physicians and currently available clinical tools.

Attempts to improve the accuracy of diagnostic tools in prostate cancer will therefore have to center on the development of new biomarkers that attempt to identify potentially life-threatening prostate cancer at a curable stage. The PCA3 urine assay has begun to show promising results in predicting the presence of prostate cancer, with sensitivities and specificities of 54% and 74%, respectively, in one study of men undergoing prostatic biopsy [48]. Technological advancements in imaging technology, such as the use of multiparametric MRI imaging, will also be central in our aim for more accurate information about the presence and nature of prostate cancer in patients [49]. Future screening efforts will undoubtedly need to utilize more accurate diagnostic tools in order to better differentiate those who harbor life-threatening cancer from indolent disease.

# References

1 NCI statistics. Available at http://www.cancer.gov/statfacts/html/prost.html. Last accessed April 13, 2013.
2 Marwick C. Global review of diet and cancer links available. *J Am Med Assoc* 1997;278:1650–1651.
3 Godley PA. Prostate cancer screening: promise and peril—a review. *Cancer Detect Prev* 1999;23:316–324.

4  Lippman SM, Klein EA, Goodman PJ, *et al.* Effect of selenium and vitamin E on risk of prostate cancer and other cancers: the Selenium and Vitamin E Cancer Prevention Trial (SELECT). *J Am Med Assoc* 2009; 301(1):39–51.

5  Musquera M, Fleshner NE, Finelli A, Zlotta AR. The REDUCE trial: chemoprevention in prostate cancer using the 5alpha-reductase inhibitor, dutasteride. *Expert Rev Anticancer Ther* 2008;8(7):1073–1079

6  Reynard J, Brewster S, Biers S. *Oxford Handbook of Urology.* Oxford: Oxford University Press; 2009.

7  Higashihara E, Nutahara K, Kojima M, *et al.* Significance of free prostate-specific antigen and gamma- seminoprotein in the screening of prostate cancer. *Prostate Suppl* 1996;7:40–47.

8  Catalona WJ, Smith DS, Ratliff TL, *et al.* Measurement of prostate-specific antigen in serum as a screening test for prostate cancer. *N Engl J Med* 1991;324(17):1156–1161.

9  Ghann PH, Hennekens CH, Stampfer MJ. A prospective evaluation of plasma prostate-specific antigen for detection of prostatic cancer. *J Am Med Assoc* 1995; 273(4):289.

10  Stamey TA, Yang N, Hay AR, *et al.* Prostate-specific antigen as a serum marker for adenocarcinoma of the prostate. *N Engl J Med* 1987;317(15):909–916.

11  Mettlin C, Lee F, Drago J, Murphy GP. The American Cancer Society National Prostate Cancer Detection Project. Findings on the detection of early prostate cancer in 2425 men. *Cancer* 1991;67(12):2949.

12  Potosky AL, Miller BA, Albertsen PC, Kramer BS. The role of increasing detection in the rising incidence of prostate cancer. *J Am Med Assoc* 1995;273(7):548.

13  Crawford ED, DeAntoni EP, Etzioni R, *et al.* Serum prostate-specific antigen and digital rectal examination for early detection of prostate cancer in a national community-based program. The Prostate Cancer Education Council. *Urology* 1996;47(6): 863.

14  Wolf AM, Wender RC, Etzioni RB, *et al.* American Cancer Society Prostate Cancer Advisory Committee. American Cancer Society guideline for the early detection of prostate cancer: update 2010. *CA Cancer J Clin* 2010;60(2):70.

15  Meigs JB, Barry MJ, Oesterling JE, Jacobsen SJ. Interpreting results of prostate-specific antigen testing for early detection of prostate cancer. *J Gen Intern Med* 1996;11(9):505.

16  Schröder FH, van der Cruijsen-Koeter I, de Koning HJ, *et al.* Prostate cancer detection at low prostate specific antigen. *J Urol* 2000;163(3):806.

17  Catalona WJ, Richie JP, Ahmann FR, *et al.* Comparison of digital rectal examination and serum prostate specific antigen in the early detection of prostate cancer: results of a multicenter clinical trial of 6,630 men. *J Urol* 1994;151(5):1283.

18  Smith RA, von Eschenbach AC, Wender R, *et al.* ACS Prostate Cancer Advisory Committee, ACS Colorectal Cancer Advisory Committee, ACS Endometrial Cancer Advisory Committee. American Cancer Society guidelines for the early detection of cancer: update of early detection guidelines for prostate, colorectal, and endometrial cancers. Also: update 2001–testing for early lung cancer detection. *CA Cancer J Clin* 2001;51(1):38.

19  Bretton PR. Prostate-specific antigen and digital rectal examination in screening for prostate cancer: a community-based study. *South Med J* 1994;87(7):720.

20 Galić J, Karner I, Cenan L, *et al.* Comparison of digital rectal examination and prostate specific antigen in early detection of prostate cancer. *Coll Antropol* 2003; 27(Suppl. 1):61–66.

21 Hammerer P, Huland H. Systematic sextant biopsies in 651 patients referred for prostate evaluation. *J Urol* 1994;151:99–101.

22 Catalona WJ. Radical surgery for advanced prostate cancer and for radiation failures. *J Urol* 1993;147:916.

23 D'Amico AV, Whittington R, Malkowicz SB. Biochemical outcome after radical prostatectomy, external beam radiation therapy or interstitial radiation therapy for clinically localized prostate cancer. *J Am Med Assoc* 1998;280:969–974.

24 Wilson JMG, Jungner G. *Principles and Practice of Screening for Disease.* Geneva: WHO; 1968.

25 Wilt TJ, Brawer MK, Jones KM, *et al.* Radical prostatectomy versus observation for localized prostate cancer. *N Engl J Med* 2012 Jul 19;367(3):203–213.

26 Benoit RM, Grönberg H, Naslund MJ. A quantitative analysis of the costs and benefits of prostate cancer screening. *Prostate Cancer Prostatic Dis* 2001;4(3):138–145.

27 Labrie F, Candas B, Dupont A, *et al.* Screening decreases prostate cancer death: first analysis of the 1988 Quebec Prospective Randomized Controlled Trial. *Prostate* 1999;38(2):83–91.

28 Andriole GL, Grubb RL, Buys SS, *et al.* Mortality results from a randomized prostate cancer screening trial. *N Engl J Med* 2009;360(13):1310–1319.

29 Schroder FH, Hugosson J, Roobol MJ, *et al.* Screening and prostate-cancer mortality in a randomized European study. *N Engl J Med* 2009;360(13):1320–1328.

30 Boer R, Schroder FH. Quebec randomized controlled trial on prostate cancer screening shows no evidence for mortality reduction – letter to the editor. *Prostate* 1999;40(2):130–131.

31 Andriole GL, Crawford ED, Grubb RL 3rd, *et al.* Prostate cancer screening in the randomized Prostate, Lung, Colorectal, and Ovarian Cancer Screening Trial: mortality results after 13 years of follow-up. *J Natl Cancer Inst* 2012;104(2):125.

32 Schröder FH, Hugosson J, Roobol MJ, *et al.* ERSPC Investigators. Prostate-cancer mortality at 11 years of follow-up. *N Engl J Med* 2012;366(11):981–990.

33 Roobol MJ, Kerkhof M, Schröder FH, *et al.* Prostate cancer mortality reduction by prostate-specific antigen-based screening adjusted for nonattendance and contamination in the European Randomised Study of Screening for Prostate Cancer (ERSPC). *Eur Urol* 2009;56(4):584.

34 Loeb S, Vonesh EF, Metter EJ, *et al.* What is the true number needed to screen and treat to save a life with prostate-specific antigen testing. *J Clin Oncol* 2011;29(4):464.

35 Barry MJ. Screening for prostate cancer–the controversy that refuses to die. *N Engl J Med* 2009;360(13):1351.

36 Hugosson J, Carlsson S, Aus G, *et al.* Mortality results from the Göteborg randomised population-based prostate-cancer screening trial. *Lancet Oncol* 2010;11(8):725.

37 Wilt TJ, Brawer MK, Barry MJ, *et al.* The Prostate Cancer Intervention versus Observational Trial VA/NCI/AHRQ Cooperative Studies Program 407 (PIVOT): design and baseline results of a randomized controlled trial comparing radical prostatectomy to watchful waiting for men with clinically localized prostate cancer. *Contemp Clin Trials* 2009;30(1):81–87.

38  Chou R, LeFevre ML. Prostate cancer screening–the evidence, the recommendations, and the clinical implications. *J Am Med Assoc* 2011;306(24):2721–2722.

39  Greene KL, Albertsen PC, Babaian RJ, *et al.* Prostate specific antigen best practice statement: 2009 update. *J Urol* 2009;182(5):2232–2241.

40  Screening for prostate cancer: draft recommendation statement. Rockville, MD: U.S. Preventive Services Task Force. Available at http://www.uspreventiveservicestask force.org/draftrec3.htm. Last accessed October 7, 2011.

41  Moyer VA. On behalf of the U.S. Preventive Services Task Force. Screening for Prostate Cancer: U.S. Preventive Services Task Force Recommendation Statement. *Ann Intern Med* 2012;157(2):120–134.

42  Rosario DJ, Lane JA, Metcalfe C, *et al.* Short term outcomes of prostate biopsy in men tested for cancer by prostate specific antigen: prospective evaluation within ProtecT study. *Br Med J* 2012;344:d7894.

43  Schröder FH. Stratifying risk–the U.S. Preventive Services Task Force and prostate-cancer screening. *N Engl J Med* 2011;365(21):1953–1955.

44  Abrahamsson P, Artibani W, Chapple CR, Wirth M. European Association of Urology position statement on screening for prostate cancer. *Eur Urol* 2009;56(2):270–271.

45  Logan R, Fougere G, Hague K, *et al.* Prostate cancer screening in New Zealand. New Zealand National Health Committee. Available at http://nhc.health.govt.nz/ publications/nhc-publications-pre-2011/prostate-cancer-screening-new-zealand. Last accessed April 17, 2013.

46  Burford DC, Austoker KM. Prostate cancer risk management programme information for primary care; PSA testing in asymptomatic men. Evidence document. NHS Cancer Screening Programmes, 2010. Available at http://www.cancerscreening. nhs.uk/prostate/pcrmp02.pdf. Last accessed April 17, 2013.

47  Committee for Establishment of the Guidelines on Screening for Prostate Cancer; Japanese Urological Association. Updated Japanese Urological Association Guidelines on prostate-specific antigen-based screening for prostate cancer in 2010. *Int J Urol* 2010;17(10):830–838.

48  Deras IL, Aubin SM, Blasé A, *et al.* PCA3: a molecular urine assay for predicting prostate biopsy outcome. *J Urol* 2008;179:1587–1592.

49  Kirkham AP, Emberton M, Allen C. How good is MRI at detecting and characterising cancer within the prostate? *Eur Urol* 2006;50:1163–1174.

# CHAPTER 3
# Understanding the Histopathology

*Jon Oxley*
Southmead Hospital, North Bristol NHS Trust, Bristol, UK

## Histological variants of prostate cancer

Prostate cancer can be divided into tumors derived from the epithelial component and the nonepithelial/stromal component. The epithelial derived tumors are further subdivided based on their morphological appearances. The most common appearance is acinar, comprising 90% of tumors and has variants such as microacinar, atrophic, pseudohyperplastic, and signet ring. The other group is the so-called non-acinar and this includes ductal, sarcomatoid, and small cell carcinoma, as well as urothelial carcinoma [1]. The acinar variants can be graded with a Gleason score, as can be ductal adenocarcinoma, and from the point of view of management this should be used as a guide to treatment. Ductal adenocarcinoma often occurs with a microacinar component [2] and appears to behave as a high-grade tumor (Gleason pattern 4). Occasionally, small cell carcinomas are seen and this is most common after hormone therapy for a microacinar tumor. Often this is associated with hormone refractory disease and has a poor prognosis. Very rarely it occurs *de novo* and the differential diagnosis would be a small cell carcinoma of the bladder involving the prostate, as small cell carcinomas in the bladder are not infrequent.

The rarer nonepithelial/stromal tumors occurring in the prostate include leiomyosarcomas and solitary fibrous tumors, and there is often involvement of the prostate in patients with chronic lymphocytic leukemia but these will not be discussed further.

---

*Prostate Cancer: Diagnosis and Clinical Management*, First Edition.
Edited by Ashutosh K. Tewari, Peter Whelan and John D. Graham.
© 2014 John Wiley & Sons, Ltd. Published 2014 by John Wiley & Sons, Ltd.

# Histology of the prostate and immunohistochemistry

The majority of prostate cancers are derived from the luminal cells of the prostatic glands. These cells express prostate-specific antigen (PSA) and are surrounded by a basal layer of cells. The basal cells express high molecular cytokeratins. Cytokeratins are the structural proteins that make up epithelial cells and different epithelium expresses different cytokeratins. These cytokeratins can be detected using a technique called immunohistochemistry. In this technique, antibodies are labeled with enzymes that precipitate pigment in the sites that the antibodies bind. These pigments can be either red or brown and are visible under the microscope. This technique has particularly revolutionized prostate pathology, as now the absence of basal cells can be shown by the absence of staining for high-molecular-weight cytokeratin. This technique was developed in the 1980s, but by the 1990s it became widely used. The commonest marker for high-molecular-weight cytokeratin is 34betaE12 but more recently antibodies to p63, which is a protein in the nuclei responsible for epithelial proliferation and differentiation, have been utilized. In 2002, the use of genetic testing of prostate cancer revealed an increase in a protein called alpha-methylacyl-CoA racemase (AMACR) [3]. This protein was increased in most prostate cancers. Antibodies to this marker are now available and the loss of basal cells and the expression of AMACR is now an extremely useful confirmatory test in borderline cases (Figure 3.1, Plate 3.1). The use of immunohistochemistry has helped the pathologist reach a diagnosis, but there are pitfalls such as high-grade prostatic intraepithelial neoplasia (PIN) which expresses AMACR [4].

# Prostate cores

The nature of prostate histopathology specimens has changed over the past 20 years due to the increase in prostate core biopsies as well as radical prostatectomies, and the decrease in the number of transurethral resections. There has been a trend in pathology to standardize reports and diagnoses used in all cancers as illustrated by datasets being published by the Royal College of Pathologists in the early 2000s [5]. Noncancer diagnoses that are widely used are PIN, PINAtyp, atypia suspicious for malignancy, and atypical small acinar proliferation (ASAP).

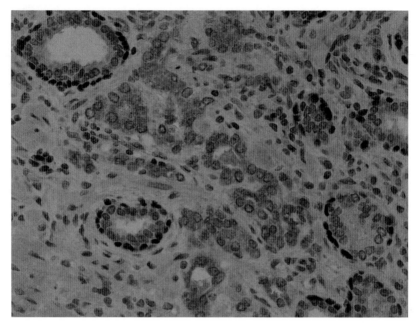

**Figure 3.1** Immunohistochemistry for AMACR and p63: The benign glands around the edge have basal cells that show nuclear staining for p63 (brown), the cancer glands centrally lack these basal cells but show positive staining for AMACR (red). (See also Plate 3.1.)

PIN was divided into high and low grade but it has become clear that low-grade PIN has poorly defined features and shows poor reproducibility among pathologists. As a result, this terminology has fallen out of favor. Today the term PIN refers to high-grade PIN. This describes nuclear crowding in the glands, prominent nucleoli but a maintained basal cell layer. Early studies suggested that repeat biopsies following a diagnosis of PIN had a high yield of prostate cancer but these studies used sextant biopsy protocols. With today's 10 or 12 core protocols, this risk appears to be similar to a negative set of cores [6], though multifocal PIN does appear to have increased risk of prostate cancer on subsequent cores.

*Atypia suspicious for prostate cancer/ASAP* is used when a pathologist finds a group of glands that lack basal layer cells but either has insufficient number of glands or lacks nuclear changes of prostate cancer. It is clear that different pathologists will have different thresholds for atypia and number of glands required. A more experienced pathologist may have a lower threshold but there can be interobserver variation as well. One major problem is that atrophic glands can lose their basal cells and there is a variant of prostate cancer that can mimic this, and as a result atrophic glands can often be labeled as ASAP. It can be useful to explain to clinicians whether the failure to reach a malignant diagnosis is based on a lack in the number of suspicious glands that have typical features of prostate cancer or concerns over atrophic mimics. There is good evidence that repeat biopsies are warranted as they can detect prostate cancer in 40% of cases [6].

Another pattern that is often placed in this category is so-called PINAtyp or outpouching of PIN. The section on the slide is a two-dimensional cut through a three-dimensional gland. If this gland has PIN with an attenuated basal layer and the gland bulges out, then the section may show a gland with no basal layer but the nuclear features of prostate cancer. As a result, atypical glands seen next to a focus of PIN are labeled PINAtyp. Studies seem to suggest that the risk of prostate cancer in subsequent cores is higher than PIN and similar to ASAP [7].

*Prostatic adenocarcinoma*—the diagnosis of prostate cancer requires the combination of morphology, architecture, and cytology. Immunohistochemistry can be used to support the diagnosis. Currently, molecular techniques play no role in the diagnosis of prostate cancer. All prostate cancer reports should contain as a minimum: the Gleason score, number of cores involved, and the volume of cancer. Perineural invasion is reported by most pathologists and is a data item in the RCPath dataset [5].

## Gleason score

Gleason developed his scoring system for prostate cancer in the 1960s looking at TURP specimens and found that patients with a one architectural pattern had a different prognosis to a patient with a mixture of this pattern and another. This lead to a scoring system using two grades— the predominant pattern and the second commonest pattern. These grades were assigned a number from 1 to 5 and when combined gave a Gleason score, for example, $3 + 3 = 6$. When core biopsies became commonplace in the 1990s, pathologists started assigning Gleason scores to these. This became a problem as Gleason pattern 2 was defined as a well-demarcated noninfiltrative focus of cancer, which in a core was difficult to assess. Many pathologists called small foci of tumor pattern 2 and as a result Gleason scores of 4 and 5 were common. When the radical prostatectomies specimens from these patients were examined, they had higher-grade tumors as the infiltrative nature became apparent. By the late 1990s, it became clear that Gleason pattern 2 could not be reliably diagnosed in core biopsies. The Gleason shift of Gleason score 5 to Gleason score 6 then occurred. This led to a problem that clinical studies/nomograms using the older classification of Gleason could no longer be used.

Another problem noted was that Gleason pattern 3 contained a cribriform pattern which was difficult to separate from cribriform pattern 4. As a result, most pathologists assigned this cribriform pattern to Gleason pattern 4. Occasionally, three patterns were present and this lead to the use of tertiary grade, for example, 3 + 4 = tertiary 5. Tertiary grade 5 implies that there was less pattern 5 than either 3 or 4. Studies looking at the tertiary scores found that these were prognostically significant and so the presence of a small amount of a higher-grade tumor should appear in the Gleason score, the argument being that this was likely to be present in the radical prostatectomy specimen. As a result of this, the Gleason score was changed to have the commonest pattern plus the highest grade present regardless of the amount of this grade present. A consensus meeting in 2005 published these recommendations [8]. With the implementation of these recommendations any pattern 4 appearing in the score and the next significant shift in Gleason scores have occurred as there was a shift from Gleason score 3 + 3 to 3 + 4. This has a major implication for risk stratification as low-risk groups typically exclude Gleason score 7, but these risk-group studies used the older definition of Gleason score.

Gleason scoring is not reliable after hormonal/radiotherapy treatment as these treatments shrink the glands so making Gleason pattern 3 look like Gleason pattern 4, that is, artificially upgrading. There is a suggestion that we should grade prostate cancer that shows no treatment affect but it is not widely performed [9].

## Volume of cancer in cores

As prostatic core biopsies are not normally directed at suspicious foci, the volume of tumor in the cores normally reflects the volume of tumor in the prostate. There are some significant exceptions to this, very large prostates are poorly sampled and tumors in the anterior zone can be missed [10]. The number of involved cores can normally be easily given by the pathologist, but when multiple cores are embedded in a single block these cores can fragment or overlap and then counting involved cores can become a problem. When a single core is examined on a slide, this helps but with increasing number of cores being taken this technique would greatly increase the workload for laboratories. There is more variation in how the volume of tumor in the cores is calculated. Some centers use overall percentage, which is easier to assess if multiple cores are embedded together, others measure the length of tumor in millimeters and then give the longest length and total length. It is recommended to give this information, but no system has proved to be superior.

## Perineural invasion

Prostate cancer has a propensity to invade the perineural spaces and uses this as a method for extending outside the prostate. There is a degree of subjectivity when this is interpreted by pathologists and this probably explains the wide variation of incidence from 11% to 33% [11]. As the majority of nerves within the prostate lie just beneath the capsule, the presence of tumor in perineural spaces in core biopsies would suggest that tumor was close to the capsule. Whether the presence of perineural invasion can predict extraprostatic extension has been extensively studied and meta-analysis suggests that on univariate analysis it does but when factors such as Gleason score are accounted for then it does not predict T3 disease but there is some evidence that it predicts PSA recurrence following surgery or radiotherapy [11].

## Core quality

The diagnosis of prostate cancer is dependent on good-quality core biopsies. The quality of the cores can be affected at many stages of the process. Understanding the processes can help to improve quality of cores. Simple changes can have an impact on the quality and it is useful for clinicians to get feedback on the adequacy of their biopsies. Comparison between operators and centers is useful and there are UK guidelines describing this [12]. The cores should not be removed from the Tru-cut needle with a needle, it is better to roll them onto blotting paper and place them into formalin. Mesh cassettes are used in some departments and these are excellent for gastrointestinal biopsies but they cause crush artefact. Also if multiple cores are placed in these, they get tangled and counting the number of cores involved becomes very difficult as they overlap on the final histology slide. Whether a single core is embedded in a single histological block is another debate—single-core embedding allows a better section to be cut which aids the diagnostic process but the increase in workload for a pathology department moving from multiple-core embedding to single-core embedding combined with newer protocols of more biopsies has meant that this has not been widely adopted in the United Kingdom.

## Reporting errors

The advent of DNA testing has meant that specimens that are mislabeled can be matched with patients but the diagnosis of prostate cancer still relies on a pathologist who is interpreting morphology. Sometimes this can be missed or incorrectly diagnosed. Prostate core biopsies are one of the commonest causes of litigation for pathologists in the United States, but there has been a change over the past 20 years from false positives to false negatives. The decrease in false-positive cases has probably occurred due to the increasing use of immunohistochemistry to confirm the diagnosis in subtle cases and the increasing use of review by another pathologist either by double reporting or reviewing the slides at multidisciplinary meetings. Most laboratories do not review their negative cores, and immunohistochemistry is not performed on all biopsies, so some small foci can be missed, which are only detected when these biopsies are reviewed later. The actual false-negative rate is difficult to measure but we reviewed all biopsies prior to the multidisciplinary team (MDT) meeting, and our overall false-negative rate was 1.7% (PSA screening population 2.1%, non-screening 1.5%). The overall false-positive rate was 0.5% (screening 0.9%, non-screening 0.4%). These error rates varied among pathologists, with the false-negative rate ranging from 0% to 9.3%, and the false-positive rate ranging from 0% to 3.8% [13]. The increasing subspecialization by pathologists will probably lower these rates. There is also evidence that central review helps detect errors with a false-positive rate of approximately 1% [14].

## Transurethral resection specimens

In order to manage the workload of histopathology laboratories, these specimens are normally sampled when there is clinically benign hyperplasia, though the methodology used varies. The RCPath recommends embedding the entire specimen up to 12 g (six blocks) and a further 2 g (one block) for every additional 5 g [5]. If the specimen is from a patient with known prostate cancer, then they recommend embedding the whole specimen, as these tend to be small-volume resections. In patients treated with hormones/radiotherapy, Gleason grading is not performed if the tumor responds to treatment because it is unreliable (see Gleason Score section above).

## Radical prostatectomies

The number of radical prostatectomies performed in the United Kingdom has greatly increased over the past decade, and with better surgical techniques offering decreased morbidity, this trend is likely to continue over the next decade.

### Fresh specimens for tumor banking

Ideally, the specimens should be sent fresh to the pathology department to enable fresh tissue to be sampled but there are problems in sampling fresh prostates. The most significant problem is that tumors are often not visible macroscopically—so a technique of systematic rather than targeted sampling is entailed. Another significant problem is that the capsule of the prostate maintains the integrity of the organ—as soon as you cut this the benign hyperplastic nodules expand, so distorting the margins. This expansion is magnified during fixation. A simple technique is to take a single slice through the middle of the prostate and then core out disks of tissue. The slice is then pinned to a cork board to maintain its shape while it is fixed [15]. The other halves are also pinned to maintain their shape. When the section with the holes is examined, there may be tumor around the holes and by inference there will be tumor in the frozen sample. If no tumor is found in the remaining prostate, the frozen samples can be examined.

### Processing the radical prostatectomy specimens

In order to make histological slides, the prostate needs to be cut into slices no thicker than 5 mm and ideally 3 mm. Clearly a prostate weighing 150 g will produce many slices and as a result many glass slides. To minimize workload, but without decreasing the prognostic information, several sampling techniques have been developed but these in themselves can be complex. Modern pathology laboratories use large blocks and this enables a whole slice of an average prostate to be embedded in one block, so decreasing the workload. Most laboratories in the United Kingdom use these large blocks and embed the whole prostate.

Before the specimen can be processed it needs to be fixed in formalin. Injecting with formalin or heating in a microwave speeds up this process, but these methods are not widely used. The larger the prostate, the longer it takes to fix; for example, a prostate weighing more than 50 g takes more than 24 hours to be fixed. Slicing the prostate before it is fixed will result in expanding of benign nodules leading slices of varying thickness. When sections are taken from these slices, holes can appear as the thicker areas are cut first.

Before the prostate is sliced, the outer surface is painted with different inks. These inks are visible on the slides. By using various colors, the left and right side can be identified. The ink has been applied to the outer surface and this correlates with the surgical margin, but one major problem is that if the capsule has been incised by the surgeon, then the benign nodules can expand. This expansion can widen the incision and a small nick can become a much larger defect following fixation but before the specimen is inked. This is particularly relevant in the apex, as the capsule is always breached around the urethra—this may explain why apical margins are often positive but are not thought to be clinically as important as other margins.

The prostate is sliced perpendicular to the posterior surface, with the slices from the apex and base normally cut into smaller slices perpendicular to this slice again [16]. This allows the margins to be assessed at the apex, base, and circumference. The seminal vesicles are sectioned either longitudinally or transversely. The slices are then processed and wax blocks are formed. This processing normally takes between 14 and 22 hours. From the wax blocks, 6 $\mu$m sections are taken and placed onto the glass slides, stained, and finally coverslipped, ready for reading on the microscope.

## Radical prostatectomy data

A large amount of data can be obtained from the radical prostatectomy specimen. Most prostates contain more than one focus of tumor and as a result the location of the tumors, Gleason score, volume, stage, perineural/vascular invasion, and margin status are all recorded.

### Location and multiplicity

There is no standard technique for recording the location of the tumor, but simple methods of left/right and anterior/posterior/lateral/basal/apical and combinations are normally employed. The location in itself has probably no prognostic value, though basal tumors have been shown to be worse. Anterior tumors are known to be underestimated in TRUS biopsies [10]. The number of tumors is recorded and this is of interest with the increasing debate over focal therapy [17], but to the patient it has little prognostic relevance.

## Gleason score

Gleason score has proved to be the best predictor of outcome but there is still debate about how to apply this to the radical prostatectomies. Gleason grading of each focus is performed by some centers, whereas others give the grade of the worse focus and yet others give a global score as if all the tumors were one. This can make a difference if there is a small focus of high-grade tumor (e.g., 4 + 4) and a much larger low-grade tumor (e.g., 3 + 3), as the overall score would be 3 + 4 but the prognosis is more likely to be related to the focus of 4 + 4. Fortunately, this scenario is uncommon. The rules for Gleason scoring in the radical prostatectomy are slightly different from the prostate cores; if a Gleason pattern is less than 5% of the tumor volume, then it should not appear in the score, unlike in the cores where there is no such cut off. With the current increase in 3 + 4 cores there may be a decrease in the concordance with the radical prostatectomies as small-volume pattern 4 in the radical prostatectomy may not appear in the score.

## Volume

There is no standardized approach to measuring volume of tumor in the prostate and there is conflicting data to its prognostic significance. There is concordance between volume in the cores and volume in the radical prostatectomy specimen. The methods involved in measuring volume of tumor in the prostates are varied—some use computer analysis, whereas others use estimation methods based on measurements of the tumor foci. There will always be a degree of estimation as the pathologist is only examining a 6 μm section of a 3–5 mm slice. Categorization into "clinically insignificant," low-, medium-, and high-volume tumor seems to be the most useful bearing in mind the limitations of the methodology.

## Stage

The stage and Gleason score are the best predictors of outcome. The TNM staging system was updated in 2009 but there was only a minor change and this related to pT3a. There had been debate about the staging of tumor when it involved the base margin—that is, bladder neck. This would have been considered as pT4 in the TNM6 system but studies had shown that the prognosis was much better than pT4 elsewhere. As a result, microscopic involvement of the bladder neck is now considered as pT3a. The problem the pathologist faces with this is that the bladder neck is not a well-defined pathological structure. Benign hyperplasia can lead to expansion of the median lobe obscuring the transition from detrusor muscle of the bladder to the muscle of the prostatic stroma. Often this is not a problem as tumors involving the bladder neck often have extracapsular extension elsewhere.

The other area which causes the pathologist difficulty is defining extra-capsular extension. There is no definite capsule to the prostate but we assume that fat demarcates extracapsular tissue, though rare examples of intraprostatic fat have been described. The presence of tumor in fat thus equates to pT3a. Unfortunately, sometimes there is tumor in tissue at the same plane as the fat but not actually in the fat (particularly when the tumor is anterior) and in other cases tumor bulges out and is surrounded by a fibrous capsule. This leads to a degree of subjectivity and often a con-sensus is reached among pathologists working together. In these difficult cases, cutting further sections into the wax blocks can help as it may show a more obvious focus of extraprostatic extension. Most pathologists cate-gorize the extent of capsular breach as focal or established, though once again, there are no strict criteria [18].

The substaging of pT2 appears less important and there are even differ-ences in how pathologists apply this. Some pathologists use pT2c when there are tumors in both lobes regardless of size, while others only use this when a tumor focus extends from one side to another.

The use of pT2+ has become established and it is used when there is an involved intraprostatic margin (see Margin Status section). When this margin is involved, the pathologist is uncertain whether there was pT3a disease in this area. Clearly this becomes less relevant if there is pT3a dis-ease elsewhere.

### Perineural invasion and vascular invasion

Perineural invasion in the radical prostatectomy specimen is so common that it is not a significant prognostic factor. On the other hand, vascular invasion is rare and is associated with a poor prognosis [19]. Identifying vascular invasion can be extremely subjective as retraction artefact is com-mon and this can mimic vascular invasion.

### Margin status

The definition of each type of margin reported by the pathologist is the single most common question asked by surgeons and cancer nurses when

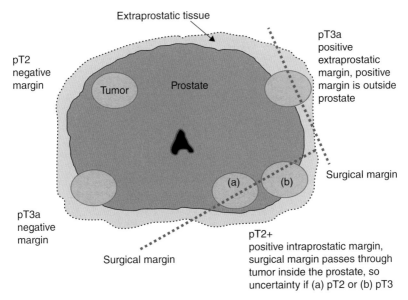

Extraprostatic tissue

pT3a
positive
extraprostatic
margin, positive
margin is outside
prostate

pT2
negative
margin

Tumor          Prostate

Surgical margin

pT3a
negative
margin

Surgical margin

pT2+
positive intraprostatic margin,
surgical margin passes through
tumor inside the prostate, so
uncertainty if (a) pT2 or (b) pT3

**Figure 3.2** Surgical margins: Diagram demonstrating the difference between intra- and extraprostatic margins.

confronted by a pathology report. Pathologists define an involved margin by the presence of tumor at ink—the ink having been applied prior to slicing of the prostate by the pathologist (see above). Other pathology specialities, such as colorectal, consider an involved margin when tumor is within a certain distance of the ink, but in the prostate, tumor has to be at the ink.

The prostate is sliced in such a way that we can assess three margins— apex, base, and circumferential. The circumferential margin is all around the prostate between the apex slice and the base slice. If there is a defect in the circumferential capsule and there is tumor in this area, this is defined as intraprostatic (Figure 3.2). If, on the other hand, tumor penetrates the capsule and extends into fat and to a margin, this is called extraprostatic (Figure 3.2). The apex and base margins are not normally divided into extra or intraprostatic, but some studies have shown that there is some value in doing this in the apex, though this is not widely done [20].

The significance of positive margins is also greatly debated but it is clear that extraprostatic margin involvement is more significant than intraprostatic, and base margin involvement is worse than apex margin involvement. There are studies to suggest that the Gleason grade at the involved margin is also important but this is not widely reported by pathologists [20].

## Lymph nodes

Lymphadenectomies are performed in high-risk patients in the United Kingdom. The tissue submitted to the pathologist consists of fatty tissue with poorly defined lymph nodes. These lymph nodes are normally fibrotic and have extensive fat infiltration unlike the nodes seen in other sites, for example, bowel mesentery. Some pathologists use node visualization liquids to help see these nodes, while others submit all the tissue. The difference in techniques may explain the difference in reported numbers of nodes present but it is unconvincing that one can accurately count these nodes [21].

It has become clear that the preprostatic fat—often disposed of at the time of surgery—can contain lymph nodes [22], and it has become common practice in our center to process this as well.

Lymph node involvement at radical prostatectomy is rare due to selection of patients based on clinical, radiology, and core biopsy data, but this may increase as surgery is offered to higher-risk or post-radiotherapy patients. When there is involvement of the lymph nodes, the pathologist can separate this into micrometasasis pN1 mi, when the tumor deposit is less than 2 mm. Immunohistochemistry can be used to detect even smaller deposits but its role is not advocated [23]. When tumor is present outside the capsule of the lymph node, this is defined as extracapsular spread. This has been shown to be a poor prognostic factor in bladder cancers but not in prostate cancer where tumor volume appears to be more significant [24, 25]. The capsule of the lymph node can be difficult to define in these fatty nodes and once again there can be a degree of subjectivity.

## Prognostic markers

The ability to predict which prostate cancer will kill a patient and which will have a more benign course is the holy grail of prostate cancer research. Many markers have been examined but in multivariate analysis Gleason score and PSA level appear better. One problem that we face is the multiplicity of prostate cancer—a set of core biopsies may detect one tumor but not the more clinically significant one—so a test may show a low-grade tumor but this may not be truly representative. The advent of template biopsies to truly map the prostate may mean that this is overcome. Better imaging techniques, such as parametric MRI, may also help overcome this problem.

The increasing use of inhibitors in other organ sites, such as BRAF inhibitors in melanoma patients with BRAF mutations, means that the pathologist is key in defining which patients receive the correct therapy. One marker that may prove useful is the TMPRSS2:ERG gene fusion which was thought to occur in advanced prostate cancer but is detected in 50% of prostate cancers [26]. It is clear that any marker used needs to be applied to all the cores containing tumor due to the reasons discussed above.

## Conclusion

The histopathology of prostate cancer is an evolving science and still there are areas of controversy—not least Gleason scoring. Any clinician involved in giving results to patients should have a good understanding of the pathology report. Also, a short time spent in a histopathology department seeing how these specimens are dealt with is strongly advised.

## References

1  Humphrey PA. Histological variants of prostatic carcinoma and their significance. *Histopathology* 2012;60(1):59–74.

2  Oxley JD, Abbott CD, Gillatt DA, MacIver AG. Ductal carcinomas of the prostate: a clinicopathological and immunohistochemical study. *Br J Urol* 1998;81(1):109–115.

3  Jiang Z, Wu CL, Woda BA, *et al.* P504S/alpha-methylacyl-CoA racemase: a useful marker for diagnosis of small foci of prostatic carcinoma on needle biopsy. *Am J Surg Pathol* 2002;26(9):1169–1174.

4  Brimo F, Epstein JI. Immunohistochemical pitfalls in prostate pathology. *Hum Pathol* 2012;43(3):313–324.

5  Standards and Datasets for Reporting Cancers Dataset for histopathology reports for prostatic carcinoma (2nd edition). Available at http://www.rcpath.org/Resources/RCPath/Migrated%20Resources/Documents/G/g084datasetprostaticcarcinomaoct09.pdf. Last accessed October 10, 2012.

6  Epstein JI, Herawi M. Prostate needle biopsies containing prostatic intraepithelial neoplasia or atypical foci suspicious for carcinoma: implications for patient care. *J Urol* 2006;175(3 Pt 1):820–834.

7  Kronz JD, Shaikh AA, Epstein JI. High-grade prostatic intraepithelial neoplasia with adjacent small atypical glands on prostate biopsy. *Hum Pathol* 2001;32(4):389–395.

8  Epstein JI, Allsbrook WC Jr, Amin MB, Egevad LL; ISUP Grading Committee. The 2005 International Society of Urological Pathology (ISUP) Consensus Conference on Gleason Grading of Prostatic Carcinoma. *Am J Surg Pathol* 2005;29(9):1228–1242.

9  Srigley JR, Delahunt B, Evans AJ. Therapy-associated effects in the prostate gland. *Histopathology* 2012;60(1):153–165.

10 Bott SR, Young MP, Kellett MJ, Parkinson MC; Contributors to the UCL Hospitals' Trust Radical Prostatectomy Database. Anterior prostate cancer: is it more difficult to diagnose? *BJU Int* 2002;89(9):886–889.

11 Harnden P, Shelley MD, Clements H, *et al.* The prognostic significance of perineural invasion in prostatic cancer biopsies: a systematic review. *Cancer* 2007 ;109(1):13–24.

12 Undertaking a transrectal ultrasound guided biopsy of the prostate. (Prostate Cancer Risk Management Programme 2006). Available at www.cancerscreening. nhs.uk/prostate/pcrmp01.pdf. Last accessed October 10, 2012.

13 Oxley JD, Sen C. Error rates in reporting prostatic core biopsies. *Histopathology* 2011;58(5):759–765.

14 Brimo F, Schultz L, Epstein JI. The value of mandatory second opinion pathology review of prostate needle biopsy interpretation before radical prostatectomy. *J Urol* 2010;184(1):126–130.

15 Warren AY, Whitaker HC, Haynes B, *et al.* Method for sampling tissue for research which preserves pathological data in radical prostatectomy. *Prostate* 2013;73(2):194–202.

16 Srigley JR. Key issues in handling and reporting radical prostatectomy specimens. *Arch Pathol Lab Med* 2006;130(3):303–317.

17 Catto JW, Robinson MC, Albertsen PC, *et al.* Suitability of PSA-detected localised prostate cancers for focal therapy: experience from the ProtecT study. *Br J Cancer* 2011;105(7):931–937.

18 Fine SW, Amin MB, Berney DM, *et al.* A contemporary update on pathology reporting for prostate cancer: biopsy and radical prostatectomy specimens. *Eur Urol* 2012;62(1):20–39.

19 van den Ouden D, Kranse R, Hop WC, *et al.* Microvascular invasion in prostate cancer: prognostic significance in patients treated by radical prostatectomy for clinically localized carcinoma. *Urol Int* 1998;60(1):17–24.

20 Tan PH, Cheng L, Srigley JR, *et al.* International Society of Urological Pathology (ISUP) Consensus Conference on Handling and Staging of Radical Prostatectomy Specimens. Working Group 5: surgical margins. *Mod Pathol* 2011;24(1):48–57.

21 Sivalingam S, Oxley J, Probert JL, *et al.* Role of pelvic lymphadenectomy in prostate cancer management. *Urology* 2007;69(2):203–209.

22 Yuh B, Wu H, Ruel N, *et al.* Analysis of regional lymph nodes in periprostatic fat following robot assisted radical prostatectomy. *BJU Int* 2012;109:603.

23 Deng FM, Mendrinos SE, Das K, *et al.* Periprostatic lymph node metastasis in prostate cancer and its clinical significance. *Histopathology* 2012;60:1004.

24 Cheng L, Pisansky TM, Ramnani DM, *et al.* Extranodal extension in lymph node-positive prostate cancer. *Mod Pathol* 2000;13(2):113–118.

25 Cheng L, Bergstralh EJ, Cheville JC, *et al.* Cancer volume of lymph node metastasis predicts progression in prostate cancer. *Am J Surg Pathol* 1998;22(12):1491–1500.

26 Kristiansen G. Diagnostic and prognostic molecular biomarkers for prostate cancer. *Histopathology* 2012;60(1):125–141.

## CHAPTER 4

# Markers in Prostate Cancer

*Philippa J. Cheetham*
Department of Urology, Winthrop University Hospital, New York

## Tumor markers

A tumor marker is a substance found in blood, urine, or tissues that can be elevated in cancer, among other tissue types, and is used to help detect the presence of cancer. Prostate cancer (PCa) cells produce specific markers and disease progression involves activation of signaling pathways controlling cell proliferation, apoptosis, angiogenesis, and metastasis. Tumor markers in PCa can thus be produced directly by the tumor or by nontumor cells as a response to the presence of neoplastic tissue. Most tumor markers are tumor antigens, but not all tumor antigens can be used as tumor markers.

## Currently available markers for prostate cancer

Prostate-specific antigen (PSA) is still the most commonly used and important biomarker for screening, detection, and follow-up of PCa. PSA was first quantitatively measured in the blood by Papsidero in 1980. Stamey carried out the initial work on the clinical use of PSA as a marker of PCa. In 1986, the US Food and Drug Administration (FDA) initially approved the PSA test for monitoring the progression of PCa in men who had already been diagnosed with the disease. In 1994, the FDA approved the use of the PSA test in conjunction with a digital rectal examination (DRE) to screen asymptomatic men for PCa. The reference range of <4 ng/mL for the first commercial PSA test (the Hybritech Tandem-R PSA test), released in 1986, was based on a study that found 99% of 472 apparently healthy men had a total PSA (tPSA) level below 4 ng/mL, the upper limit of normal being much less than 4 ng/mL [1].

*Prostate Cancer: Diagnosis and Clinical Management*, First Edition.
Edited by Ashutosh K. Tewari, Peter Whelan and John D. Graham.
© 2014 John Wiley & Sons, Ltd. Published 2014 by John Wiley & Sons, Ltd.

The widespread use of the PSA test during the past two decades has revolutionized the detection and management of men with PCa, reducing disease-specific mortality. Yet, despite widespread screening for PCa and major advances in the treatment of metastatic disease, PCa remains the second leading cause of cancer death in men (with 28 170 PCa-related deaths in the United States in 2012 accounting for 29% of all male cancers and 9% of male cancer-related deaths) exceeded only by lung cancer.

## Total PSA

PSA, also known as gamma-seminoprotein or kallikrein-3 (KLK3), is a glycoprotein enzyme encoded in humans by the KLK3 gene. PSA is a member of the kallikrein-related peptidase family and is secreted by the epithelial cells of the prostate gland. PSA is produced for the ejaculate, where it liquefies semen in the seminal coagulum and allows sperm to swim freely.

Total PSA (tPSA) has been shown to be superior to percent-free PSA (fPSA), PSA velocity (PSAV), and human kallikrein (hK2), the most studied kallikrein protein after PSA (hK3) itself.

## Problems with the PSA test

The PSA test is responsible for the increased incidence of PCa, with a marked increase in the number of men diagnosed with PCa and a profound migration toward earlier-stage disease at the time of diagnosis [2]. There is strong evidence in support of the growing concern that such "stage migration" causes overdiagnosis and overtreatment of men with indolent low-grade clinically insignificant cancers, which pose little threat to the life or health of the patient [3].

The current PSA test also has limitations in both sensitivity and specificity for the diagnosis of PCa, both of which have been examined and published extensively. Furthermore, the inherent biological variability of tPSA levels affects the interpretation of any single result. This is particularly true when serum concentrations are only modestly elevated [4], that is, tPSA is <10 ng/mL.

PSA is prostate specific, but not PCa specific. Thus, elevations in PSA can be seen in other conditions such as benign prostatic hyperplasia (BPH), prostatitis, irritation, and recent ejaculation [5] producing a false-positive result. DRE has also been shown in several studies [6] to produce an increase in PSA. The effect, however, is probably clinically insignificant, since DRE causes the most substantial increases in patients with PSA levels already elevated over 4.0 ng/mL.

The well-documented lack of sensitivity and specificity has led not only to unnecessary prostate biopsies (an invasive test that is not without risks such as bleeding, sepsis (which can be life-threatening), and hospitalization) but also to the limited ability to accurately distinguish patients with and without PCa, as well as those who harbor an aggressive form of the disease. This is especially true when the aggressive treatment of these indolent cancers has caused significant morbidity without clinical benefit in many cases. Currently, the United States Preventative Task Force (USPSTF) panel has recommended against PSA testing as a screening method because of low specificity and has questioned the benefit of PSA. The American Urologic Association (AUA), The American Society of Clinical Oncology (ASCO), and the American Cancer Society (ACS) maintain previous recommendations.

So far, a limited value for the PSA derivatives (including PSAV, density, free and pro-isoforms, and doubling time) has been recognized. Further research for the development and validation of more specific biomarkers for early cancer detection is warranted to help overcome the limitations of PSA and improve PCa detection substantially.

Numerous studies of potential serum, urine, and tissue biomarkers of PCa have been presented in the last ten years. These new biomarkers have the potential to provide an opportunity to better define groups of men at high risk of developing PCa, to improve screening techniques, to discriminate indolent versus aggressive disease (to ascertain whether the patient needs immediate or deferred treatment), and to improve therapeutic strategies in patients with advanced disease. In theory, these biomarkers should therefore result in improved diagnostic and prognostic accuracy, improve survival, reduce unnecessary investigations, and benefit the health economy.

Factors responsible for the delay in development of useful biomarkers and their use in clinical practice today include lack of standardized methodology for performance and interpretation of immunohistochemistry, cancer heterogeneity, poor study design with insufficient biomaterial, sampling errors, inappropriate statistical analysis, and lack of appropriate cohorts to test PCa biomarkers. These can be overcome by categorizing prognostic factors into particular gene pathways or by supplementing biopsy information with blood- or urine-based biomarkers. Unsuccessful integration of new biomarkers in nomograms can also be explained by the good performance of the clinical and pathological base model with serum PSA as the only independent biomarker. A new biomarker must be powerful enough to improve this prediction model and not merely a replacement. Significant efforts are now underway to develop research findings into clinically useful diagnostic tests in order to improve clinical decision-making.

A single biomarker is unlikely to provide comprehensive prognostic information about a newly diagnosed PCa. Used alone, assays detecting these biomarkers have their respective shortcomings, and biomarkers for identifying the most aggressive subsets of this malignancy are still missing. Several newer studies evaluating the clinical utilization of multiple biomarkers show promising results in improving PCa profiling (including its presence, stage, metastatic potential, and prognosis). Predictive nomograms that have been constructed using a panel of biomarkers still require further validation of their utility, and accuracy at the biopsy level is needed. Genetic profiling may also allow for the targeting of high-risk populations for screening and may offer the opportunity to combine biomarker results with genotype to aid risk assessment.

Current research is focusing on more specific biomarkers and therapeutic targets. At least 236 individual biomarkers have been identified, of which 29 were predictive on multivariate analysis in at least 2 independent cohorts. These can be categorized as: (1) circulating biomarkers found in serum or whole blood, (2) molecular urine markers, and (3) cellular markers. This chapter discusses the current understanding of these tumor markers for the diagnosis and therapeutic response of PCa. The hope is that increasing use of these biomarkers will not only result in PCa being more accurately diagnosed (with improved sensitivity and specificity over PSA), characterized, staged, and targeted with inhibitory antitumor agents but also will lead to improvement in PCa prognosis and management of the therapeutic response of PCa patients. At the present time, most of these newer biomarkers have not yet been evaluated in prospective trials for providing useful prognostic or predictive information or improvement upon clinicopathological parameters already in use. For the majority, further validation in independent studies is required.

## Serum or whole-blood biomarkers

Several modifications to PSA biomarker detection have been suggested to improve its sensitivity and selectivity including PSA density, fPSA:tPSA, PSAV/PSA doubling time (PSADT), and different PSA isoforms.

## Percent free PSA

Most PSA in the blood is bound to serum proteins. A small amount is not protein bound and is called free PSA (fPSA). Percent fPSA (%fPSA, i.e., fPSA/tPSA × 100) is a commercially available PSA marker approved by the FDA and has been used to stratify the risk of PCa in men with tPSA levels of 4–10 ng/mL and a negative DRE. In men with PCa, the ratio of free (unbound) PSA to tPSA is decreased. The risk of PCa increases if the fPSA to tPSA ratio is less than 25%. The lower the ratio, the greater the probability of PCa. Measuring the ratio of free to tPSA appears to be particularly promising for eliminating unnecessary biopsies in men with PSA levels between 4 and 10 ng/mL [7]. With a fPSA:tPSA threshold of <0.1, PCa was detected in 56% of men on biopsy compared with 8% of men with a fPSA:tPSA level >0.25 [8]. A large-scale study has recently reported the value of %fPSA to reduce the risk of overdiagnosis [9]. The diagnostic performance of %fPSA among men with a tPSA of 2–10 ng/mL compared with tPSA alone was shown to be improved in one meta-analysis [10]. There are limitations to the use of fPSA in that it is unstable at 4°C and room temperature [11] and can produce conflicting results in men with BPH and large prostates [12]. A comparison of 10 different fPSA assay kits has been reported showing that there was variability in the values recorded that impacted the fPSA:tPSA measure [13]. Consequently, it is important that combinations of free and tPSA assays be carefully selected based on validated diagnostic performance.

## PSAV and PSADT

PSAV and PSADT have been used to measure the change in PSA level with time, the former recording the change per year and the latter a specific value increase. PSAV has been shown on a multivariate analysis including age, date of diagnosis, and PSA to significantly improve the ability to detect high-risk PCa, unlike PSADT [14]. Nevertheless, a systematic review published in 2009 of 87 papers suggested that there was scant evidence to show that PSAV or PSADT provided predictive information that was better than PSA level alone [15].

## Inactive PSA

Proteolytically active PSA has been shown to have an anti-angiogenic effect [16] and certain inactive subforms may be associated with PCa, as shown by MAb 5D3D11, an antibody able to detect forms abundantly represented in sera from PCa patients [17]. The presence of inactive proenzyme forms of PSA is another potential indicator of disease [17].

# Precursor forms of PSA (PROPSAS) (protein)

## PSA isoforms

Retrospective studies have suggested that an isoform of proenzyme PSA called [−2]proenzyme PSA (p2PSA) may enhance the specificity of PSA-based screening [18]. Other studies suggest that p2PSA and its derivatives, namely %p2PSA and the Beckman Coulter Prostate Health Index (phi), a mathematical combination of tPSA, fPSA, and p2PSA, may significantly improve the accuracy of tPSA and %fPSA in predicting the presence of PCa [19]. The test was granted FDA approval in 2012. A recent prospective study has compared the diagnostic accuracy of serum tPSA, %PSA, PSA density (PSAD), p2PSA, %p2PSA ([p2PSA/fPSA] x 100) and phi in a group of 268 patients of whom 107 (39.9%) were diagnosed with PCa at prostate biopsy [20]. Univariate analysis indicated that phi and %p2PSA were the most accurate predictors of PCa followed by PSAD, %fPSA and tPSA. In multivariate accuracy analyses, both phi and %p2PSA significantly improved the accuracy of established predictors in determining the presence of PCa at biopsy.

## ProPSA (protein)

ProPSA is an isoform of fPSA that is used in combination with tPSA and fPSA to calculate Prostate Health Index (phi). Phi has yielded promising results and appears superior to tPSA and fPSA in predicting those patients with PCa. Increased phi levels also seem to preferentially detect patients harboring more aggressive disease. Further studies in the form of large, multicenter prospective trials with detailed health economic analyses are required to evaluate the true clinical applicability of these novel markers.

## [−2]ProPSA

Studies to date suggest that [−2]proPSA, a truncated form of proPSA, is the most cancer-specific form of all, being preferentially expressed in cancerous prostatic epithelium and being significantly elevated in serum of men with PCa. There is evidence to suggest that %[−2]proPSA measurement ([−2]proPSA/fPSA [fPSA] × 100) improves the specificity of both tPSA and fPSA in detecting PCa.

## Nucleic acid detection immunoassay (NADIA) ProsVue (protein: PSA immuno-polymerase chain reaction)

NADIA ProsVue is an immuno-polymerase chain reaction (PCR) assay for total serum PSA. It detects PSA levels as low as 0.00065 ng/mL

(0.65 pg/mL) in serum, more than an order of magnitude lower than the most sensitive commercial PSA assays. NADIA ProsVue incorporates a double-stranded DNA label for high-sensitivity analyte detection and resists nonspecific binding to improve precision. The assay also uses a calculation of the PSA slope (PSA change over time) as a unique prognostic factor and is the first assay based on the linear slope of tumor marker concentrations over time to receive FDA clearance, which was granted in 2011.

In pilot studies using NADIA PSA, 90% of men without biochemical recurrence had a serum PSA concentration <5 pg/mL in the first several months after radical prostatectomy (RP) [21]. In addition, the superior sensitivity and precision of this assay have provided a unique opportunity to evaluate the kinetics of PSA at these very low post-RP concentrations.

These studies determined that a ProsVue result was the most powerful indicator of a reduced risk of clinical recurrence and added prognostic value to established risk factors. It has thus been postulated that men with a PSA slope of ≤2.0 pg/mL/month after RP could be at a reduced risk of clinical recurrence. ProsVue testing could possibly reduce healthcare costs by reducing the intensity of follow-up examinations in men identified at a reduced risk of recurrence. Additional studies will assess method performance and define the role of the assay in risk models and nomograms [21].

Several novel blood-based biomarkers such as human glandular kallikrein 2 (hK2), urokinase plasminogen activator (uPA) and its receptor (uPAR), transforming growth factor-beta 1 (TGF-β1), and interleukin-6 (IL-6) and its receptor (IL-6R) may help PCa diagnosis, staging, prognostication, and monitoring. Panels of biomarkers that capture the biologic potential of PCa are in the process of being validated for PCa prognostication.

## Human glandular kallikrein 2

Human glandular kallikrein 2 (hK2) and KLK3 (also known as PSA) share 80% of their amino acid sequence with each other—they form 2 of the 15 genes on the *KLK* gene locus on chromosome 19q13-4 [22].

hK2 is produced in prostatic epithelium at concentrations 50–100 times less than PSA. hK2 is also overexpressed in PCa [23] and is more sensitive than PSA at detecting extracapsular extension [23]. It has been shown that the ratio of hK2/PSA mRNA increases with grade of tumor.

Other members of the kallikrein family are being studied for their prognostic significance in PCa.

## Urokinase plasminogen activator

Urokinase plasminogen activator (uPA) is involved in various phases of tumor development and progression. The suggested mechanism involves first binding to the uPAR and then converting plasminogen to plasmin, which in turn activates proteases that degrade extracellular matrix proteins [24]. Aggressive PCa recurrence has been associated with overexpression of uPA and its inhibitor, plasminogen activator inhibitor 1 (PAI-1) [25]. Other studies show that uPA and uPAR are linked to PCa stage and bone metastases [26, 27]. Further large-scale studies are being conducted.

## Transforming growth factor-beta 1

Transforming growth factor-beta 1 (TGF-β1) is involved in proliferation of immune response, differentiation, and angiogenesis along with regulation of other cellular mechanisms [28]. In PCa, TGF-β1 promotes cell progression, and is linked with higher tumor grade, invasion, and metastasis [29].

## Interleukin-6 and its receptor

Interleukin-6 (IL-6) is involved in the regulation of various cellular functions: proliferation, apoptosis, angiogenesis, differentiation, and regulation of the immune response [30]. Elevated levels of IL-6 and IL-6R have been linked with metastatic and hormone-refractory PCa [31], suggesting its potential as a predictor for disease progression and mortality.

## Insulin-like growth factor and insulin-like growth binding protein

Insulin-like growth factors (IGFs) have potent proliferative and anti-apoptotic effects and thus have a role in tumorigenesis. IGF-1 has been shown to stimulate the proliferation of human prostate epithelial cells in culture and to be necessary for normal prostate growth and development. Epidemiological studies have established a link between high circulating serum IGF-1 levels and the risk of later developing advanced PCa. Overexpression of IGF-1 in the prostate basal epithelial layer of transgenic mice results in PCa. Thus, IGF-1 action appears to be important for PCa initiation. On the other hand, decreased IGF action, subsequent to the downregulation of IGF-1 receptor expression, is associated with advanced, metastatic disease. This decrease in receptor expression may confer a survival advantage to PCa cells that have entered the circulation by making them resistant to the effects of IGF-1 at metastatic sites such as bone [32].

Insulin-like growth factor binding protein-3 (IGFBP-3) is a pro-apoptotic, anti-metastasic, and anti-angiogenic protein. Low serum IGFBP-3 has been associated with risk of more aggressive PCa. In patients with low-grade cancer, IGFBP-3 nuclear positivity was a better predictor of recurrence than baseline PSA, tumor margin status, TNM tumor stage, or presence of capsular invasion. High nuclear IGFBP-3 is amongst the strongest predictors of cancer recurrence in patients with low-grade PCa and may therefore play an important role in risk stratification [33].

*Neuron-specific enolase* (NSE) is a specific marker for neuroendocrine tumors that express proteins or enzymes that are reflective of a de-differentiated tumor cell population, such as small cell PCa.

*Chromogranin A* (CGA) is a neuropeptide expressed in high-grade PCa, whose levels are related to the neuroendocrine differentiation of the cancer. When both NSE and CGA are elevated, PCa is usually unresponsive to hormone deprivation therapy and thus carries a poor prognosis [34].

*Prostatic acid phosphatase* (PAP) is an enzyme measured in the blood whose levels may be elevated in patients with PCa that has invaded or metastasized elsewhere. PAP is not elevated unless the tumor has spread outside the anatomic prostatic capsule. Serum PAP noted at the time of diagnosis of PCa is usually associated with extra-prostatic spread. Although a persistently elevated serum PAP is considered evidence of metastatic disease, only 75% of patients with metastatic disease have elevated serum PAP.

Prior to the introduction of serum PSA, PAP was used widely to indicate advanced PCa, but fell into disuse. However, a number of publications have promoted a renewed role for this enzyme as a prognostic indicator in early disease. Moul *et al.* [35] reported on 295 patients who underwent RP and compared the value of pretreatment serum PSA and PAP. The authors concluded that PAP testing added prognostic information to pretreatment PSA values and that PAP was an independent predictor of PCa recurrence.

## Molecular urine markers

Urine-based testing is noninvasive and provides a rich source of cancer products. Biomarker development using urine has been accelerating in recent years, with numerous studies identifying DNA, RNA, protein, and metabolite-based biomarkers in the urine. Testing for the biomarker involves collection of urine samples after a DRE is conducted to increase sensitivity.

Advanced clinical studies have identified PCA3 and TMPRSS2:ERG fusion transcripts, among others, as promising RNA markers for cancer detection. Few markers, however, have been validated in multiple large sample sets. Prospective studies in a multivariate setting, including larger sample sizes and avoiding attribution bias caused by preselection on the basis of serum PSA are now urgently required. The ability to identify aggressive subsets of PCa as promising markers for prognosis also requires further development. DNA methylation analysis of multiple genes improves specificity and represents a promising platform for the development of clinical-grade assays.

## RNA markers in urine

RNA-based urine biomarkers are by far the most developed. RNA profiling using microarray-based technologies has been particularly useful in tracking changes in gene expression during tumorigenesis. To date, the two most prominent candidate RNA biomarkers are the PCA3 gene and the TMPRSS2-ERG fusion gene. Transcript expression levels of GOLPH2, SPINK1, and their combination have also been subject of many studies showing encouraging results.

### Prostate cancer antigen 3 (RNA) PROGENSA®
The prostate cancer antigen 3 (PCA3) gene (previously known as DD-3) is a prostate-tissue-specific noncoding gene, whose RNA is highly overexpressed in specific PCa cell lines in comparison to non-neoplastic prostate [36]. These attributes make it a promising PCa-specific marker and it has been extensively reviewed [37]. The urine assay measures the ratio of mRNA for PCA3 and PSA in urine collected after prostate massage; the ratio of the two normalizes for the variable number of PCa cells collected [38]. The sensitivity of the optimal PCA3/PSA ratio has been shown to be 67% and the specificity 83% [38].

PCA3 was discovered in 1999. In 2006, a simple and robust quantitative urine test for PCA3 (PROGENSA PCA3 developed by Gen-Probe, Inc, San Diego, California, USA.) became commercially available and received FDA approval in 2012 for its ability to predict cancer in patients with increased PSA and negative biopsy. A PCA3 score cut-off of 35 has resulted in the best balance of sensitivity and specificity [39].

The largest double-blind study to evaluate the performance of PCA3 to date was the REDUCE (Reduction by Dutasteride of Prostate Cancer

Events) trial involving PCA3 analysis of 1140 participants [40]. The PCA3 score was shown to correlate with the percentage of biopsy-positive men, and the sensitivity and specificity reported were 48% and 79%, respectively. Furthermore, a predictive model incorporating PCA3, serum PSA level, and %fPSA improved the diagnostic accuracy compared with PSA level and %fPSA [39]. If confirmed in further studies, using PCA3 together with established staging risk factors in novel biopsy nomograms or risk stratification tools could assist clinicians in specific pretreatment decision-making.

PCA3 independently predicts low-volume disease and pathologically insignificant PCa but is not associated with locally advanced disease and is limited in the prediction of aggressive cancer. Some studies have indicated that PCA3 is correlated with prostatectomy Gleason score [41], although other studies dispute this [42]. The evidence for the usefulness of PCA3 in active surveillance programs remains controversial. Combining PCA3 with other new biomarkers almost certainly will further improve diagnostic and prognostic accuracy. Finally, findings of the first PCA3-Gene-ViroTherapy study suggest therapeutic potential by exploiting PCA3 overexpression.

## TMPRSS2:ERG fusion gene or *ERG* (RNA)

Gene fusions of two distinct gene transcripts can occur after chromosomal translocation or deletion of segments of the genome, and such rearrangements are frequently the trigger point in oncogenesis [43].

The most commonly studied gene fusion in PCa involves the prostate-specific gene transmembrane protease, serine2 (*TMPRSS2*) and members of the erythroblastosis virus E26 oncogene homolog (avian) transforming sequence (ETS) family of transcription factors. The biological function of *ERG* in PCa is involvement in invasion, differentiation, and inflammation. This gene fusion has been identified in most PSA-screened PCa [44, 45]. The gene fusion TMPRSS2:ETV1 is rare and occurs in 1–10% of PCa [46], whereas the TMPRSS2:ERG fusion is present in up to 50% of PCa [46].

Evaluation in 1312 men in a multi-center study in the United States showed that higher levels of the TMPRSS2-ERG mRNA in post-DRE urine are associated with indicators of clinically significant cancer at biopsy and prostatectomy. TMPRSS2-ERG in combination with PCA3 improved the PCa risk. Data are soon to be published on a recently completed clinical trial assessing the change in PCA3and TMPRSS2:ERG expression during hormone therapy.

## GOLPH2

GOLPH2/GP73, elevated in PCa tissues, is detectable in postprostatic massage urine from PCa patients. GOLPH2 immunohistochemical staining indicates a perinuclear Golgi-type pattern that is more intense in PCa glands compared with normal glands [47]. In a large study, upregulation of GOLPH2 protein was reported in 567 of 614 tumors (92.3%) and alpha-methylacyl-coenzyme A racemase (AMACR) in 583 of 614 tumors (95%) (correlation coefficient 0.113, $p = .005$) [47]. Importantly, GOLPH2 immunohistochemical analysis indicates a lower level of intratumoral heterogeneity (25% vs. 45%). Further, GOLPH2 upregulation was detected in 26 of 31 (84%) AMACR-negative PCa cases. Using PCR analysis, increased GOLPH2 levels have been demonstrated in postprostatic massage urine as a significant predictor of PCa when multiplexed with PCA3 and SPINK1 [48].

## SPINK1

SPINK1 is a serine peptidase inhibitor, which encodes a 6-kD trypsin inhibitor. It is a biomarker for PCa that can be detected in prostatic massage sedimented urine. It is overexpressed in 10% of PCa, and these have an adverse prognosis. The aggressive 22RV1 PCa cell line expresses SPINK1 and the expression of the latter in urine has been shown to outperform PSA or PCA3 alone in patients presenting for biopsy or prostatectomy, as well as being an independent predictor of biochemical recurrence after resection [48].

## Telomerase activity

Telomerase reverse transcriptase (TERT) is detectable in the vast majority of PCa but not in benign prostate tissue. Improved methods of telomerase detection may make this marker useful for early detection of PCa in tissue samples or in urine and is currently undergoing evaluation.

## DNA-based urine biomarkers

Studies on DNA-based urine biomarkers focus on hypermethylation of gene panels. Several have been investigated. Hypermethylation of panel markers in combination with histology may aid in PCa diagnosis and aberrant methylation profiles in prostate tissue samples have also correlated with clinicopathological features of poor prognosis. Loss of glutathione-S-transferase-p1 (GSTP1) expression is the most common hypermethylated gene studied and the most promising individual marker undergoing evaluation in a clinical trial.

GSTP1 protects cells from oxidative damage, reduced expression in PCa due to hypermethylation of its promoter region. In theory, GSTP1 distinguishes between BPH and PCa; methylation status of GSTP1 gene promoter quantified in prostatic tissue; cells derived from serum, urine, and seminal plasma PCR. Results, however, are conflicting [49].

8-Hydroxy deoxyguanosine (8-OHDG) is another potential DNA-based urine marker for monitoring PCa.

More recently a panel of markers, GSTP1, retinoic acid receptor β2 (RARβ2), and adenomatous polyposis coli (APC), have been assessed but no increased predictive value was shown compared with tPSA level and DRE alone [50]. Larger prospective clinical studies of single DNA-based markers and gene panels are needed to validate their clinical utility.

## Protein markers in urine

Several protein-based biomarkers for PCa in urine have been studied. These include annexin 3 [51], matrix metalloproteinases (MMP9) [52], delta-catenin [53], hepatocyte growth factor (c-met) [54], thymosin β15a (TMSB15A) [55], minichromosome maintenance complex component 5 (MCM5), basic human urinary arginine amidase (BHUAE), coagulation factor III (thromboplastin tissue factor), prostatic inhibin-like peptide (PIP), S100 calcium binding protein (S100A9), steroid 5-alpha-reductase type 2 (SRD5A2), vascular endothelial growth factor (VEGF), and the urinary PSA. Some show contradictory results. Further studies are thus warranted to be able to assess their clinical value and cost-effectiveness.

### Annexin A3

Annexin A3 (ANXA3), a calcium and phospholipid binding protein, implicated in cell differentiation and migration, immunomodulation, bone formation, and mineralization in PCa metastasis is a recently identified PCa protein biomarker. ANXA3 has an inverse relationship to PCa progression and Gleason score (with decreased production in PCa compared to BPH) and can be detected in the urine of PCa patients [56]. Improved sensitivities have been noted when ANXA3 was used in conjunction with PSA [56]. ANXA3 has been quantified by western blot in the urine samples of patients with negative DRE findings and low tPSA (2–10 ng/mL), which is the clinically relevant group facing the biopsy dilemma. Combined readouts of PSA and urinary ANXA3 gave the best results [51].

## Matrix metalloproteinases 9

Matrix metalloproteinases (MMPs) have a role in growth, invasion, and metastatic spread in a number of tumors including PCa [52]. The detection of any MMP in urine as predictive of PCa has an 82% specificity and a 74% sensitivity [57]. Further studies are required to fully assess the clinical value of protein-based urinary markers in PCa.

## Microseminoprotein-beta gene

As one of the most abundant prostatic proteins, microseminoprotein-beta (MSMB) can be reliably detected in tissue and serum. Members of the cysteine-rich secretory protein family and laminin receptors have been shown to bind MSMB at the cell surface and in serum thereby regulating apoptosis. Thus, in the benign prostate, MSMB regulates cell growth, but when MSMB is lost during tumorigenesis, cells are able to grow in a more uncontrolled manner. Both full-length MSMB and a short peptide comprised of amino acids 31–45 have been tested for potential therapeutic benefit in mouse models and humans. It has been consistently shown that MSMB expression is high in normal and benign prostate tissue and lowered or lost in PCa, suggesting MSMB has potential as a biomarker of PCa development, progression, and recurrence and potentially as a target for therapeutic intervention.

## Metabolite urine markers

Metabolomics seek to distinguish the metabolite content of PCa cells from normal cells. A recent study of more than 1126 metabolite profiles in urine, blood plasma, and surgical tissue samples of benign, PCa, and metastatic PCa characterized levels of a large number of metabolites.

## N-methylglycine

N-methylglycine is a lead candidate sarcosine, which can be detected in urine by gas chromatography/mass spectrometry using a commercial biomarker for the early detection of PCa and for prediction of tumor aggressiveness. The median sarcosine:creatinine ratio in urine was 13% lower in PCa patients than in those with no evidence of malignancy (NEM). Yet, sarcosine values were not associated with tumor stage (pT2 vs. pT3) or grade (Gleason score <7 vs. >7). Subsequent analysis proved that the discrimination between PCa and NEM patients was not improved by sarcosine in comparison with tPSA, but it was significantly worse than the %fPSA. The role of sarcosine as a urinary biomarker is still controversial. Further validation studies are thus required before it can be considered as a suitable marker to differentiate between patients with and without PCa. Even so, the finding of a link with more aggressive disease is promising [58].

## Genetic markers

### Nucleotide polymorphism

Several new genomic-based biomarkers for PCa have been identified and 35 single nucleotide polymorphisms (SNPs) have been independently validated as being associated with PCa [59]. It is estimated that these markers explain 20% of the familial risk of PCa. The SNPs associated with PCa so far are not associated with disease stage or outcome. A large-scale study evaluated seven SNPs in 7370 patients with PCa and 5742 controls, and found no association with tumor grade [60]. Another study reported an association between two variants, rs10993994 and rs5945619, and Gleason score [61].

## Cellular markers

Multiple groups have developed gene expression signatures from primary prostate tumors correlating with poor prognosis, and attempts to improve and standardize these signatures as diagnostic tests are presented. Massive sequencing efforts are underway to define important somatic genetic alterations (amplifications, deletions, point mutations, translocations) in PCa, and these alterations hold great promise as prognostic markers and for predicting response to therapy. There is also a rationale for assessing genetic markers in metastatic disease for guiding choice of therapy and for stratifying patients in clinical trials.

Circulating prostate cells, RT-PCR gene targets PSA, hK2, and PSMA mRNAs

Much has been published describing a range of tissue biomarkers for PCa characterization. These include apoptotic factors such as p53 and Bcl-2; the androgen receptor (AR); signal transduction factors within the EGF receptor family; cell-cycle regulators exemplified by c-myc, p16, p27, pRb, and Ki67; cell adhesion and cohesion factors; and factors involved in neo-angiogenesis, such as VEGF, VEGF receptors, and nitric oxide. Measurements of the frequency in the shedding of circulating prostate/tumor cells in blood using RT-PCR assays for PSA and/or systemic disease stage has also been evaluated in clinical trials.

The following are all undergoing evaluations.

## Cytokeratin

High-molecular-weight cytokeratin present in the basal cells of prostatic glandular epithelium can be labeled with antibodies. Invasive PCa is lacking in a basal cell layer, although there is low incidence of incorrect labeling [62]. Adding to the inaccuracy is the fact that benign lesions may sometimes be negative for the marker [63]. Staining for the marker should be examined in conjunction with conventional morphology.

## p63

p63 is another marker for the basal cell layer and can be used in conjunction with high-molecular-weight cytokeratin [64]. This marker does have the same inaccuracies as cytokeratin, and the sensitivities of the two are similar [65].

## Alpha-methylacyl-coenzyme A racemase

Alpha-methylacyl-coenzyme A racemase (AMACR) is a mitochondrial and peroxisomal enzyme involved in oxidation. AMACR is differentially expressed in PCa and is usually negative in benign glands [66]. It is a very commonly used immunohistochemical marker for PCa. In conjunction with loss of basal cell markers, staining for AMACR can improve the accuracy of needle biopsy samples with a sensitivity of 80–100% in small atypical foci [67, 68]. A correlation between AMACR staining and increased Gleason score has also been reported [68]. However, AMACR is also positive in prostatic intraepithelial neoplasia and occasionally in benign lesions. Thus, its usefulness as a biomarker in urine remains controversial and further evaluation is required [68].

## PTEN and loss of heterozygosity (e.g., loss of PTEN)

PTEN is a lipid phosphatase that functions as a tumor suppressor by inhibiting the phosphatidylinositol 3-kinase/ protein kinase B (pl3K/Akt) signaling pathway. The gene can be deleted or mutated in some PCa and its decreased levels are associated with higher grade and stage of disease.

Chromosomal aberrations are very common in prostate tumors and may act together in the progression of the disease. For example, the loss of both the PTEN gene on chromosome 10q and a recurrent 30Mb deletion on 21q, which leads to the fusion of TMPRSS2, are common aberrations which appear to act together in disease progression.

## Cyclin-dependent kinase inhibitor 1B (p27)

Cyclin-dependent kinase inhibitor 1B (CDKN1B) (p27) is an important regulator of cell-cycle progression to S-phase during mitosis. This tumor suppressor protein is decreased in PCa. Furthermore, increased loss of this gene and gene product correlate well with both tumor stage and grade, thus CDKN1B levels appear to predict a worse prognosis. Patients with PCa who have low p27 have a nearly fivefold increased relative risk of disease recurrence, regardless of Gleason score or preoperative PSA level, after RP [69].

## Ki-67

Immunohistochemical methods have been used to quantify the expression of the Ki-67 antigen, a marker of cellular proliferation, thus providing an estimate of the growth fraction [70]. Ki-67 staining index has consistently been correlated with poor prognosis for patients with PCa treated definitively with RP or radiotherapy [71, 72].

## Prostate-specific membrane antigen

Prostate-specific membrane antigen (PSMA) is a cell-surface membrane protein that is localized to the prostate and overexpressed in all tumor stages [73]. The protein has been researched in recent years from the perspective of both PCa diagnosis and therapy. High levels of PSMA expression, identified through radioisotope-labeled antibody, have been associated with advanced tumor stage [74], androgen-independent tumor growth [75], presence of metastases [76], and early PSA recurrence [76], which could have implications for treatment decisions.

## Chromosome 8p22 loss and 8q24 (c-myc) gain

8q24 overrepresentation, especially in combination with loss of 8p22 using a FISH assay, is associated with PCa progression with stage pT2N0M0, pT3N0M0, and pT23N1-3M0. Gain and amplification of the myc gene on 8q24 is of great interest.

## Prostate stem cell antigen

Prostate stem cell antigen (PSCA) is a cell-surface protein found primarily in the prostate. Its increased expression is seen in many higher-grade PCa and most metastatic lesions, and is correlated with late-stage disease.

# Circulating tumor cells

Assays detecting circulating tumor cells (CTCs) in the peripheral blood have been developed and approved for clinical use by the FDA to provide prognostic information in women with node-positive breast cancer [77].

Detection of CTCs in the blood of PCa patients has continued to evolve over the years with more streamlined technology. CTCs have been largely analyzed for prognostic potential but studies also showed diagnostic potential [78]. The Cell Search System (Veridex, LLC, Raritan, New Jersey, USA) to determine CTC count received FDA clearance in 2008 for evaluation in Castrate Resistant Prostate Cancer (CRPC), and subsequent studies have shown the utility of the system in clinical trials [79, 80].

A correlation between the number of CTCs in blood and survival has been reported [81]. Median overall survival and progression-free survival was significantly shorter in patients with CTC level of $\geq 5/7.5$ mL compared with those with a CTC level of $<5/7.5$ mL. Although initial results of the correlation of CTC counts with mRNAs for PSA or PSMA and available clinical predictors [82] are encouraging, the techniques for measuring circulating PCa cells in peripheral blood are not yet sufficiently validated to warrant recommendations for their application in routine clinical practice.

CTC evaluation at baseline and posttreatment appears prognostic of survival. Large phase III trials of novel anti-androgen therapies (MDV3100; Abiraterone) are in progress to assess the utility of CTCs as biomarker for treatment efficacy.

# Conclusions

PSA is a strong prognostic marker for long-term risk of clinically relevant PCa. The questionable specificity and potential for the overdiagnosis of nonthreatening PCa with PSA screening has resulted in a need for novel biomarkers that aid clinical decision-making about biopsy, initial treatment, and prognosis. A range of biomarkers is under intense investigation, some of which show potential in not only diagnosis but also prognosis after treatment. The requirement of a marker with both high sensitivity and specificity is still unmet at present, and the use of multiple markers in combination with other clinical factors appears promising. There is no doubt that progress will continue to be made, based on the integrated collaboration of researchers, clinicians, and biomedical firms.

## References

1 Thompson IM, *et al.* Prevalence of prostate cancer among men with a prostate-specific antigen level < or =4.0 ng per milliliter. *N Engl J Med* 2004;350(22):2239–46.
2 Makinen T, *et al.* Tumor characteristics in a population-based prostate cancer screening trial with prostate-specific antigen. *Clin Cancer Res* 2003;9(7):2435–2439.
3 Draisma G, *et al.* Lead times and overdetection due to prostate-specific antigen screening: estimates from the European Randomized Study of Screening for Prostate Cancer. *J Natl Cancer Inst* 2003;95(12):868–878.
4 Punglia RS, *et al.* Effect of verification bias on screening for prostate cancer by measurement of prostate-specific antigen. *N Engl J Med* 2003;349(4):335–342.
5 Nadler RB, *et al.* Effect of inflammation and benign prostatic hyperplasia on elevated serum prostate specific antigen levels. *J Urol* 1995;154(2 Pt 1):407–413.
6 Crawford ED, *et al.* The effect of digital rectal examination on prostate-specific antigen levels. *J Am Med Assoc* 1992;267(16):2227–2228.
7 Catalona WJ, Smith DS, Ornstein DK. Prostate cancer detection in men with serum PSA concentrations of 2.6 to 4.0 ng/mL and benign prostate examination. Enhancement of specificity with free PSA measurements. *J Am Med Assoc* 1997;277(18):1452–1455.
8 Catalona WJ, *et al.* Use of the percentage of free prostate-specific antigen to enhance differentiation of prostate cancer from benign prostatic disease: a prospective multicenter clinical trial. *J Am Med Assoc* 1998;279(19):1542–1547.
9 Pepe P, Aragona F. Incidence of insignificant prostate cancer using free/total PSA: results of a case-finding protocol on 14,453 patients. *Prostate Cancer Prostatic Dis* 2010;13(4):316–319.
10 Roddam AW, *et al.* Use of prostate-specific antigen (PSA) isoforms for the detection of prostate cancer in men with a PSA level of 2–10 ng/ml: systematic review and meta-analysis. *Eur Urol* 2005;48(3):386–399; discussion 398–399.
11 Sokoll LJ, *et al.* Short-term stability of the molecular forms of prostate-specific antigen and effect on percent complexed prostate-specific antigen and percent free prostate-specific antigen. *Urology* 2002;60(4 Suppl. 1):24–30.
12 Stephan C, *et al.* The influence of prostate volume on the ratio of free to total prostate specific antigen in serum of patients with prostate carcinoma and benign prostate hyperplasia. *Cancer* 1997;79(1):104–109.
13 Oberpenning F, *et al.* Combining free and total prostate specific antigen assays from different manufacturers: the pitfalls. *Eur Urol* 2002;42(6):577–582; discussion 582.

14  Loeb S, *et al.* PSA doubling time versus PSA velocity to predict high-risk prostate cancer: data from the Baltimore Longitudinal Study of Aging. *Eur Urol* 2008;54(5):1073–1080.

15  Vickers AJ, *et al.* Systematic review of pretreatment prostate-specific antigen velocity and doubling time as predictors for prostate cancer. *J Clin Oncol* 2009;27(3):398–403.

16  Mattsson JM, *et al.* Structural characterization and anti-angiogenic properties of prostate-specific antigen isoforms in seminal fluid. *Prostate* 2008;68(9):945–954.

17  Stura EA, *et al.* Crystal structure of human prostate-specific antigen in a sandwich antibody complex. *J Mol Biol* 2011;414(4):530–544.

18  Catalona WJ, *et al.* Serum pro-prostate specific antigen preferentially detects aggressive prostate cancers in men with 2 to 4 ng/ml prostate specific antigen. *J Urol* 2004;171(6 Pt 1):2239–2244.

19  Le BV, *et al.* [−2]Proenzyme prostate specific antigen is more accurate than total and free prostate specific antigen in differentiating prostate cancer from benign disease in a prospective prostate cancer screening study. *J Urol* 2010;183(4):1355–1359.

20  Guazzoni G, *et al.* Prostate-specific antigen (PSA) isoform p2PSA significantly improves the prediction of prostate cancer at initial extended prostate biopsies in patients with total PSA between 2.0 and 10 ng/ml: results of a prospective study in a clinical setting. *Eur Urol* 2011;60(2):214–222.

21  Moul JW, *et al.* NADiA ProsVue prostate-specific antigen slope is an independent prognostic marker for identifying men at reduced risk of clinical recurrence of prostate cancer after radical prostatectomy. *Urology* 2012;80(6):1319–1325.

22  Harvey TJ, *et al.* Tissue-specific expression patterns and fine mapping of the human kallikrein (KLK) locus on proximal 19q13.4. *J Biol Chem* 2000;275(48):37397–37406.

23  Lintula S, *et al.* Relative concentrations of hK2/PSA mRNA in benign and malignant prostatic tissue. *Prostate* 2005;63(4):324–329.

24  Duffy MJ. Urokinase-type plasminogen activator: a potent marker of metastatic potential in human cancers. *Biochem Soc Trans* 2002;30(2):207–210.

25  Gupta A, *et al.* Predictive value of the differential expression of the urokinase plasminogen activation axis in radical prostatectomy patients. *Eur Urol* 2009;55(5):1124–1133.

26  Hienert G, *et al.* Urokinase-type plasminogen activator as a marker for the formation of distant metastases in prostatic carcinomas. *J Urol* 1988;140(6):1466–1469.

27  Miyake H, *et al.* Elevation of serum levels of urokinase-type plasminogen activator and its receptor is associated with disease progression and prognosis in patients with prostate cancer. *Prostate* 1999;39(2):123–129.

28  Shariat SF, *et al.* Preoperative plasma levels of transforming growth factor beta(1) (TGF-beta(1)) strongly predict progression in patients undergoing radical prostatectomy. *J Clin Oncol* 2001;19(11):2856–2864.

29  Shariat SF, *et al.* Association of pre- and postoperative plasma levels of transforming growth factor beta(1) and interleukin 6 and its soluble receptor with prostate cancer progression. *Clin Cancer Res* 2004;10(6):1992–1999.

30  Culig Z, *et al.* Interleukin-6 regulation of prostate cancer cell growth. *J Cell Biochem* 2005;95(3):497–505.

31  Michalaki V, *et al.* Serum levels of IL-6 and TNF-alpha correlate with clinicopathological features and patient survival in patients with prostate cancer. *Br J Cancer* 2004;90(12):2312–2316.

32 Neuhouser ML, *et al.* Insulin-like growth factors and insulin-like growth factor-binding proteins and prostate cancer risk: results from the prostate cancer prevention trial. *Cancer Prev Res (Phila)* 2013;6(2):91–99.

33 Seligson DB, *et al.* IGFBP-3 nuclear localization predicts human prostate cancer recurrence. *Horm Cancer* 2013;4(1):12–23.

34 Isshiki S, *et al.* Chromogranin a concentration as a serum marker to predict prognosis after endocrine therapy for prostate cancer. *J Urol* 2002;167(2 Pt 1):512–515.

35 Moul JW, *et al.* The contemporary value of pretreatment prostatic acid phosphatase to predict pathological stage and recurrence in radical prostatectomy cases. *J Urol* 1998;159(3):935–940.

36 de Kok JB, *et al.* DD3(PCA3), a very sensitive and specific marker to detect prostate tumors. *Cancer Res* 2002;62(9):2695–2698.

37 Vlaeminck-Guillem V, *et al.* Urinary prostate cancer 3 test: toward the age of reason? *Urology* 2010;75(2):447–453.

38 Hessels D, *et al.* DD3(PCA3)-based molecular urine analysis for the diagnosis of prostate cancer. *Eur Urol* 2003;44(1):8–15; discussion 15–16.

39 Roobol MJ, *et al.* Performance of the prostate cancer antigen 3 (PCA3) gene and prostate-specific antigen in prescreened men: exploring the value of PCA3 for a first-line diagnostic test. *Eur Urol* 2010;58(4):475–481.

40 Andriole G, *et al.* Chemoprevention of prostate cancer in men at high risk: rationale and design of the reduction by dutasteride of prostate cancer events (REDUCE) trial. *J Urol* 2004;172(4 Pt 1):1314–1317.

41 Nakanishi H, *et al.* PCA3 molecular urine assay correlates with prostate cancer tumor volume: implication in selecting candidates for active surveillance. *J Urol* 2008;179(5):1804–1809; discussion 1809–1810.

42 Whitman EJ, *et al.* PCA3 score before radical prostatectomy predicts extracapsular extension and tumor volume. *J Urol* 2008;180(5):1975–1978; discussion 1978–1979.

43 Mitelman F, Johansson B, Mertens F. The impact of translocations and gene fusions on cancer causation. *Nat Rev Cancer* 2007;7(4):233–245.

44 Morris DS, *et al.* The discovery and application of gene fusions in prostate cancer. *BJU Int* 2008;102(3):276–82.

45 Tomlins SA, *et al.* Recurrent fusion of TMPRSS2 and ETS transcription factor genes in prostate cancer. *Science* 2005;310(5748):644–648.

46 Mehra R, *et al.* Comprehensive assessment of TMPRSS2 and ETS family gene aberrations in clinically localized prostate cancer. *Mod Pathol* 2007;20(5):538–544.

47 Kristiansen G. [Immunohistochemical algorithms in prostate diagnostics: what's new?]. *Pathologe* 2009;30(Suppl. 2):146–153.

48 Laxman B, *et al.* A first-generation multiplex biomarker analysis of urine for the early detection of prostate cancer. *Cancer Res* 2008;68(3):645–649.

49 Harden SV, *et al.* Quantitative GSTP1 methylation and the detection of prostate adenocarcinoma in sextant biopsies. *J Natl Cancer Inst* 2003;95(21):1634–1637.

50 Baden J, *et al.* Multicenter evaluation of an investigational prostate cancer methylation assay. *J Urol* 2009;182(3):1186–1193.

51 Schostak M, *et al.* Annexin A3 in urine: a highly specific noninvasive marker for prostate cancer early detection. *J Urol* 2009;181(1):343–353.

52 Egeblad M, Werb Z. New functions for the matrix metalloproteinases in cancer progression. *Nat Rev Cancer* 2002;2(3):161–174.

53 Lu Q, *et al.* Identification of extracellular delta-catenin accumulation for prostate cancer detection. *Prostate* 2009;69(4):411–418.

54 Russo AL, *et al.* Urine analysis and protein networking identify met as a marker of metastatic prostate cancer. *Clin Cancer Res* 2009;15(13):4292–4298.

55 Hutchinson LM, *et al.* Development of a sensitive and specific enzyme-linked immunosorbent assay for thymosin beta15, a urinary biomarker of human prostate cancer. *Clin Biochem* 2005;38(6):558–71.

56 Kollermann J, *et al.* Expression and prognostic relevance of annexin A3 in prostate cancer. *Eur Urol* 2008;54(6):1314–23.

57 Roy R, *et al.* Tumor-specific urinary matrix metalloproteinase fingerprinting: identification of high molecular weight urinary matrix metalloproteinase species. *Clin Cancer Res* 2008;14(20):6610–7.

58 Miyake M, *et al.* Sarcosine, a biomarker for prostate cancer: ready for prime time? *Biomark Med* 2012;6(4):513–4.

59 Aly M, Wiklund F, Gronberg H. Early detection of prostate cancer with emphasis on genetic markers. *Acta Oncol* 2011;50(Suppl. 1):18–23.

60 Kote-Jarai Z, *et al.* Multiple novel prostate cancer predisposition loci confirmed by an international study: the PRACTICAL Consortium. *Cancer Epidemiol Biomarkers Prev* 2008;17(8):2052–61.

61 Fitzgerald LM, *et al.* Analysis of recently identified prostate cancer susceptibility loci in a population-based study: associations with family history and clinical features. *Clin Cancer Res* 2009;15(9):3231–7.

62 Ali TZ, Epstein JI. False positive labeling of prostate cancer with high molecular weight cytokeratin: p63 a more specific immunomarker for basal cells. *Am J Surg Pathol* 2008;32(12):1890–5.

63 Wang W, Sun X, Epstein JI. Partial atrophy on prostate needle biopsy cores: a morphologic and immunohistochemical study. *Am J Surg Pathol* 2008;32(6):851–7.

64 Zhou M, *et al.* Basal cell cocktail (34betaE12 + p63) improves the detection of prostate basal cells. *Am J Surg Pathol* 2003;27(3):365–71.

65 Wu HH, Lapkus O, Corbin M. Comparison of 34betaE12 and P63 in 100 consecutive prostate carcinoma diagnosed by needle biopsies. *Appl Immunohistochem Mol Morphol* 2004;12(4):285–9.

66 Zhou M, *et al.* How often does alpha-methylacyl-CoA-racemase contribute to resolving an atypical diagnosis on prostate needle biopsy beyond that provided by basal cell markers? *Am J Surg Pathol* 2004;28(2):239–43.

67 Magi-Galluzzi C, *et al.* Alpha-methylacyl-CoA racemase: a variably sensitive immunohistochemical marker for the diagnosis of small prostate cancer foci on needle biopsy. *Am J Surg Pathol* 2003;27(8):1128–33.

68 Murphy AJ, *et al.* Heterogeneous expression of alpha-methylacyl-CoA racemase in prostatic cancer correlates with Gleason score. *Histopathology* 2007;50(2):243–51.

69 Yang RM, *et al.* Low p27 expression predicts poor disease-free survival in patients with prostate cancer. *J Urol* 1998;159(3):941–5.

70 van Weerden WM, *et al.* Ki-67 expression and BrdUrd incorporation as markers of proliferative activity in human prostate tumour models. *Cell Prolif* 1993;26(1):67–75.

71 Berney DM, *et al.* Ki-67 and outcome in clinically localised prostate cancer: analysis of conservatively treated prostate cancer patients from the Trans-Atlantic Prostate Group study. *Br J Cancer* 2009;100(6):888–93.

72 Khor LY, *et al.* MDM2 and Ki-67 predict for distant metastasis and mortality in men treated with radiotherapy and androgen deprivation for prostate cancer: RTOG 92-02. *J Clin Oncol* 2009;27(19):3177–84.

73 Bostwick DG. Prostatic adenocarcinoma following androgen deprivation therapy: the new difficulty in histologic interpretation. *Anat Pathol* 1998;3:1–16.

74 Ross JS, *et al.* Correlation of primary tumor prostate-specific membrane antigen expression with disease recurrence in prostate cancer. *Clin Cancer Res* 2003;9(17):6357–62.

75 Wright GL, Jr, *et al.* Upregulation of prostate-specific membrane antigen after androgen-deprivation therapy. *Urology* 1996;48(2):326–34.

76 Sweat SD, *et al.* Prostate-specific membrane antigen expression is greatest in prostate adenocarcinoma and lymph node metastases. *Urology* 1998;52(4):637–40.

77 Cristofanilli , M, *et al.* Circulating tumor cells, disease progression, and survival in metastatic breast cancer. *N Engl J Med* 2004;351(8):781–91.

78 Gao CL, *et al.* Diagnostic potential of prostate-specific antigen expressing epithelial cells in blood of prostate cancer patients. *Clin Cancer Res* 2003;9(7):2545–50.

79 Pal SK, Twardowski P, Josephson DY. Beyond castration and chemotherapy: novel approaches to targeting androgen-driven pathways. *Maturitas* 2009;64(2):61–6.

80 Scher HI, *et al.* Circulating tumour cells as prognostic markers in progressive, castration-resistant prostate cancer: a reanalysis of IMMC38 trial data. *Lancet Oncol* 2009;10(3):233–9.

81 de Bono JS, *et al.* Circulating tumor cells predict survival benefit from treatment in metastatic castration-resistant prostate cancer. *Clin Cancer Res* 2008;14(19):6302–9.

82 Rissanen M, *et al.* Novel homogenous time-resolved fluorometric RT-PCR assays for quantification of PSA and hK2 mRNAs in blood. *Clin Biochem* 2007;40(1-2):111–8.

## CHAPTER 5

# Imaging

*Jonathan Richenberg*

Department of Imaging, Royal Sussex County Hospital, Brighton, UK

## Introduction

By actively embracing modern imaging there are new opportunities to detect cancers, to improve staging, to guide management decisions, and to direct interventions, thus reducing iatrogenic complications.

## Role of imaging in prostate cancer

Imaging may be used to detect/diagnose prostate cancer, stage biopsy-proven disease, help determine the best therapy (including active surveillance (AS) or radical therapy with curative intent), modulate treatment choice, follow-up once treatment has been commenced (on AS or post-therapy), and guide focal therapy.

The mainstay of prostate imaging is directed toward soft-tissue imaging techniques, ultrasound (US), and magnetic resonance imaging (MRI). X-ray-based techniques (plain radiographs and CT) have a very limited role, either as adjunct to other imaging (dedicated plain films of spine, pelvis, and so on looking for bone lesions) or in staging when MRI is contraindicated. CT has very poor accuracy for T stage, but is equivalent for N stage. Because of the limitation, the radiographic modalities will not be further discussed.

Bone scintigraphy has a defined, albeit limited role in prostate cancer imaging, to detect skeletal metastases. This M staging is being replaced by MRI of the bony pelvis and the lumbar spine and sacrum Table 5.1.

*Prostate Cancer: Diagnosis and Clinical Management*, First Edition.
Edited by Ashutosh K. Tewari, Peter Whelan and John D. Graham.
© 2014 John Wiley & Sons, Ltd. Published 2014 by John Wiley & Sons, Ltd.

**Table 5.1** Summary of imaging modalities in aspects of detection, staging, and treating prostate cancer

|  | Ultrasound | MRI | Bone scan |
| --- | --- | --- | --- |
| Diagnosis detection | + (+) | +++ | − |
| Diagnosis tissue | +++ TRUS or TP | + MR guidance, ++ fusion | − |
| Treatment guidance | (+) | +++ | + |
| T, N, M staging | T (+) N −, M − | T +++, N +(+), M ++ | T −, N−, M++ |
| AS | − | ++ | − |
| Treatment modulation: surgical approach, type radiotherapy or field, neoadjuvant or adjuvant androgen deprivation therapy (ADT) | − | +++ | + |
| Treatment monitoring | − | + (+) | + |

## Detection and diagnosis

### Overview

At the time of diagnosis, most men (~85%) will have more than one focus of cancer within the prostate gland, commonly of differing volume and often of variable grade. There are difficulties from the outset in evaluating any disease with this degree of heterogeneity [1].

### Overview of transrectal ultrasound-guided prostate biopsy

The standards and conduct of transrectal ultrasound-guided biopsy (TRUS-Bx) have been set out in 2011 and 2012 [2, 3]. This includes advice on pre-procedure consent, preparation, and postprocedure advice. The universally accepted standard is a minimum of 10 cores obtained in a systematic fashion at least one from each peripheral sextant. Often 12–14 cores are taken, especially in glands whose volume exceeds 50 mL. Antibiotic prophylaxis and periprostatic local anesthetic should be used in all patients.

There has been a steady rise in the number of prostate biopsies in the United Kingdom, close to 20 000 men in 2011 if transperineal biopsies are included (Figure 5.1). The transperineal route is becoming more popular, having a lower risk for sepsis, and also because it provides more uniform access to the whole of the prostate. Despite the uptake of transperineal biopsy and major inherent limitations, until recently, TRUS-Bx constituted the most common pathway for prostate cancer detection.

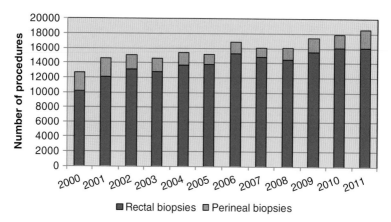

**Figure 5.1**  Number of rectal and perineal needle prostate biopsies performed as inpatient or day case procedures in England, in patients diagnosed with cancer. Identified using OPCS-4 codes M703 (rectal) and M702 (perineal). Where patients were reported to undergo both rectal and perineal biopsy in the same episode [4], was classed as perineal (*Source:* HES)

## Limitation one—over diagnosis of unimportant cancers

The first limitation is the oversampling of low-grade, low-volume tumors with attendant negatives of anxiety from diagnosis and morbidity from treatment for an indolent cancer that may not merit detection. Half the cancers detected by active prostate specific antigen (PSA) screening in combination with systematic TRUS-Bx are considered overdiagnosed [5].

## Limitation two—missing significant disease

In men presenting with PSA below 10 ng/mL, the majority of tumors will not be visible on TRUS. Therefore, TRUS primarily is a means to direct biopsy to the gland periphery, in the hope that the needle will sample any cancer present. Transrectal ultrasound-guided biopsy follows a sys-tematic approach dividing the gland into sextants and sampling 1–3 cores from each sextant (a minimum of 10 cores). Tumor detection in biopsy sets of 10–12 cores is ~30% for men presenting with serum PSA values between 4 ng/mL and 10 ng/mL, with an estimated sensitivity of only 39% in detecting tumor [6,7]. On subsequent biopsies, detection rates are estimated at 10–15% for second biopsy and 5–10% for third biopsy [8–10].

Transrectal ultrasound-guided biopsy tends to oversample the posterior and lateral peripheries of the gland, and undersamples the anterior and apical regions and the central gland [11]. The undersampling based on geometry alone leads to missing important cancers; and as the tumors are not usually visible, they cannot be targeted. Moreover, even positive biopsy results are limited since the needle may have:

- Passed through the periphery of the cancer, underestimating the tumor volume.
- Passed through a less-aggressive part of the cancer (Gleason 3 pattern) and missed higher Gleason areas, underestimating the tumor grade/risk.
- Passed through a small low-grade tumor in one sextant (reassuring histology suggesting low-risk disease) and missed a larger/more aggressive lesion elsewhere (typically in anterior or transitional zone), underestimating the true risk of prostate cancer to the patient.

In the subgroup of biopsy-positive patients who proceed to radical prostatectomy, there is a reported 35–65% upgrade in Gleason score at final histology compared with the biopsy cores [12, 13].

It is hardly surprising that clinicians have been striving for techniques to improve the conspicuity of prostate cancers on TRUS, and for methods to gauge the aggressiveness of any lesions so revealed.

## Techniques to improve conspicuity
### Prostate cancer detection on grayscale (B mode) transrectal ultrasound

Prostate cancer is typically echo poor on grayscale (B mode) ultrasound, but benign hyperplastic nodules and prostatitis may look identical; no more than half the echo-poor nodules seen on conventional ultrasound are malignant (Figure 5.2). In other words, standard TRUS is barely better than 50% accurate in detecting focal prostate cancer with a correspondingly poor positive predictive value (PPV) of 6%. Furthermore, 30–40% of cancers are isoechoic and a small percentage are echogenic. A comprehensive review of the TRUS characteristics of prostate cancer has been published recently in the British Journal of Radiology [2].

The detection rate, unsurprisingly, varies with the PSA value: when the PSA is greater than 20 ng/mL, over 75% of tumors are seen while <30% are seen at a PSA <10 ng/mL (the current situation in modern practice).

### Role of color and power Doppler [14–17]

Initial hopes for color and power Doppler in highlighting vascular asymmetry, and thereby flagging cancer foci, have foundered. Adding Doppler analysis to B mode confers no more than 10% improvement in sensitivity. While there is some sense in biopsying focal vascular areas, this does not obviate the need for established systematic (10–12 cores) sampling.

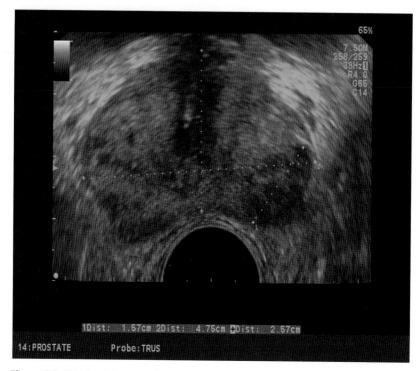

**Figure 5.2** TRUS axial section depicting left mid zone 16 mm hypoechoic lesion typical for cancer; biopsy-proven prostatitis. Low specificity of TRUS.

### Contrast-enhanced ultrasound

Ultrasound microbubble contrast agents capitalize on the chaotic prolif-eration of microvessels in prostate cancer, a behavior shared with many other soft-tissue malignancies [18]. Microbubbles are, uniquely, a true vascular agent—they do not migrate across the endothelium—so that their kinetics reliably describe the blood flow indices within a lesion [19]. They can be seen on TRUS in vessels of 50–100 $\mu$m diameter, 50 $\mu$m being the upper limit for tumor microvessels [20]. Analysis of contrast-time–intensity curves increase detection rates and classification of detected lesions, with accuracy up to 80%. Several papers have used intermittent harmonic imaging, whereby high-power ultrasound beams are used peri-odically to burst the bubbles in the prostate vessels and reappearance of the contrast bubbles are analyzed (reperfusion kinetics) to increase cancer detection sensitivity without reducing specificity [21, 22].

Contrast-enhanced ultrasound (CEUS) adds functional information in lesion characterization, and lesions targeted by CEUS tend to be of higher

Gleason grade compared to lesions "detected" by systematic biopsy, and use of contrast means that more cancers may be found *for fewer biopsies* [23, 24]. In theory, it may reduce for any particular man the number of biopsy samples, increase the discovery of cancer, and bias this increase toward aggressive cancers. CEUS would then, indeed, be an antidote to limitation one and limitation two. However, the promise has not yet been realized in day-to-day practice largely because the increased sensitivity is not yet good enough and the specificity remains low. In conjunction with developments in three-dimensional (3D) and four-dimensional (4D) imaging, it may improve to a threshold acceptable for clinical use [25–27].

### Elastography

The theory behind "elastography" is that a prostate gland infiltrated with tumor will be less compressible (stiffer) than normal parenchyma, akin to the increased firmness that raises suspicion on digital rectal examination. The transrectal probe compresses the gland, and the strain is measured and depicted as a colored region superimposed on the grayscale image, stiffer regions are traditionally portrayed as red. Some studies indicate elastography can guide biopsy and reduce the overall number of samples taken while increasing the detection rate twofold to fivefold [28, 29]. If validated, these findings will be important because potentially, as with CEUS, they overcome the limitations of TRUS-Bx while capitalizing on all the verified benefits of TRUS-Bx, and they combine seamlessly with the "approved" method of prostate sampling. The benefits to patient and to hospital budgets are manifest (Figure 5.3, Plate 5.3).

### Extended biopsy under image guidance—more of the same?
### Saturation biopsies

European Association of Urology (EAU) guidelines recommend a saturation scheme on repeat biopsy [30]. Saturation techniques have not been precisely defined, either in terms of the number of cores or regions sampled, which may explain why the urological community cannot agree whether saturation techniques confer an advantage [31, 32] or not overextended schemes [7].

A reasonable working definition of an extended biopsy scheme would be transrectal sampling, 18–24 cores, usually under general anesthesia. The central zone is included in the samples, but there is still limited sampling of the anterior gland. The sensitivity of lesion detection rises modestly [33] but inevitably there will be proportionate increased detection of low-grade clinically unimportant cancers, "limitation one" above.

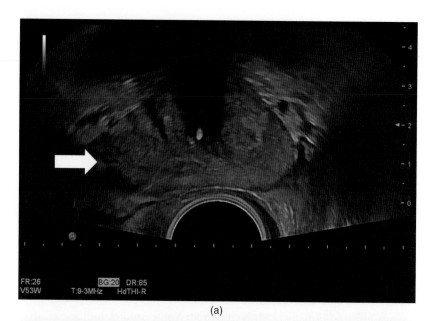

(a)

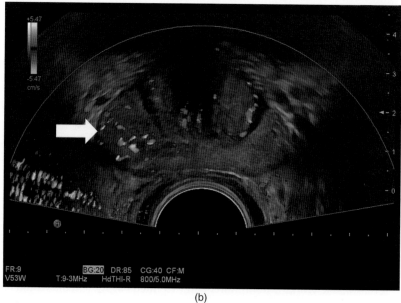

(b)

**Figure 5.3** Prostate cancer (arrows) Gleason 7 (3 + 4) biopsy confirmed on (a) grayscale, (b) color Doppler. (See also Plate 5.3.)

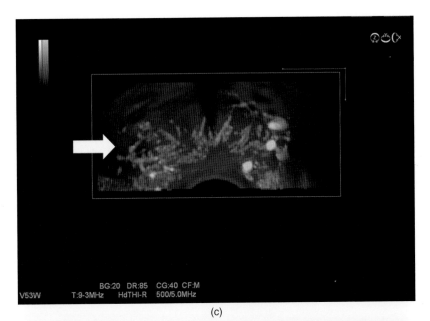

(c)

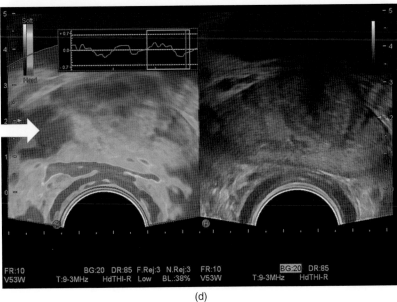

(d)

**Figure 5.3** (*Continued*) (c) 3D color Doppler, (d) seen as an area of increased stiffness on elastography. (See also Plate 5.3.)

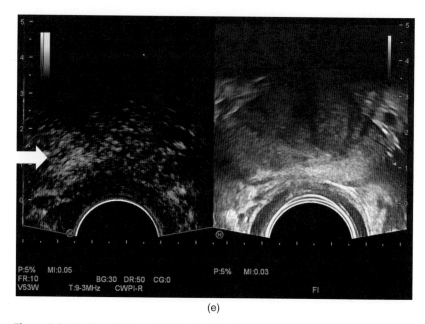

(e)

**Figure 5.3** (*Continued*) (e) as a focal enhancing lesion following intravenous Sonovue (Bracco, Italy) microbubbles using microbubble-specific imaging. Prostate cancer right mid zone shown as a focal enhancing lesion following intravenous Sonovue (Bracco, Italy) microbubbles using microbubble-specific imaging. Biopsy confirmed a Gleason 7 (3 + 4) prostate cancer. Reproduced from Reference 2 with permission from British Institute of Radiology. (See also Plate 5.3.)

## Transperineal biopsies [34, 35]

In 2000, almost one-third of prostate biopsies were by the transperineal route, falling to under 10% by 2007. The resurgence in this technique is a result of increasing awareness of the limitation of TRUS-Bx. The transperineal approach permits complete coverage of the gland, including the anterior and central parts, and has a much lower risk of sepsis. However, it entails a general anesthetic and operating theater time, and has a high rate of hemorrhage and urinary retention. Moreover, there will be overdiagnosis of unimportant diseases.

## Multiparametric magnetic resonance imaging

During the preceding decade, MRI of the prostate has come of age. It is being used increasingly alongside clinical, biochemical, and histopathological assessment to detect, stage, and follow up prostate cancers. Indeed, as the technique has matured, it has begun to supplant some of the more established diagnostic tests to determine management. The attraction of MRI to the clinician is that it tends to detect more aggressive diseases, so does not suffer from limitation one and depicts the whole gland avoiding anterior and central zone bias. The attraction to the patient is that MRI may obviate the need for multiple biopsies with their attendant complications [36].

## What is mpMRI?

The term multiparametric MRI (mpMRI) incorporates the idea of combined anatomical and functional magnetic resonance (MR) sequences acquired in a single examination. The anatomy is provided by the magnified field of view of T2-weighted sequences and functional information by one or more sequences comprising diffusion-weighted imaging (DWI), dynamic contrast enhancement (DCE), and choline-citrate spectroscopy (MRS).

Multiparametric MRI interrogates different aspects of any lesion within the prostate tissue—cell density, vascular and microvascular integrity, and metabolic activity—combining with anatomical signal changes that suggest tumor or benign gland tissue.

### Diffusion-weighted imaging

The diffusion of extracellular water molecules, Brownian motion, tends to be more restricted in malignant tissue because of the more compact cellular architecture than in "healthy" tissue. Diffusion-weighted imaging makes use of this phenomenon. A diffusion sensitizing gradient of increasing strength (b value) is applied and the time taken for the water molecules to "fall out of line" (diffuse randomly) can be presented ultimately as an apparent diffusion coefficient (ADC) map, where slower diffusion associated with pathological tissue is darker than normal tissue.

### Dynamic contrast enhancement

Dynamic contrast MRI yields information about the vascularity of the prostate. Malignant tissue typically has more abundant and chaotic low-resistance vessels than normal so tumor has rapid enhancement and rapid washout. Semiquantitative analysis can look at a region of prostate and generate a time-enhancement curve, the curve pattern being suggestive of benign or malignant tissue. The increased permeability of extravascular extracellular space means that the malignant tissue has early and brisk enhancement (15–30 seconds).

### Magnetic resonance spectroscopy

Spectroscopy relies on the relative abundance of choline and citrate in cell membranes. In cancer, the choline rises and the citrate falls. Metabolic spectra tuned to choline and citrate molecules will show a high ratio of choline and a low ratio of citrate in cancerous tissues compared with healthy tissue.

Spectroscopy can be used to predict the aggressiveness of a particular cancer [37]. However, it has several drawbacks compared to other MR techniques, including the need for an endorectal coil at 1.5 T, a lengthy scan time, limited resolution, and a high number of unusable voxels. The claimed superiority of spectroscopy over DWI and ADC measurement [38] has not been borne out [39], and the claim that magnetic resonance spectroscopy (MRS) can predict aggressiveness is not unique; T2-weighted images have signal intensity that correlates with tumor biology [40] and DWI can predict tumor aggressiveness (Gleason grade) [41–44].

### Is there a best combination?

Clinical studies are beginning to address the question of the relative benefit of the sequences using correlation with prostatectomy specimens. For example, in cases of biopsy-proven, intermediate, and high-risk prostate cancer, diffusion-weighted magnetic resonance imaging (DW MRI) is the most senstivite for tumor localisation and of particular utility in the transition zone [45]. Assessment of tumor volume also appears best on DWI. Enhanced sequences add specificity in both peripheral and transition zones, and sometimes detect tumors missed with other techniques [46].

An obsessive comparison of the different sequences, in my opinion, is futile as the clear message is that mpMRI is best when performed as a combination. If confronted, the advocates of the different sequences would argue that it is the very combination of differing tumor properties that makes mpMRI so useful. There is objective evidence to support this [47], and the most satisfactory combination seems to be T2 weighted (T2W), DWI, and DCE. Turkbey and Choyke echo this in a review of mpMRI in cancer detection and risk stratification [48] (Figure 5.4) (Table 5.2).

### The ability of mpMRI to overcome limitations of PSA–TRUS approach

The limitations of the traditional approach—overdiagnosis of insignificant disease (limitation one) and missing potentially lethal cancers (limitation two) may be countered by the uptake of mpMRI using the combined anatomical and functional information to detect and "grade" lesions.

The utility of mpMRI varies according to the definition of "significant disease". For the purposes of this chapter, *insignificant cancer* will be classed

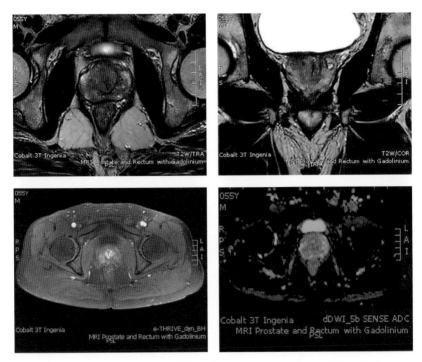

**Figure 5.4** Multiparametric MRI pelvis, right base tumour seen on T2W axial (top left), and coronal (top right), dynamic contrast early phase uptake (bottom left) and ADC map (bottom right).

as Gleason 3+3 disease or less, or volume <0.5 cm$^3$ (equivalent 10 mm diameter).[1]

## Can mpMRI counter limitation one—overdiagnosis of insignificant disease?

Studies looking at mpMRI compared with subsequent extensive biopsies and/or radical prostatectomy specimens indicate a high negative predictive value of mpMRI, that is, a "normal" MRI correlates well with the absence of clinically significant cancer. For example, using a variety of definitions of clinically significant disease based on core length and Gleason 7 in over 180 men, comparing lesions targeted by transperineal biopsy based

---

[1] Although of course some of the small lesions will be en route to becoming larger and hence significant cancers.

**Table 5.2** Minimum standards for multiparametric MRI

| Sequence | Slice thickness (mm) | In-plane resolution (mm) | Scan time (range) | Optimal |
|---|---|---|---|---|
| T2 axial, coronal | 3 | 0.7 | 3–6 min | Sagittal sequence as well. Include external sphincter and entire seminal vesicles |
| Diffusion—multi b | 5 | 1.5 | 4–7 min | At least three, typically four values (in s/mm$^2$) 0, 50, 400, 800 for ADC |
| Diffusion—long b | 5 | 1.5 | 4–6 min | 1400–1500 s/mm$^2$ on 1.5T, 2000 s/mm$^2$ on 3T. Do not include in ADC |
| Dynamic enhanced | 3 | 1 | <15 s per iteration, total 5 min | Contrast at 3 mL/s. Visualization of contrast enhancement may need to be supplemented by semiquantitative analysis using workstation to analyze curves. Formal estimation of Ktrans and other parameters not required in general clinical practice. |

Minimum standards for multiparametric MRI using a pelvic phased array coil at 1.5T, with additional notes and suggestions for optimal technique. Based on European Society of Uroradiology guidelines.

on mpMRI against systematic (nontargeted but more extensive) biopsy regimen, there was ~50% reduction in diagnosis of insignificant disease while missing only 10 significant tumors (<10% of all detected), and with fewer biopsies [49]. MRI-targeted biopsies detected less micro-focal cancers than randomized 12-core biopsies. They did not seem however to decrease the detection of clinically significant cancers [50]. Others affirm negative predictive values of ~82–86% for all cancers, and 93% for high-grade lesions [51]. If men had not been biopsied because of a negative mpMRI, 21% with no cancer and 5% with clinically insignificant cancer could have avoided a biopsy [52].

The flip side of these impressive figures, with the promise of finding fewer low-grade cancers, is a meagre sensitivity of 60–65% so any positive MRI result warrants biopsy for characterization. It is hoped but not yet affirmed that negative mpMRI may obviate biopsy but not follow-up, especially as detection of transitional zone lesion remains less accurate.

**Can mpMRI counter limitation two—missing significant disease?**
Multiparametric MRI-guided biopsy outperforms TRUS-Bx in detecting prostate cancer in men who proceed to radical prostatectomy especially in the mid and transitional zones, and in glands weighing more than 50 g [53]. Detection rates of cancer in men with one or more previous negative TRUS-Bx are in the range of 30–59% [54–58]. Based on a systematic review of the literature, the pooled sensitivity of T2 and DWI is 76% and the pooled specificity is 82% [59].

Multiparametric MRI can, because it includes functional data, shed light on the aggressiveness of individual lesions. This ability has been shown to correlate with Gleason grade assessed at prostatectomy, for example, by using ADC maps to direct biopsy [43]. Under ideal circumstances, which include prebiopsy, mpMRI has 80% detection rates of Gleason 4+3 cancers 7 mm or larger (equivalent 0.2 cm$^3$) and Gleason 3+4 cancers 10 mm or larger (equivalent 0.5 cm$^3$) throughout the gland. Current mpMRI is unreliable in identifying Gleason 6 disease, a paradoxical advantage over indiscriminate TRUS. MRI shows an additional value in biopsy detection rate in targeted TRUS-Bx, increasing the detection rate of tumors with a Gleason score >6 from 72% to 88% [60].

Diffusion-weighted imaging data correlate with Gleason grade, while DCE data highlight microvessel density but do not predict Gleason grade [61].

The benefit of MRI in detection increases with increasing aggresivenss of the lesion, and the confidence with which a lesion is singled out as being significant rises in proportion to the number of multiparametric sequences that suggest it, with PPVs rising to above 90% [62] (Figure 5.4), with lesion seen confidently on T2, DWI, and DCE.

## Biopsy new techniques
The ability of mpMRI to detect lesions, and in a way that identifies tumors by their agressivenss, means that it has a role prebiopsy. There are three strategies for using the MRI map during biopsy: cognitive, MR-guided, and fusion.

### Cognitive ultrasound-guided biopsy
Cognitive biopsy, ultrasound-guided transrectal or transperineal placement of the needle, aims for a specific region of the gland based on a mental appreciation of where a lesion shown by mpMRI resides.

If suspicious lesions are marked on a stylized prostate gland map and cores are targeted to the vicinity of the lesion on subsequent TRUS biopsy, the detection rate in the targeted cores may be as high as 75% with a proportionately high incidence of high-grade disease [63].

Ironically a recent paper by Shigemura *et al.* that concludes "systematic 12-core biopsy (sextant peripheral zone + 4 transitional zone + 2 far lateral peripheral zone) can be considered an excellent tool for [prostate cancer] detection and there may be no need for additional cores based on MRI findings" adds to the argument that prebiopsy MRI can reduce the number of samples; the MRI detected many lesions that were sampled by TRUS, and in those cases, the biopsy could have been limited to the visible disease (perhaps 2–3 cores rather than 12) [64].

## MRI-guided biopsy

Equipment has been developed to guide a needle under MR control into the lesion highlighted by mpMRI. Some centers advocate MR-guided biopsy as the method of choice after a negative TRUS-Bx and quote positivity rates of 40–50%, with 80–90% of lesions being clinically significant [54, 65].

Bearing this in mind and acknowledging the proven utility of TRUS guidance, and its unassailable dominance over MR guidances in terms of cost, convenience, and patient satisfaction, the goal must be real-time MR–TRUS fusion. I have advocated this strategy for several years and a very recent review suggests that "Supportive data are emerging for the fusion devices, two of which received U.S. Food and Drug Administration approval in the past 5 years: Artemis (Eigen, USA) and Urostation (Koelis, France)" [66].

## The grail—fusion of ultrasound-guided biopsy using mpMRI data

The Digital Imaging and Communications in Medicine (DICOM) dataset of mpMRI may be superimposed onto a live TRUS image, guiding the needle under direct vision into the lesion now conspicuous as a predefined (MR-detected) target. Work from Heidelberg using 3 Tesla MRI–biplane TRUS system in combination with transperineal biopsies has reported detection rates of 59% *in low-risk patients.* Overall, MRI correlated positively with histopathology in 69%, up to 96% in lesions regarded as highly suspicious [67] (Figure 5.5, Plate 5.5) (Figure 5.6, Plate 5.6).

Data published on over 800 men [66, 68–70] indicate that:
- Target accuracy is >95%.
- Three-dimensional deformable registration is sufficiently accurate to match TRUS and MRI volumes with a topographic precision of 1 mm.

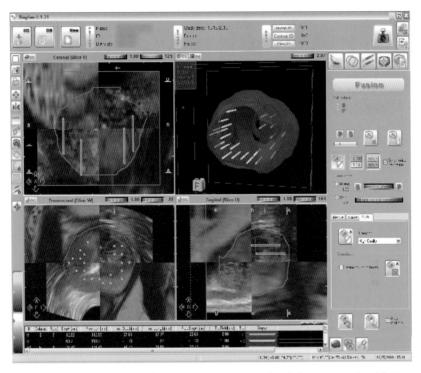

**Figure 5.5** Fusion of mpMRI dataset on TRUS as part of real-time transperineal fusion biopsy of focal lesions of the prostate gland detected on mpMRI. (See also Plate 5.5.)

- Detection rates overall are ~50%, varying from 10% for low-suspicion lesions (based on combined mpMRI findings) to over 90% for high-suspicion lesions.
- Targeted biopsies are two to three times more sensitive for detection of cancer than nontargeted systematic biopsies.
- In up to 50% of men with Gleason score of at least 7, lesion is detected on targeted biopsy but not on 12-core standard biopsy.
- In almost 40%, targeting biopsy results in an upgrade of Gleason grade when compared to corresponding lesion sampled by traditional TRUS biopsy.

### Summary

In a high-quality scientific review, 62% of biopsy-naïve men had an abnormal mpMRI, corresponding on targeted biopsy to 66% cancer

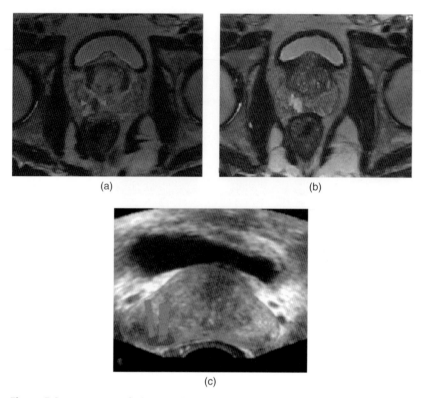

(a)   (b)

(c)

**Figure 5.6** MR transrectal ultrasound (TRUS) fusion image. (a, b) Multiparametric axial MR images with functional information (related to diffusion-weighted MRI) identifying a cancer (arrowheads) not visible on TRUS (study not shown). (c) Fused dataset, superimposing after coregistering the MR images that identify the tumor based on its reduced diffusion onto the real-time TRUS images. The red bars represent biopsy trajectories. Biopsy directed by the TRUS revealed a Gleason 7 cancer. Courtesy of Dr Erik Rud, Oslo University Hospital, Oslo, Norway. (See also Plate 5.6.)

detection. Interestingly, clinically significant cancer was reported in 43% regardless of whether the biopsy was targeted or not, but the targeted approach meant that 30% fewer men were biopsied and that the number of cores on average dropped from the standard dozen to 4% targeted, there being a 10% reduction in the detection of insignificant cancers [71].

MRI before repeat or even initial biopsy can accurately select patients who require immediate biopsies and those in whom biopsy could be deferred. MRI before biopsy helps to detect high-grade tumors to target biopsies within areas of low ADC values.

# Staging and treatment determination

## Preamble

After histological diagnosis of prostate cancer, staging may be on clinical parameters alone or may rely additionally on imaging investigations. In those who go on to radical prostatectomy, clinical staging is upgraded in ~60% following surgery. If the upgrading were possible by preoperative mpMRI, the proposed treatment may be modified, reducing iatrogenic morbidity and mortality when there is no possibility of cure by prostatectomy.

## T stage—TRUS and mpMRI

Digital rectal examination is limited in assessing T stage. Transrectal ultrasound is similarly limited, and neither technique gives any information about node involvement [72, 73]. The accuracy of TRUS for local staging is poor: for extracapsular extension (T3 disease), reported mean sensitivity is ~75%, specificity ~70%, and accuracy ~75%. TRUS signs of extracapsular extension are focal bulges, irregularity of the capsule, and echo-poor stranding of the periprostatic fat [2] (Figure 5.7). For seminal vesicle involvement (T3b) the sensitivity of TRUS is ~40%, specificity 88%, and accuracy 78% [74]; this compares badly with MRI.

T2-weighted sequences alone improve staging accuracy compared to nomograms [75, 76]. Performance for both detection of tumor and staging will likely be improved by the *addition* of an endorectal coil [77], but the benefit for routine use does not necessarily outweigh the costs: patient discomfort, extra time for placement, and field inhomogeneity.

Using more sophisticated MRI with additional functional sequences, with 3T field strengths or with endorectal coils, improves sensitivity of T-stage prediction, but often at the cost of sensitivity. The variation in reported staging performance of MRI for prostate cancer (against inevitable prostatectomy specimens) is large, 40–80% sensitivity and 75–95% specificity [78–81]. This wide variation reflects differing imaging practice, and the use of "historic" data, rapidity of advances meaning that studies become outdated quickly (Table 5.3).

A very relevant study comprised 158 men who underwent radical prostatectomy for *clinical T1c disease*. Preoperative mpMRI achieved 80% accuracy in staging—and this is very significant because within the group final (pathological) stage was T3a in 18%, T3b in 1%, and T4 in 1% [82] (Table 5.4).

With current MRI platforms, the lower-end examinations with pelvic phased array 1.5T MRI show promise in detecting the extracapsular

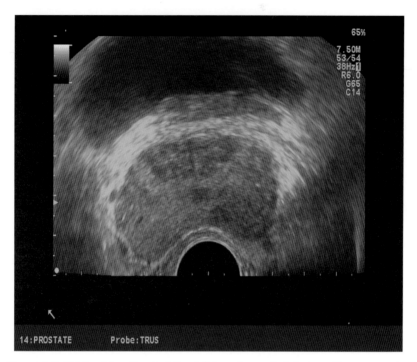

**Figure 5.7** TRUS axial section depicting left bases hypoechoic lesion with extracapsular spread, stage T3a. Reproduced from Reference 2 with permission from British Institute of Radiology.

extension of tumors to a level that has clinical worth/creditability, with the most significant factor being radiological reader experience [83]. There are morphologic predictors of extracapsular disease (T3a) and seminal vesicle (T3b) involvement [84]. See Table 5.4. MRI sensitivity and specificity to detect extracapsular extension (ECE) is reported as 55% and 96% if direct signs of ECE are used; and 84% and 89% if both direct and indirect signs are combined on 1-mm section endorectal 3T [79, 85] (Table 5.5) (Figures 5.8, 5.9, 5.10).

**Table 5.3** Indicative parameters of mpMRI for T and N stage assessment measured against radical prostatectomy in 32 patients

|  | Tumor (2 × 32) | EPE = T3a | SV = T3b (%) | PLN = N1 (%) |
| --- | --- | --- | --- | --- |
| Tumor | 53/64 83% | 17/64 27% | 19 | 11 |
| Sensitivity | 94 | 82 | 83 | 71 |
| Specificity | 82 | 87 | 92 | 95 |

Thirty-two men (64 prostate lobes) who underwent radical prostatectomy following mpMRI [33].

**Table 5.4** Direct and indirect signs on mpMRI for evaluating the T stage of prostate cancer

**Extracapsular extension**
Abutment
Bulge of capsule
*Irregularity and neurovascular bundle thickening* (3)
*Filling in of rectoprostatic angle*
*Measurable extracapsular disease = SI in periprostatic fat* (5)
**Seminal vesicles (coronal views)**
Expansion (1)
Low T2 signal (2)
*Filling in of angle* (4)
*Enhancement and restricted diffusion* (5)
**Distal sphincter**
Adjacent tumor (2)
Effacement of low signal sphincter muscle (3)
*Abnormal enhancement extending into sphincter* (5)
**Bladder neck**
Adjacent tumor (2)
Loss of low T2 signal in bladder muscle (4)
*Abnormal enhancement extending into bladder neck* (5)

Direct signs are in italics. Numbers in parentheses give an indication of probability (on a scale of 1–5) for T3 disease.

**Table 5.5** Predicted and observed rates of T2 and T3 disease based on preoperative mpMRI and surgical resection specimens depending on the D'Amico risk group

See also Table 13 for definition of D'Amico risk groups

|  | Low risk (%) | Intermediate (%) | High (%) |
|---|---|---|---|
| T2 MRI | 80 | 65 | 40 |
| T2 surgery | 75 | 40 | 20 |
| T3 MRI | 20 | 35 | 60 |
| T3 surgery | 25 | 60 | 80 |
| Sensitivity | 60 | 50 | 65 |
| Specificity | 90 | 90 | 70 |
| NPV | 85 | 60 | 40 |
| PPV | 70 | 90 | 90 |

Personal data.

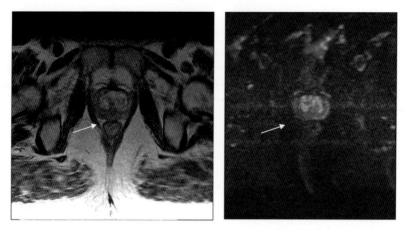

**Figure 5.8** PSA 6–9.2 ng/mL in 8 months, previous TRUS biopsy negative. mpMRI before second biopsy. (a) Axial T2W MRI pelvis and (b) ADC map, right T3a disease with low-signal tumor and in filling of the recto-prostatic angle (arrow).

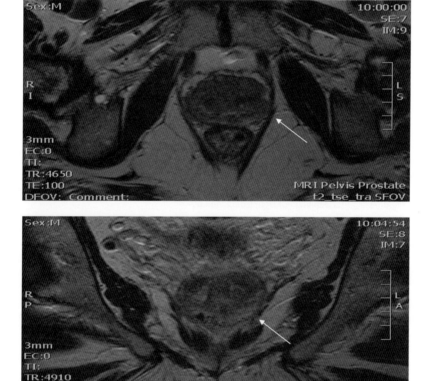

**Figure 5.9** (a) Axial T2W MRI pelvis and (b) coronal T2, left T3a disease with low-signal tumor extending beyond the capsule (arrows).

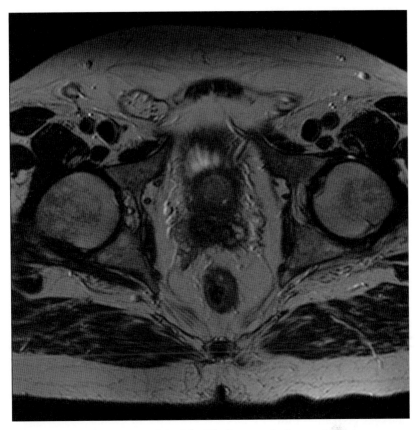

**Figure 5.10** Axial T2W MRI pelvis, right T3b disease and adjacent right base cancer as low signal mass.

The cost–benefit of any imaging will vary between particular patient groups (PSA, PSA velocity, Gleason grade, number, and extent of cores positive) [84, 86, 87] (Table 5.6).

### Reporting and Pi-RADS

A scoring system similar to that employed successfully by breast radiologists (breast imaging-reporting and data system (Bi-RADS) for X-ray mammography and MRI) has been developed and validated for prostate mpMRI. The prostate should be divided into 12–27 regions of interest; 16 sectors may be the best balance between detail and reporting burden, and such a scheme was described in 2011 in a consensus meeting [36]. Scoring criteria for T2W, DWI, DCE, and MRS are summarized in

**Table 5.6** Pi-RADS T2W scoring

Peripheral Zone

| Score | Criteria |
|---|---|
| 1 | Uniform high signal intensity |
| 2 | Linear, wedge-shaped, or geographic areas of lower SI, usually not well demarcated |
| 3 | Intermediate appearances not in categories 1/2 or 4/5 |
| 4 | Discrete, homogeneous low signal focus/mass confined to the prostate |
| 5 | Discrete, homogeneous low signal intensity focus with extracapsular extension/invasive behavior or mass effect on the capsule (bulging) or broad (<1.5 cm) contact with the surface |

Transitional Zone

| Score | Criteria |
|---|---|
| 1 | Uniform high signal intensity or with well-defined margins; "organized chaos" |
| 2 | Areas of more homogeneous low SI, however well marginated, originating from the TZ/BPH |
| 3 | Intermediate appearances not in categories 1/2 or 4/5 |
| 4 | Areas of more homogeneous low SI, ill defined: "erased charcoal sign" |
| 5 | Same as 4, but involving the anterior fibromuscular stroma or the anterior horn of the peripheral zone (PZ), usually lenticular or water-drop shaped |

Tables 5.7, 5.8, 5.9, 5.10, and 5.11, based on the European Society of Uro-radiology guidelines [88].

Two studies have reported on using the scheme in men who proceeded to mpMRI–TRUS fusion biopsies, with pre-evaluation of each lesion using prostate imaging-reporting and data system (Pi-RADS) [89, 90]. Lesions

**Table 5.7** Pi-RADS diffusion-weighted imaging scoring

DWI scoring

| Score | Criteria |
|---|---|
| 1 | No reduction in ADC compared to normal glandular tissue. No increase in SI on any high b-value image (≥b800) |
| 2 | Diffuse hyper SI on ≥b800 image with low ADC; no focal features; however, linear, triangular, or geographical features are allowed |
| 3 | Intermediate appearances not in categories 1/2 or 4/5 |
| 4 | Focal area(s) of reduced ADC but isointense SI on high b-value images (≥b800) |
| 5 | Focal area/mass of hyper SI on the high b-value images (≥b800) with reduced ADC |

**Table 5.8** Pi-RADS dynamic contrast enhancement imaging scoring

DCE–MRI scoring

| Score | Criteria |
|---|---|
| 1 | Type 1 enhancement curve |
| 2 | Type 2 enhancement curve |
| 3 | Type 3 enhancement curve |
| +1 | For focal enhancing lesion with curve types 2–3 |
| +1 | For asymmetric lesion or lesion in an unusual place with curve types 2–3 |

with a total score <10 points are very unlikely to be malignant [90] (Table 5.12).

The individual scores may be combined into an aggregate score for each sextant, based on a 5-point likelihood scale—after all, what matters clinically is the final assessment of the likelihood of disease: the "overall impression" score.

"This first step in collating all methods of scoring and reporting mpMRI will ultimately lead to consensus approaches to develop a standardized reporting scheme that can be widely adopted and validated to ensure comparability of research outputs and optimal clinical practice" [91].

Score 1 = Clinically significant disease is highly unlikely to be present

Score 2 = Clinically significant cancer is unlikely to be present

Score 3 = Clinically significant cancer is equivocal

Score 4 = Clinically significant cancer is likely to be present

Score 5 = Clinically significant cancer is highly likely to be present

**Table 5.9** Pi-RADS magnetic resonance spectroscopy imaging scoring (MRSI)

Qualitative MRSI

In qualitative analysis, the relative peak heights of citrate and choline are visually compared (pattern analysis), rather than quantified.

The following criteria apply for 1.5T magnet: looking at the choline and citrate peaks for at least three adjacent voxels, apply scores 1–5:

| Score | Criteria |
|---|---|
| 1 | Citrate peak height exceeds choline peak height >2 times |
| 2 | Citrate peak height exceeds choline peak height >1, <2 times |
| 3 | Choline peak height equals citrate peak height |
| 4 | Choline peak height exceeds citrate peak height >1, <2 times |
| 5 | Choline peak height exceeds citrate peak height >2 times |

**Table 5.10** Pi-RADS magnetic resonance spectroscopy imaging scoring (MRSI)

Quantitative MRSI

The (choline + creatinine)/citrate ratio for any region, using two or more adjacent voxels can be compared to the mean value for the gland (eliminating inter-MRI variation). The following criteria apply for 1.5 T:

- >4 standard deviations from the mean normal value: 5 points
- >3–4 standard deviations from the mean normal value: 4 points
- >2–3 standard deviations from the mean normal value: 3 points
- >1–2 standard deviations from the mean normal value: 2 points
- ≤1 standard deviations from the mean normal value: 1 point

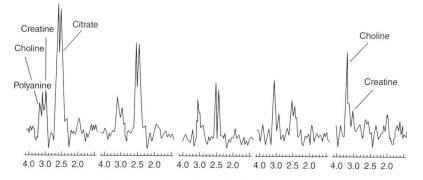

TABLE 1.   Choline + Creatine/Citrate Ratios for the Different Tissues in the Prostate on a 5-Point Scale

| Rating | Peripherul Zone | Central Gland |
|---|---|---|
| 1. Definitely benign tissue | ≤0.44 | ≤0.52 |
| 2. Probably benign tissue | 0.44–0.58 | 0.52–0.66 |
| 3. Possible malignant tissue | 0.58–0.72 | 0.66–0.80 |
| 4. Probably malignant tissue | 0.72–0.86 | 0.80–0.94 |
| 5. Definitely malignant tissue | >0.86 | >0.94 |

**Table 5.11** Pi-RADS scoring validation studies for different thresholds of total score

| ESUR-score | Sensitivity (%) | Specificity (%) | PPV (%) | NPV (%) |
|---|---|---|---|---|
| ≥9 (1514 cores) | 74 | 82 | 38 | 95 |
| ≥10 (47 lesions) | 94 | 43 | 49 | 93 |

**Table 5.12** Regional lymph nodes (N1) for prostate cancer and indicative short axis diameters in brackets, above which the node may be regarded as suspicious

| Regional = N1 | Nonregional = M1 |
|---|---|
| Perivisceral | Common iliac |
| Internal iliac (7 mm) | Para-aortic |
| Obturator (8 mm) | Inguinal |
| External iliac (10 mm) | |

The unanimous opinion of a UK expert group (recommendations in press, Clin Radiol) is that any report of a prostate should document the likelihood of a tumor measuring >0.2 cc or Gleason 3+4 or higher. Widely available image analysis software can, based on axial and coronal sequences, map out a lesion; the volume of any worrying lesion should be estimated, the recognised error rate notwithstanding [92], volume correlates well with histological grade [93].

### Timing and prebiopsy MRI

Hemorrhage is inevitable after biopsy and the blood products can influence the performance of the MRI [94]. The duration of effect is not known with certainty, but runs to months, especially on dynamic contrast-enhanced sequences. To avoid the deleterious effects of blood on the MR's accuracy, staging scans would have to be delayed by many weeks, which is not clinically justifiable, and runs in the face of strict national timelines from diagnosis to treatment. In such cases (scans <10 weeks after biopsy), the dynamically enhanced sequences are so degraded that they are likely to add little value, and a limited staging scan using the T1, T2, and diffusion-weighted parts of the protocol should be performed. However, a study dedicated to assess the impact of hemorrhage and delay after biopsy on prostate tumor detection highlighted a reduction of senstivity for tumor detection in sextants with hemorrhage on T2W; accuracy, sensitivity, and specificity were otherwise similar for sextants with and without extensive hemorrhage for all sessions. Postponement of MRI after biopsy of over 4 weeks did not improve accuracy [95].

### N stage
#### MRI and CT

Routine cross-sectional imaging, CT, and MRI have a disappointing performance in nodal assessment. The techniques rely heavily on the size of the lymph nodes visualized, but there is a wide crossover in morphology of lymph nodes that are benign and that are malignant. The sensitivity of nodal staging is no better than 60% and specificity is also underwhelming. A meta-analysis of 24 studies showed no difference between CT and MR in the detection of malignant lymph nodes from prostate cancer with pooled sensitivity ~40% and sensitivity ~80% [96].

The criteria for diagnosis of nodal metastases, and their limitations, are elegantly summarized by McMahon *et al.* [97]. The article refers to a study on healthy volunteers by Vinnicombe *et al.* [98], and using a cutoff of 6 mm for short-axis diameter corresponds to sensitivity 78%, specificity 97% for prostate cancer malignant node detection.

Evaluation may be refined by looking at the shape of individual nodes, spherical rather than ovoid nodes suggesting malignant involvement and on MRI particularly, the node contour and internal architecture (on T2-weighted images).

On a more positive note, nodal involvement is rare in patients with PSA <20 ng/mL and the pelvic nodes are involved first in the great majority. Therefore, acknowledging the limitations of cross-sectional imaging, MR of pelvic nodes is still advocated in selected cases [88]. The pelvic nodes are adequately imaged on the T2 coronal sequence of the pelvis, and large field of view T1 or T2 sequences are not necessary in routine practice if the PSA is <20. On the other hand, almost 2/5 of high-risk patients will have detectable lymph node involvement and this knowledge may influence planning radiotherapy fields, use of antiandrogen therapy, and helps in gauging prognosis [1, 99].

## Magnetic resonance lymphangiography

Ferromagnetic agents that are ingested by macrophages have shown promise in detecting micrometastases from prostate cancer in lymph nodes. The contrast agents consist of iron oxide nanoparticles suspended in colloid, and where they collect, their magnetic effect causes signal reduction on T2-weighted sequences. If the contrast collects in a lymph node, the node turns from high to low signal on T2 sequences. These agents may suggest involvement of nodes inside and outside the standard lymph node dissection area irrespective of size (i.e., <6–8 mm) [100, 101]. In a multicenter Dutch study looking at men with prostate cancer who had an intermediate or high risk (risk of >5% according to routinely used nomograms) of having lymph node metastases, MR lymphography (MRL) showed 82% sensitivity and 96% Negative predictive value (NPV), leading to the assertion that "after a negative MRL, the post-test probability of having lymph-node metastases is low enough to omit pelvic lymph node dissection" [102, 103]. Refinement of use of these agents, driven by difficulties with inconsistent diagnostic accuracy and interpretation, came by combining contrast use with diffusion-weighted MRI [104].

Unfortunately the agents are costly, inconvenient to use demanding pre- and post-contrast MR acquisitions 24 hours apart, and have notable side effects. Therefore, the manufacturers have withdrawn marketing authorization application more than 6 years ago, and currently there are no available suitable MR lymphangiographic contrast agents.

## M stage

Prostate cancer metastases have a proclivity for cortical bone, usually pelvis and lower spine as the first sites. Traditional technetium-based bone scintigraphy, recommended by European Association of Urology (2011), American Urology Association (2007), and the National Comprehensive Cancer Network Guidelines (2011), is now being supplemented or replaced by other nuclear medicine studies, and also by MRI. Recommendations for instigating a radionuclide bone scan are well established. Patients with PSA $\leq 20$ ng/mL and Gleason score $<8$ have a 1–13% rate of positive bone scans.

### Conventional bone scan

Technetium-based bone scintigraphy remains the mainstay for assessing skeletal involvement in prostate cancer, although specificity is low. Osteoblastic lesion detection can be improved by using combinations of nuclear medicine and CT techniques (single-photon emission computed tomography (SPECT)) [105]; SPECT–CT bone scan has sensitivity of ~90% and sensitivity of over 80%. Equally, plain radiographs and more recently CT or MRI directed to suspicious/indeterminate "hot spots" on bone scans can increase specificity of bone imaging.

Conventional positron emission tomography–computed tomography (PET-CT) using fludeoxyglucose (18F) ($^{18}$F-FDG) has been disappointing, with overall poor sensitivity, and inaccuracy because of the "noise" from the tracer in urine in the ureters and bladder. Moreover, FDG signal in sclerotic metastases of prostate cancer seems to be obscured by the bone reaction. Another tracer under scrutiny is $^{18}$F-sodium fluoride: specificity of the tracer is low but this limitation may be overcome by using PET-CT, the CT imaging helping to distinguish benign from malignant foci of tracer uptake. $^{18}$F-sodium fluoride PET-CT is more accurate than bone scintigraphy but at a considerable cost.

## MRI

In a comparison of spinal MRI to bone scintigraphy for several cancer types, MR outperformed bone scintigraphy and MR imaging added value in planning treatment such as radiation therapy or systemic chemotherapy [4]. The superiority of MRI over scintigraphy in detecting bone lesions in prostate cancer is even more apparent (MRI: sensitivity 100% and specificity 80%, scintigraphy + conventional plain films: sensitivity 63% and specificity 64%) [106].

Even if nuclear medicine proponents refute the findings and insist whole-body MRI and radionuclide bone scintigraphy have similar specificity and sensitivity [107, 108], MRI has the advantage of cost, convenience (a single combined test rather than two), and avoidance of radiation. Whole-body diffusion-weighted MRI (WB-DWI) has the added advantage of imaging the soft tissues as well as cortical bone, WB-DWI is better at detecting bone metastases than combined scintigraphy and dedicated plain radiography, and can match CT in assessing N stage [109].

The attraction of combined N and M stages (single acquisition) is obvious and MRI limited to the pelvis (T, N, and M staging with additional axial T1W sequence) and axial skeleton (M staging) is a realistic single 45-minute complete staging investigation. Visualization of the pelvic and axial skeleton is sufficient, as isolated metastases in the nonaxial skeleton is a very rare situation and the cost-effectiveness of bone scintigraphy for examination of the *entire* skeleton becomes irrelevant [110]. When available, there is a cogent argument to use WB-DWI as a single investigation in high-risk prostate cancer at presentation or in men post-treatment with a PSA doubling time <12 months [111] (Figure 5.11).

## Choline-based nuclear medicine studies in staging

The choline molecule is phosphorylated with great avidity by malignant prostate cancer cells and transported to the outer membrane; as a result choline is abundant on the surface of prostate cancers. Radionuclide choline tracers are therefore a logical tool to use in tumor detection, and may detect bone and nodal disease in a single examination.

Choline may be labeled with $^{11}C$ or $^{18}F$; the radiopharmaceuticals have sensitivity of over 90% for detection of cancer cells, but low specificity with overlap in benign hyperplasia. Conversely, for lymph node involvement, sensitivity is poor but specificity is high; in other words, the labels have a high PPV for the N stage. PET-CT using choline is more accurate than standard MRI for lymph node evaluation. Some advocate fluoride–choline PET-CT for the evaluation of patients with prostate

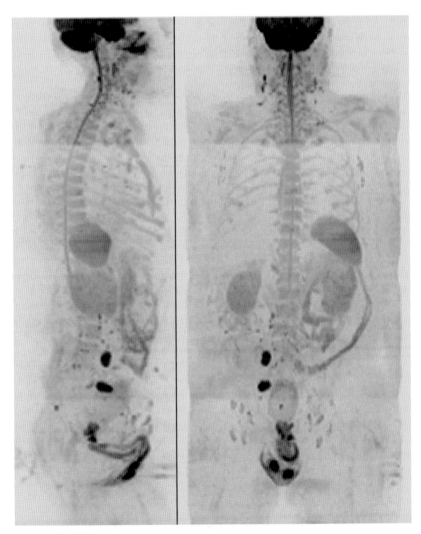

**Figure 5.11** Whole-body diffusion-weighted scan b900 69 M. Prostate cancer treated with external beam radiotherapy, RT. Rising PSA. Note atrophy of pelvic bone marrow due to RT. Nodal metastases in right hypogastric and common iliac nodes. Presacral node also. Note persistent active disease in treated prostate gland. Images provided courtesy of Prof. Anwar Padhani, Paul Strickland Scanner Centre, Mount Vernon Cancer Centre, London.

cancer who are at high risk for extracapsular disease, and it could be used to preoperatively exclude distant metastases—especially in aggressive disease associated with bone destruction as uptake is higher with lytic (destructive) deposits than with sclerotic deposits [112]. Nevertheless the technique is expensive, and, in practice, limited to centers with on-site cyclotron to manufacture the tracer. In any case, DWI appears to be as effective as $^{11}$C–choline PET/CT in the detection of bone metastases [113]. In short, choline–PET/CT and whole-body MRI are both highly accurate in the detection of bone and lymph node metastases: "the strength of MRI is excellent image quality providing detailed anatomical information whereas the advantage of Choline-PET/CT is high image contrast of pathological foci" [114]. Early results are promising, with increasing interest in $^{18}$F–choline for lesion detection [115].

## Modifying treatment by image-derived stage (over clinical stage)

Following diagnosis of prostate cancer, treatment choice is usually determined by a complex process involving patient and a multidisciplinary team dedicated to prostate cancer care, and much of the decision making up to now has been influenced by D'Amico risk groups. Table 5.13 As imaging, effectively mpMRI and some of the new radionuclide tests, become more accepted, imaging is replacing clinically based D'Amico assessment as the key determinant for selecting best treatment option.

### Imaging in men planned for active surveillance

Performing mpMRI (if not already done) at 4 months after enrolment in AS may help ensure that there has not been undergrading of histology of the index lesion, volume of the index lesion, or undersampling of cancer elsewhere in the gland. Delaying the examination by 4 months means that the postbiopsy effect is minimized [116]. In the future, mpMRI may contribute to follow-up. For example, a repeat of mpMRI at 18 months

**Table 5.13** D'Amico risk groups

D'Amico and the risk groups
Low-risk – PSA < 10 ng/mL and biopsy Gleason score ≤6 and clinical stage T1-T2a
Intermediate-risk – PSA 10.1–20 ng/mL, or biopsy Gleason score 7, or clinical stage T2b
High-risk – PSA ≥20 ng/mL, or Gleason score 8–10, or clinical stage T2c or T3 or T4.

allows comparison with the study suggested for 4 months: if there is no change, repeat (protocol-driven) biopsy may be avoided.

### The index lesion—confirming (low) volume and (low) aggressiveness

As stated, ADC value on preoperative DW MRI correlates with final Gleason grade tumor such that tumors with more than 20% of high Gleason grades can be predicted by measurement of the ADC value. In 388 men with clinically low-risk prostate cancer, who underwent endorectal MRI before confirmatory biopsy, MRI was highly sensitive for upgrading on confirmatory biopsy. mpMRI in AS may help detect lesions that have been undergraded by TRUS biopsy core, helping decide who needs rebiopsy, who can continue on AS, and who should consider early radical intervention rather than AS [117].

### Identifying other sites of disease

MpMRI offers improved detection of cancer, especially anterior and apical cancers, over TRUS diagnosis, which may lead to upgrading of patient risk suggested by TRUS biopsy alone, and move patients away from AS toward earlier active intervention. Based on D'Amico low-risk men undergoing prostatectomy, in whom TRUS suggested unilateral cancer but whole-specimen pathology showed bilateral tumor in one-third, preoperative mpMRI predicted bilateral tumors in 80% of these cases [118] (Figure 5.12).

The current thinking that many such low-grade cancers are overtreated may wane as focal therapies improve and iatrogenic complications of cancer removal decrease, so that even small Gleason 6 tumors will be targeted. There is of course an economic aspect to this as much as a medical one [119, 120].

### Imaging in men planned for surgery
#### Modified approach

Recent shift in surgical practice has meant that T3 disease is now considered operable in some men. The T stage battleground has altered; preoperative mpMRI may identify early T3a disease still amenable to surgical cure, but inform the surgeon of the need for wider margins. An abnormality near the neurovascular bundle may not preclude surgery but does mean a nerve-sparing approach would be ill advised; the patient is then able to make a more informed choice about treatment options. Note, T2-weighted imaging with a pelvic phased array coil, even when combined with biopsy findings, is not sufficiently accurate and the benefits come with addition of functional sequences [121–124].

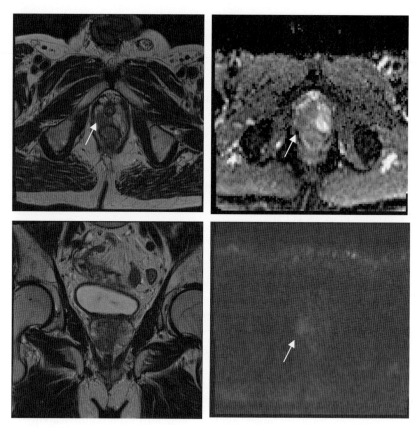

**Figure 5.12**  64-year-old starting active surveillance. Entry PSA 8.6 ng/ml, TRUS biopsy sinage 4 mm core Gleason 6 cancer focus, LMZ biopsy. (a) Axial T2W MRI pelvis and (b) ADC map, (c) coronal T2, and (d) axial DWI with b = 1400. Right apical cancer that has characteristics of Gleason 7+ disease, confirmed on repeat biopsy (arrows).

## Imaging in men planned for DXT

In a similar manner, if mpMRI suggests extensive T3 disease or nodal disease, the radiotherapy field may be better planned and the dose modulated.

## Follow-up of known cancer under treatment

### Active surveillance—see above
### Follow-up after radical therapy (biochemical recurrence)

A sustained rise, post-treatment, in serum PSA level indicates a biochemical recurrence; however, only one-third of these patients will go on to a clinical (symptomatic) recurrence [125]. The primary role of imaging in follow-up is to identify those with nodal or metastatic disease rather than local recurrence. DWI and DCE sequences can detect recurrent disease, but the sensitivity of mpMRI at values PSA <0.2 ng/mL (the biochemical definition of recurrence and the level at which palliation is considered) is not good enough to date.

Choline- and acetate-based PET-CT show promise in identifying local recurrence and regional lymph node involvement after radical therapy, although the studies are expensive and site limited. Bone scanning has been addressed already, and the sodium fluoride nuclear medicine techniques or WB-DWI are likely to dominate in the near future.

## Focal therapies [126, 127]

Akin to breast "lumpectomy" there is a great attraction to treat prostate cancer by focal, lesion-directed ablation with organ preservation. However, there are two obvious barriers: the multifocal nature of prostate cancer and poor visualization of focal lesions. As PSA screening becomes more widespread, men are presenting earlier and the expectation is that the proportion of isolated tumors will rise. Recent pathology literature indicates, however, that up to 25% of prostate cancers are solitary and unilateral [128]. mpMRI and the choline-based radionuclide examinations promise to improve localization of cancers, and fusion of mpMRI and US mean that needles to deliver thermal energy may be placed within the cancer [129].

Onik *et al.* report experience of cryotherapy, concluding a "male lumpectomy" in which the prostate tumor region itself is destroyed, appears to preserve potency in a majority of patients and limits other complications (particularly incontinence), without compromising cancer control [128]. Other techniques under consideration include photodynamic laser ablation [130], high-intensity focused ultrasound (HIFU), and radiofrequency ablation, reviewed following a consensus summary in 2007 [131]. More recently, the benefit of functional sequences as part of mpMRI in the follow-up of men looking for local recurrence after cryotherapy or HIFU has been described [132].

## Prediction—prostate paradigm

Many aspects of prostate cancer—diagnosis and treatment and screening—have come to a crucial point, like a critical astrological event with the aligning of planets. With the promise of a dramatic and widespread change in patient care, it seems opportune to make some predictions:

Multiparametric MRI will become dominant in diagnosis, preferably before biopsy [133]. Need for biopsy; currently an mpMRI examination that does not detect significant tumour has a negative predictive value at least as good as 12 core TRUS biopsy for clinically important prostate cancer. Multiparametric MRI, which will comprise T2-weighted imaging and DWI in all and dynamic contrast sequences in many, will generate a probability map identifying likelihood of significant tumor in specific region of the prostate (probably 16-sextant model). Reporting will be by specialists involved with urology cancer multidisciplinary teams who have the opportunity to view and discuss and receive feedback on at least 50 cases per year.

1 MRI when detecting lesions will focus on most aggressive, and capitalize on functional sequences that select more significant disease, that is, higher Gleason grade, larger, or extracapsular disease. A modified form of Pi-RADS, with an overall probability 1–5 derived from the different sequences, will be validated. Biopsy will be targeted using MRI–US fusion, or, less commonly, MR-guided biopsy. Transperineal approach will take over from TRUS approach but both will be used—TRUS if obvious peripheral focus, transperineal biopsy for anterior or central disease. Most biopsies will be directed to focal lesions and performed under local anesthesia as an outpatient procedure. Extended/template approach may be limited to indeterminate MRI or where clinical concern remains despite ostensibly normal mpMRI.

2 In AS, MRI will be used at 3–6 months (assuming no prebiopsy MRI) to ensure that biopsy has not underestimated extent, grade, or volume of cancer, and there will be another mpMRI at 18 months, avoiding need for biopsy if imaging and PSA values are stable.

3 In staging, T3a and even T3b stage will not be synonymous with inoperability, placing onus on MRI to improve accuracy in subdividing extracapsular disease into likely "margin positive" or "margin negative."

4 Focal therapy and its utter reliance on lesion detection by imaging will become standard practice, in line with nephron-sparing and breast-sparing treatments.

## References

1  Kelloff GJ, Choyke P, Coffey DS. Challenges in clinical prostate cancer: role of imaging. *AJR Am J Roentgenol* 2009;192(6):1455–1470.

2  Harvey CJ, Pilcher J, Richenberg J, *et al.* Applications of transrectal ultrasound in prostate cancer. *Br J Radiol* 2012;85(Spec No 1):S3–S17.

3  Turner BA, Aslet P, Drudge-Coates L, Forristal H, Gruschy L, Hieronymi S, Mowle K, Pietrasik M, Vis A. *Transrectal Ultrasound Guided Biopsy of the Prostate.* European Association of Urology Nurses; 2011. Available at http://www.uroweb. org/fileadmin/EAUN/guidelines/EAUN_TRUS_Guidelines_EN_2011_LR.pdf.    Last accessed September 14, 2013.

4  Chiewvit P, Danchaivijitr N, Sirivitmaitrie K, *et al.* Does magnetic resonance imaging give value-added than bone scintigraphy in the detection of vertebral metastasis? *J Med Assoc Thai* 2009;92(6):818–829.

5  Draisma G, Boer R, Otto SJ, *et al.* Lead times and overdetection due to prostate-specific antigen screening: estimates from the European Randomized Study of Screening for Prostate Cancer. *J Natl Cancer Inst* 2003;95(12):868–878.

6  Roehl KA, Antenor JA, Catalona WJ. Serial biopsy results in prostate cancer screening study. *J Urol* 2002;167(6):2435–2439.

7  Pepe P, Aragona F. Saturation prostate needle biopsy and prostate cancer detection at initial and repeat evaluation. *Urology* 2007;70(6):1131–1135.

8  Lujan M, Paez A, Santonja C, *et al.* Prostate cancer detection and tumor characteristics in men with multiple biopsy sessions. *Prostate Cancer Prostatic Dis* 2004;7(3):238–242.

9  Mian BM, Naya Y, Okihara K, *et al.* Predictors of cancer in repeat extended multisite prostate biopsy in men with previous negative extended multisite biopsy. *Urology* 2002;60(5):836–840.

10  Djavan B, Milani S, Remzi M. Prostate biopsy: who, how and when. An update. *Can J Urol* 2005;12(Suppl. 1):44–48.

11  Ouzzane A, Puech P, Lemaitre L, *et al.* Combined multiparametric MRI and targeted biopsies improve anterior prostate cancer detection, staging, and grading. *Urology* 2011;78(6):1356–1362.

12  Rajinikanth A, Manoharan M, Soloway CT, *et al.* Trends in Gleason score: concordance between biopsy and prostatectomy over 15 years. *Urology* 2008;72(1):177–182.

13  Kvale R, Moller B, Wahlqvist R, *et al.* Concordance between Gleason scores of needle biopsies and radical prostatectomy specimens: a population-based study. *BJU Int* 2009;103(12):1647–1654.

14  Turgut AT, Olcucuoglu E, Kosar P, *et al.* Power Doppler ultrasonography of the feeding arteries of the prostate gland: a novel approach to the diagnosis of prostate cancer? *J Ultrasound Med* 2007;26(7):875–883.

15  Turgut AD. Prostatic cancer: evaluation using transrectal sonography. In: *Methods of Cancer Diagnosis, Therapy and Prognosis,* 1st edn (ed. M Hayat). New York: Elsevier; 2008. pp 499–520.

16  Halpern EJ, Strup SE. Using gray-scale and color and power Doppler sonography to detect prostatic cancer. *AJR Am J Roentgenol* 2000;174(3):623–627.

17  Pallwein L, Mitterberger M, Pelzer A, *et al.* Ultrasound of prostate cancer: recent advances. *Eur Radiol* 2008;18(4):707–715.

18  Bigler SA, Deering RE, Brawer MK. Comparison of microscopic vascularity in benign and malignant prostate tissue. *Hum Pathol* 1993;24(2):220–226.

19  Cosgrove D, Eckersley R, Blomley M, Harvey C. Quantification of blood flow. *Eur Radiol* 2001;11(8):1338–1344.

20  Leen E, Averkiou M, Arditi M, *et al.* Dynamic contrast enhanced ultrasound assessment of the vascular effects of novel therapeutics in early stage trials. *Eur Radiol* 2012;22(7):1442–1450.

21  Halpern EJ, Rosenberg M, Gomella LG. Prostate cancer: contrast-enhanced us for detection. *Radiology* 2001;219(1):219–225.

22  Halpern EJ, Frauscher F, Rosenberg M, Gomella LG. Directed biopsy during contrast-enhanced sonography of the prostate. *AJR Am J Roentgenol* 2002;178(4): 915–919.

23  Mitterberger M, Pinggera GM, Horninger W, *et al.* Comparison of contrast enhanced color Doppler targeted biopsy to conventional systematic biopsy: impact on Gleason score. *J Urol* 2007;178(2):464–468.

24  Mitterberger MJ, Aigner F, Horninger W, *et al.* Comparative efficiency of contrast-enhanced colour Doppler ultrasound targeted versus systematic biopsy for prostate cancer detection. *Eur Radiol* 2010;20(12):2791–2796.

25  Wink M, Frauscher F, Cosgrove D, *et al.* Contrast-enhanced ultrasound and prostate cancer; a multicentre European research coordination project. *EurUrol* 2008;54(5):982–992.

26  Strazdina A, Krumina G, Sperga M. The value and limitations of contrast-enhanced ultrasound in detection of prostate cancer. *Anticancer Res* 2011;31(4):1421–1426.

27  Piscaglia F, Nolsoe C, Dietrich CF, *et al.* The EFSUMB guidelines and recommendations on the clinical practice of contrast enhanced ultrasound (CEUS): update 2011 on non-hepatic applications. *Ultraschall Med* 2012;33(1):33–59.

28  Pallwein L, Mitterberger M, Struve P, *et al.* Comparison of sonoelastography guided biopsy with systematic biopsy: impact on prostate cancer detection. *Eur Radiol* 2007;17(9):2278–2285.

29  Aigner F, Pallwein L, Junker D, *et al.* Value of real-time elastography targeted biopsy for prostate cancer detection in men with prostate specific antigen 1.25 ng/ml or greater and 4.00 ng/ml or less. *J Urol* 2010;184(3):913–917.

30  Heidenreich A, Bastian PJ, Bellmunt J, Bolla M, Joniau S, Mason MD, Matveev V, Mottet N, van der Kwast TH, Wiegel T, Zattoni F. *Guidelines on Prostate Cancer*. European Association of Urology; 2012. Available at http://www.uroweb.org/gls/pdf/ 08%20Prostate%20Cancer_LR%20March%2013th%202012.pdf. Last accessed September 14, 2013.

31  Guichard G, Larre S, Gallina A, *et al.* Extended 21-sample needle biopsy protocol for diagnosis of prostate cancer in 1000 consecutive patients. *Eur Urol* 2007;52(2):430–435.

32  Scattoni V, Raber M, Abdollah F, *et al.* Biopsy schemes with the fewest cores for detecting 95% of the prostate cancers detected by a 24-core biopsy. *Eur Urol* 2010;57(1):1–8.

33  Kim B, Breau RH, Papadatos D, *et al.* Diagnostic accuracy of surface coil magnetic resonance imaging at 1.5 T for local staging of elevated risk prostate cancer. *Can Urol Assoc J* 2010;4(4):257–262.

34  Takenaka A, Hara R, Ishimura T, *et al.* A prospective randomized comparison of diagnostic efficacy between transperineal and transrectal 12-core prostate biopsy. *Prostate Cancer Prostatic Dis* 2008;11(2):134–138.

35  Hara R, Jo Y, Fujii T, *et al.* Optimal approach for prostate cancer detection as initial biopsy: prospective randomized study comparing transperineal versus transrectal systematic 12-core biopsy. *Urology* 2008;71(2):191–195.

36 Dickinson L, Ahmed HU, Allen C, *et al.* Magnetic resonance imaging for the detection, localisation, and characterisation of prostate cancer: recommendations from a European consensus meeting. *Eur Urol* 2011;59(4):477–494.

37 Kobus T, Hambrock T, Hulsbergen-van de Kaa CA, *et al.* In vivo assessment of prostate cancer aggressiveness using magnetic resonance spectroscopic imaging at 3 T with an endorectal coil. *Eur Urol* 2011;60(5):1074–1080.

38 Nagarajan R, Margolis D, Raman S, *et al.* MR spectroscopic imaging and diffusion-weighted imaging of prostate cancer with Gleason scores. *J Magn Reson Imaging* 2012;36(3):697–703.

39 Mazaheri Y, Shukla-Dave A, Hricak H, *et al.* Prostate cancer: identification with combined diffusion-weighted MR imaging and 3D 1H MR spectroscopic imaging–correlation with pathologic findings. *Radiology* 2008;246(2):480–488.

40 Wang L, Mazaheri Y, Zhang J, *et al.* Assessment of biologic aggressiveness of prostate cancer: correlation of MR signal intensity with Gleason grade after radical prostatectomy. *Radiology* 2008;246(1):168–176.

41 Turkbey B, Shah VP, Pang Y, *et al.* Is apparent diffusion coefficient associated with clinical risk scores for prostate cancers that are visible on 3-T MR images? *Radiology* 2011;258(2):488–495.

42 Verma S, Rajesh A, Morales H, *et al.* Assessment of aggressiveness of prostate cancer: correlation of apparent diffusion coefficient with histologic grade after radical prostatectomy. *AJR Am J Roentgenol* 2011;196(2):374–381.

43 Hambrock T, Hoeks C, Hulsbergen-van de Kaa C, *et al.* Prospective assessment of prostate cancer aggressiveness using 3-T diffusion-weighted magnetic resonance imaging-guided biopsies versus a systematic 10-core transrectal ultrasound prostate biopsy cohort. *Eur Urol* 2012;61(1):177–184.

44 Yamamura J, Salomon G, Buchert R, *et al.* MR Imaging of Prostate Cancer: Diffusion Weighted Imaging and (3D) Hydrogen 1 (H) MR Spectroscopy in Comparison with Histology. *Radiol Res Pract* 2011;2011:616852.

45 Park BK, Lee HM, Kim CK, *et al.* Lesion localization in patients with a previous negative transrectal ultrasound biopsy and persistently elevated prostate specific antigen level using diffusion-weighted imaging at three Tesla before rebiopsy. *Invest Radiol* 2008;43(11):789–793.

46 Iwazawa J, Mitani T, Sassa S, Ohue S. Prostate cancer detection with MRI: is dynamic contrast-enhanced imaging necessary in addition to diffusion-weighted imaging? *Diagn Interv Radiol* 2010;17:243–248.

47 Isebaert S, Van den Bergh L, Haustermans K, *et al.* Multiparametric MRI for prostate cancer localization in correlation to whole-mount histopathology. *J Magn Reson Imaging* 2012;37:1392–1401.

48 Turkbey B, Choyke PL. Multiparametric MRI and prostate cancer diagnosis and risk stratification. *Curr Opin Urol* 2012;22(4):310–315.

49 Kasivisvanathan V, Dufour R, Moore CM, *et al.* Transperineal magnetic resonance image targeted prostate biopsy versus transperineal template prostate biopsy in the detection of clinically significant prostate cancer. *J Urol* 2013;189(3):860–866.

50 Belas O, Klap J, Cornud F, *et al.* Prebiopsy multiparametric MRI of the prostate: the end of randomized biopsies?. *Prog Urol* 2012;22(10):583–589.

51 Rosenkrantz AB, Mussi TC, Borofsky MS, *et al.* 3.0 T multiparametric prostate MRI using pelvic phased-array coil: utility for tumor detection prior to biopsy.

*Urol Oncol* 2012. Available at http://www.urologiconcology.org/article/S1078-1439(12)00081-6/abstract. Last accessed September 14, 2013.

52 Rouse P, Shaw G, Ahmed HU, *et al.* Multi-parametric magnetic resonance imaging to rule-in and rule-out clinically important prostate cancer in men at risk: a cohort study. *Urol Int* 2011;87(1):49–53.

53 Goris Gbenou MC, Peltier A, Addla SK, *et al.* Localising prostate cancer: comparison of endorectal magnetic resonance (MR) imaging and 3D-MR spectroscopic imaging with transrectal ultrasound-guided biopsy. *Urol Int* 2012;88(1):12–17.

54 Hoeks CM, Schouten MG, Bomers JG, *et al.* Three-Tesla magnetic resonance-guided prostate biopsy in men with increased prostate-specific antigen and repeated, negative, random, systematic, transrectal ultrasound biopsies: detection of clinically significant prostate cancers. *Eur Urol* 2012;62(5):902–909.

55 Hambrock T, Somford DM, Hoeks C, *et al.* Magnetic resonance imaging guided prostate biopsy in men with repeat negative biopsies and increased prostate specific antigen. *J Urol* 2010;183(2):520–527.

56 Engelhard K, Hollenbach HP, Kiefer B, *et al.* Prostate biopsy in the supine position in a standard 1.5-T scanner under real time MR-imaging control using a MR-compatible endorectal biopsy device. *Eur Radiol* 2006;16(6):1237–1243.

57 Franiel T, Stephan C, Erbersdobler A, *et al.* Areas suspicious for prostate cancer: MR-guided biopsy in patients with at least one transrectal US-guided biopsy with a negative finding–multiparametric MR imaging for detection and biopsy planning. *Radiology* 2011;259(1):162–172.

58 Lee SH, Chung MS, Kim JH. Magnetic resonance imaging targeted biopsy in men with previously negative prostate biopsy results. *J Endourol* 2012;26(7):787–791.

59 Wu LM, Xu JR, Ye YQ, *et al.* The clinical value of diffusion-weighted imaging in combination with T2-weighted imaging in diagnosing prostate carcinoma: a systematic review and meta-analysis. *AJR Am J Roentgenol* 2012;199(1):103–110.

60 Haffner J, Lemaitre L, Puech P, *et al.* Role of magnetic resonance imaging before initial biopsy: comparison of magnetic resonance imaging-targeted and systematic biopsy for significant prostate cancer detection. *BJU Int* 2011;108(8 Pt 2):E171–E178.

61 Oto A, Yang C, Kayhan A, *et al.* Diffusion-weighted and dynamic contrast-enhanced MRI of prostate cancer: correlation of quantitative MR parameters with Gleason score and tumor angiogenesis. *AJR Am J Roentgenol* 2011;197(6):1382–1390.

62 Rosenkrantz AB, Deng FM, Kim S, *et al.* Prostate cancer: multiparametric MRI for index lesion localization–a multiple-reader study. *AJR Am J Roentgenol* 2012;199(4):830–837.

63 Arsov C, Quentin M, Rabenalt R, *et al.* Repeat transrectal ultrasound biopsies with additional targeted cores according to results of functional prostate MRI detects high-risk prostate cancer in patients with previous negative biopsy and increased PSA – a pilot study. *Anticancer Res* 2012;32(3):1087–1092.

64 Shigemura K, Motoyama S, Yamashita M. Do additional cores from MRI cancer-suspicious lesions to systematic 12-core transrectal prostate biopsy give better cancer detection? *Urol Int* 2012;88(2):145–149.

65 Roethke M, Anastasiadis AG, Lichy M, *et al.* MRI-guided prostate biopsy detects clinically significant cancer: analysis of a cohort of 100 patients after previous negative TRUS biopsy. *World J Urol* 2012;30(2):213–218.

66  Marks L, Young S, Natarajan S. MRI-ultrasound fusion for guidance of targeted prostate biopsy. *Curr Opin Urol* 2013;23(1):43–50.

67  Hadaschik BA, Kuru TH, Tulea C, *et al.* A novel stereotactic prostate biopsy system integrating pre-interventional magnetic resonance imaging and live ultrasound fusion. *J Urol* 2011;186(6):2214–2220.

68  Vourganti S, Rastinehad A, Yerram NK, *et al.* Multiparametric magnetic resonance imaging and ultrasound fusion biopsy detect prostate cancer in patients with prior negative transrectal ultrasound biopsies. *J Urol* 2012;188(6):2152–2157.

69  Durmus T, Stephan C, Grigoryev M, *et al.* Detection of prostate cancer by real-time MR/ultrasound fusion-guided biopsy: 3T MRI and state of the art sonography. *RoFo* 2013;185:428–433.

70  Rud E, Baco E, Eggesbo HB. MRI and ultrasound-guided prostate biopsy using soft image fusion. *Anticancer Res* 2012;32(8):3383–3389.

71  Moore CM, Robertson NL, Arsanious N, *et al.* Image-guided prostate biopsy using magnetic resonance imaging-derived targets: a systematic review. *Eur Urol* 2013;63(1):125–140.

72  Ward JF, Slezak JM, Blute ML, *et al.* Radical prostatectomy for clinically advanced (cT3) prostate cancer since the advent of prostate-specific antigen testing: 15-year outcome. *BJU Int* 2005;95(6):751–756.

73  Mullerad M, Hricak H, Kuroiwa K, *et al.* Comparison of endorectal magnetic resonance imaging, guided prostate biopsy and digital rectal examination in the preoperative anatomical localization of prostate cancer. *J Urol* 2005;174(6):2158–2163.

74  Patel U. The prostate and seminal vesicles. In: *Clinical Ultrasound*, 3rd edn (eds P Allan, G Baxter, M Weston). Edinburgh: Churchill-Livingsone Elsevier; 2011 pp 572–592.

75  Wang L, Hricak H, Kattan MW, *et al.* Prediction of organ-confined prostate cancer: incremental value of MR imaging and MR spectroscopic imaging to staging nomograms. *Radiology* 2006;238(2):597–603.

76  Augustin H, Fritz GA, Ehammer T, *et al.* Accuracy of 3-Tesla magnetic resonance imaging for the staging of prostate cancer in comparison to the Partin tables. *Acta Radiol* 2009;50(5):562–569.

77  Heijmink SW, Futterer JJ, Hambrock T, *et al.* Prostate cancer: body-array versus endorectal coil MR imaging at 3 T–comparison of image quality, localization, and staging performance. *Radiology* 2007;244(1):184–195.

78  Beyersdorff D, Taymoorian K, Knosel T, *et al.* MRI of prostate cancer at 1.5 and 3.0 T: comparison of image quality in tumor detection and staging. *AJR Am J Roentgenol* 2005;185(5):1214–1220.

79  Cornud F, Rouanne M, Beuvon F, *et al.* Endorectal 3D T2-weighted 1mm-slice thickness MRI for prostate cancer staging at 1.5Tesla: should we reconsider the indirects signs of extracapsular extension according to the D'Amico tumor risk criteria? *Eur J Radiol* 2012;81(4):e591–e597.

80  Wang L, Zhang J, Schwartz LH, *et al.* Incremental value of multiplanar cross-referencing for prostate cancer staging with endorectal MRI. *AJR Am J Roentgenol* 2007;188(1):99–104.

81  Futterer JJ, Engelbrecht MR, Jager GJ, *et al.* Prostate cancer: comparison of local staging accuracy of pelvic phased-array coil alone versus integrated

endorectal-pelvic phased-array coils. Local staging accuracy of prostate cancer using endorectal coil MR imaging. *Eur Radiol* 2007;17(4):1055–1065.

82  Zhang J, Hricak H, Shukla-Dave A, *et al.* Clinical stage T1c prostate cancer: evaluation with endorectal MR imaging and MR spectroscopic imaging. *Radiology* 2009;253(2):425–434.

83  Renard-Penna R, Rouprot M, Comperat E, *et al.* Accuracy of high resolution (1.5 tesla) pelvic phased array magnetic resonance imaging (MRI) in staging prostate cancer in candidates for radical prostatectomy: Results from a prospective study. *Urol Oncol* 2013;31(4):448–454.

84  Wang L, Hricak H, Kattan MW, *et al.* Prediction of seminal vesicle invasion in prostate cancer: incremental value of adding endorectal MR imaging to the Kattan nomogram. *Radiology* 2007;242(1):182–188.

85  Ruprecht O, Weisser P, Bodelle B, *et al.* MRI of the prostate: interobserver agreement compared with histopathologic outcome after radical prostatectomy. *Eur J Radiol* 2012;81(3):456–460.

86  Spahn M, Briganti A, Capitanio U, *et al.* Outcome predictors of radical prostatectomy followed by adjuvant androgen deprivation in patients with clinical high risk prostate cancer and pT3 surgical margin positive disease. *J Urol* 2012;188(1):84–90.

87  Jager GJ, Severens JL, Thornbury JR, *et al.* Prostate cancer staging: should MR imaging be used?–A decision analytic approach. *Radiology* 2000;215(2):445–451.

88  Barentsz JO, Richenberg J, Clements R, *et al.* ESUR prostate MR guidelines 2012. *Eur Radiol* 2012;22(4):746–757.

89  Portalez D, Mozer P, Cornud F, *et al.* Validation of the European Society of Urogenital Radiology scoring system for prostate cancer diagnosis on multiparametric magnetic resonance imaging in a cohort of repeat biopsy patients. *Eur Urol* 2012;62(6):986–996.

90  Arsov C, Blondin D, Rabenalt R, *et al.* Standardised scoring of a multi-parametric 3-T MRI for a targeted MRI-guided prostate biopsy. *Urologe A* 2012;51(6):848–856.

91  Dickinson L, Ahmed HU, Allen C, *et al.* Scoring systems used for the interpretation and reporting of multiparametric MRI for prostate cancer detection, localization, and characterization: could standardization lead to improved utilization of imaging within the diagnostic pathway? *J Magn Reson Imaging* 2013;37(1):48–58.

92  Bastian PJ, Carter BH, Bjartell A, *et al.* Insignificant prostate cancer and active surveillance: from definition to clinical implications. *Eur Urol* 2009;55(6):1321–1330.

93  Song SY, Kim SR, Ahn G, Choi HY. Pathologic characteristics of prostatic adenocarcinomas: a mapping analysis of Korean patients. *Prostate Cancer Prostatic Dis* 2003;6(2):143–147.

94  Tamada T, Sone T, Jo Y, *et al.* Prostate cancer: relationships between postbiopsy hemorrhage and tumor detectability at MR diagnosis. *Radiology* 2008;248(2):531–539.

95  Rosenkrantz AB, Mussi TC, Hindman N, *et al.* Impact of delay after biopsy and postbiopsy haemorrhage on prostate cancer tumour detection using multi-parametric MRI: a multi-reader study. *Clin Radiol* 2012;67(12):e83–e90.

96  Hovels AM, Heesakkers RA, Adang EM, *et al.* The diagnostic accuracy of CT and MRI in the staging of pelvic lymph nodes in patients with prostate cancer: a meta-analysis. *Clin Radiol* 2008;63(4):387–395.

97  McMahon CJ, Rofsky NM, Pedrosa I. Lymphatic metastases from pelvic tumors: anatomic classification, characterization, and staging. *Radiology* 2010;254(1): 31–46.

98  Vinnicombe SJ, Norman AR, Nicolson V, Husband JE. Normal pelvic lymph nodes: evaluation with CT after bipedal lymphangiography. *Radiology* 1995;194(2):349–355.

99  Swanson GP, Thompson IM, Basler J. Current status of lymph node-positive prostate cancer: incidence and predictors of outcome. *Cancer* 2006;107(3):439–450.

100 Bellin MF, Roy C. Magnetic resonance lymphography. *Curr Opin Urol* 2007; 17(1):65–69.

101 Heesakkers RA, Jager GJ, Hovels AM, *et al.* Prostate cancer: detection of lymph node metastases outside the routine surgical area with ferumoxtran-10-enhanced MR imaging. *Radiology* 2009;251(2):408–414.

102 Heesakkers RA, Hovels AM, Jager GJ, *et al.* MRI with a lymph-node-specific contrast agent as an alternative to CT scan and lymph-node dissection in patients with prostate cancer: a prospective multicohort study. *Lancet Oncol* 2008;9(9):850–856.

103 Barentsz JO, Futterer JJ, Takahashi S. Use of ultrasmall superparamagnetic iron oxide in lymph node MR imaging in prostate cancer patients. *Eur J Radiol* 2007;63(3):369–372.

104 Thoeny HC, Triantafyllou M, Birkhaeuser FD, *et al.* Combined ultrasmall superparamagnetic particles of iron oxide-enhanced and diffusion-weighted magnetic resonance imaging reliably detect pelvic lymph node metastases in normal-sized nodes of bladder and prostate cancer patients. *Eur Urol* 2009;55(4):761–769.

105 Lee Z, Sodee DB, Resnick M, Maclennan GT. Multimodal and three-dimensional imaging of prostate cancer. Computerized medical imaging and graphics : the official *journal of the Computerized Medical Imaging Society* 2005;29(6):477–486.

106 Ketelsen D, Rothke M, Aschoff P, *et al.* Detection of bone metastasis of prostate cancer – comparison of whole-body MRI and bone scintigraphy. *RoFo* 2008;180(8):746–752.

107 Venkitaraman R, Cook GJ, Dearnaley DP, *et al.* Whole-body magnetic resonance imaging in the detection of skeletal metastases in patients with prostate cancer. *J Med Imaging Radiat Oncol* 2009;53(3):241–247.

108 Gutzeit A, Doert A, Froehlich JM, *et al.* Comparison of diffusion-weighted whole body MRI and skeletal scintigraphy for the detection of bone metastases in patients with prostate or breast carcinoma. *Skeletal Radiol* 2010;39(4):333–343.

109 Lecouvet FE, El Mouedden J, Collette L, *et al.* Can whole-body magnetic resonance imaging with diffusion-weighted imaging replace Tc 99m bone scanning and computed tomography for single-step detection of metastases in patients with high-risk prostate cancer? *Eur Urol* 2012;62(1):68–75.

110 Lecouvet FE, Simon M, Tombal B, *et al.* Whole-body MRI (WB-MRI) versus axial skeleton MRI (AS-MRI) to detect and measure bone metastases in prostate cancer (PCa). *Eur Radiol* 2010;20:2973–2982.

111 Padhani AR, Koh DM, Collins DJ. Whole-body diffusion-weighted MR imaging in cancer: current status and research directions. *Radiology* 2011;261(3):700–718.

112 Beheshti M, Imamovic L, Broinger G, *et al.* 18F choline PET/CT in the preoperative staging of prostate cancer in patients with intermediate or high risk of extracapsular disease: a prospective study of 130 patients. *Radiology* 2010;254(3):925–933.

113 Luboldt W, Kufer R, Blumstein N, *et al.* Prostate carcinoma: diffusion-weighted imaging as potential alternative to conventional MR and 11C-choline PET/CT for detection of bone metastases. *Radiology* 2008;249(3):1017–1025.

114 Eschmann SM, Pfannenberg AC, Rieger A, *et al.* Comparison of 11C-choline-PET/CT and whole body-MRI for staging of prostate cancer. *Nuklearmedizin* 2007; 46(5):161–168.

115 Pucar D, Sella T, Schoder H. The role of imaging in the detection of prostate cancer local recurrence after radiation therapy and surgery. *Curr Opin Urol* 2008;18(1):87–97.

116 Margel D, Yap SA, Lawrentschuk N, *et al.* Impact of multiparametric endorectal coil prostate magnetic resonance imaging on disease reclassification among active surveillance candidates: a prospective cohort study. *J Urol* 2012;187(4):1247–1252.

117 Vargas HA, Akin O, Afaq A, *et al.* Magnetic resonance imaging for predicting prostate biopsy findings in patients considered for active surveillance of clinically low risk prostate cancer. *J Urol* 2012;188(5):1732–1738.

118 Delongchamps NB, Beuvon F, Eiss D, *et al.* Multiparametric MRI is helpful to predict tumor focality, stage, and size in patients diagnosed with unilateral low-risk prostate cancer. *Prostate Cancer Prostatic Dis* 2011;14(3):232–237.

119 Parker C, Muston D, Melia J, *et al.* A model of the natural history of screen-detected prostate cancer, and the effect of radical treatment on overall survival. *Br J Cancer* 2006;94(10):1361–1368.

120 Wolters T, Roobol MJ, van Leeuwen PJ, *et al.* A critical analysis of the tumor volume threshold for clinically insignificant prostate cancer using a data set of a randomized screening trial. *J Urol* 2011;185(1):121–125.

121 Jeong CW, Ku JH, Moon KC, *et al.* Can conventional magnetic resonance imaging, prostate needle biopsy, or their combination predict the laterality of clinically localized prostate cancer? *Urology* 2012;79(6):1322–1327.

122 McClure TD, Margolis DJ, Reiter RE, *et al.* Use of MR imaging to determine preservation of the neurovascular bundles at robotic-assisted laparoscopic prostatectomy. *Radiology* 2012;262(3):874–883.

123 Hricak H, Wang L, Wei DC, *et al.* The role of preoperative endorectal magnetic resonance imaging in the decision regarding whether to preserve or resect neurovascular bundles during radical retropubic prostatectomy. *Cancer* 2004;100(12):2655–2663.

124 Masterson TA, Touijer K. The role of endorectal coil MRI in preoperative staging and decision-making for the treatment of clinically localized prostate cancer. *MAGMA* 2008;21(6):371–377.

125 Pound CR, Partin AW, Eisenberger MA, *et al.* Natural history of progression after PSA elevation following radical prostatectomy. *JAMA* 1999;281(17):1591–1597.

126 Turkbey B, Pinto PA, Choyke PL. Imaging techniques for prostate cancer: implications for focal therapy. *Nat Rev Urol* 2009;6(4):191–203.

127 Mouraviev V, Madden JF. Focal therapy for prostate cancer: pathologic basis. *Curr Opin Urol* 2009;19(2):161–167.

128 Onik G, Vaughan D, Lotenfoe R, *et al.* The "male lumpectomy": focal therapy for prostate cancer using cryoablation results in 48 patients with at least 2-year follow-up. *Urol Oncol* 2008;26(5):500–505.

129  Jayram G, Eggener SE. Patient selection for focal therapy of localized prostate cancer. *Curr Opin Urol* 2009;19(3):268–273.

130  Lindner U, Weersink RA, Haider MA, *et al.* Image guided photothermal focal therapy for localized prostate cancer: phase I trial. *J Urol* 2009;182:1371–1377.

131  Eggener SE, Scardino PT, Carroll PR, *et al.* Focal therapy for localized prostate cancer: a critical appraisal of rationale and modalities. *J Urol* 2007;178(6):2260–2267.

132  De Visschere PJ, De Meerleer GO, Futterer JJ, Villeirs GM. Role of MRI in follow-up after focal therapy for prostate carcinoma. *AJR Am J Roentgenol* 2010;194(6):1427–1433.

133  Ahmed HU, Kirkham A, Arya M, *et al.* Is it time to consider a role for MRI before prostate biopsy? *Nat Rev Clin Oncol* 2009;6(4):197–206.

## CHAPTER 6

# Counseling the Patient with Newly Diagnosed Prostate Cancer, Stage by Stage

*Nicholas James Smith and William Richard Cross*
Department of Urology, St James's University Hospital, Leeds Teaching Hospitals NHS Trust, Leeds, UK

> *Fully informing men about their prostate cancer treatment options involves honestly telling men what we do not know as well as the little we do.*
>
> Michael J. Barry

On receiving a diagnosis of prostate cancer, patients are often faced with the difficult and confusing process of selecting their treatment preference. To allow the patient to take an active role in making an informed choice requires close collaboration between healthcare provider and patient. The shared decision-making process aims to take into account the patient's (and their family's) values and preferences as well as the best available scientific evidence.

The Salzburg statement on shared decision-making [1] calls on clinicians to:

1 Recognize that they have ethical imperative to share important decisions with patients.

2 Stimulate a two-way flow of information and encourage patients to ask questions, explain their circumstances, and express their personal preferences.

3 Provide accurate information about the options and uncertainties, benefits, and harms of treatment in line with best practice for risk communication.

4 Tailor information in individual patient needs and allow them sufficient time to consider their options.

---

*Prostate Cancer: Diagnosis and Clinical Management*, First Edition.
Edited by Ashutosh K. Tewari, Peter Whelan and John D. Graham.
© 2014 John Wiley & Sons, Ltd. Published 2014 by John Wiley & Sons, Ltd.

**5**  Acknowledge that most decisions do not have to be taken immediately, and give patients and families the resources to help reach decisions.

However, there is a challenge to healthcare providers to ensure that the Salzburg statement is followed. In particular, allowing enough time to ensure adequate patient counseling can be difficult in healthcare systems driven by government targets.

Shared decision-making in prostate cancer management has been shown to be associated with increased patient satisfaction [2], preferred by both patient and clinician [3] and leads to low levels of treatment decision regret [4]. This chapter highlights important aspects that require consideration for the decision-making process. In keeping with the principles of shared decision-making, the weight of influence for these factors will vary considerably between patients.

## Decision-making complicated by lack of level one evidence

Central to treatment counseling is informing the patient what we do know and what we currently do not know regarding comparative therapeutic outcomes. Patients diagnosed with prostate cancer inherently want to know which treatment will give the best chance of cure with least impact on quality of life. However, there is a lack of level one evidence to inform the decision-making process. To date, the only published randomized control trials comparing radical prostatectomy with watchful waiting are the Scandinavian Prostate Cancer Group-4 (SPCG-4) and Radical Prostatectomy versus Observation for Localized Prostate Cancer (PIVOT) studies [5,6]. The SPCG-4 study has reassured the urological surgeon since its first publication that radical prostatectomy can reduce prostate cancer mortality [5]. However, the recent initial analysis of PIVOT questions the role of radical prostatectomy, particularly in low-risk disease [6]. The SPCG-4 study has shown an absolute reduction of 6.1% in prostate cancer mortality in the prostatectomy group at 15 years follow-up [5]. This reduction in mortality is confined to men aged less than 65 years with a number requiring treatment of 7 [5]. One of the limitations of the SPCG-4 study in application with modern-day practice is that few patients were detected by prostate-specific antigen (PSA) screening. In the PIVOT study, 50% of patients were diagnosed with T1c disease, which more closely reflects the current patient cohort presenting through opportunist PSA screening [6]. PIVOT did not show a significant difference in all-cause and prostate cancer mortality between radical prostatectomy and watchful waiting groups at a follow-up of 10 years [6]. In subgroup analysis, overall mortality was reduced in patients with a PSA level of >10 ng/mL, suggesting that patients with intermediate- and high-risk disease may benefit from radical treatment [6].

With the lack of evidence of which treatment offers the best long-term survival to help guide the patient, treatment decisions in prostate cancer are, therefore, very individual. Many different factors influence a patient's decision and specialists need to be aware of these potential influences to provide effective counseling.

## Factors that influence decision-making

### Stage of disease, chance of cure, and risk of recurrence
The stage of disease has obvious implications in determining which therapy is recommended to the patient, and published guidelines (discussed later) aim to give evidence-based direction.

In addition to clinical guidelines, predictive tables and nomograms have been developed to estimate various outcome measures pre- and post-treatment [7]. Predictive tools have been shown to be more accurate than a physician's clinical judgment alone [8] and generate individualized quantitative information to help aid decision-making. One possible limitation of predictive tools is that they may lose accuracy if applied to cohorts of patients from different geographical areas [9]. In addition, there is a paucity of studies that assess to what extent predictive nomograms influence treatment decision-making, patient anxiety, or decisional regret. Despite these limitations, however, predictive tools are important evidence-based adjuncts for patient counseling.

### Age and co-morbidity
A life expectancy of more than 10 years is often quoted as the benchmark prior to considering radical therapy in localized prostate cancer. As life expectancy is central to decision-making in prostate cancer, the accuracy in its prediction is obviously paramount. Predicting life expectancy however can be difficult and clinician accuracy is at best modest [10, 11]. It is therefore intuitive that tools, which include life tables, co-morbidity indices, and statistical modeling to aid the clinician in predicting life expectancy, should be considered for routine use.

A life table shows the probabilities of a member of a particular population living to or dying at a particular age, and from this the remaining life expectancy for people at different ages is derived. Life tables may, however, be no more accurate than clinician accuracy [10]. Life expectancy, derived from life tables, has been predicted in men undergoing radical prostatectomy and compared to actual 10-year survival (corrected for prostate cancer mortality) in these patients [12]. Life tables were shown to overestimate life expectancy, with predicted 10-year life expectancy of 97% versus 81% observed [12]. Therefore, the use of life tables may lead to a propensity to overtreatment in prostate cancer. Life tables make adjustments for average co-morbidities; therefore indices have been developed to predict life expectancy based on the individual's co-morbidities. One such co-morbidity index is the Charlson co-morbidity index [13], which has a number of variations. The overestimation of life expectancy by life tables has been shown to be predictably worse in patients with higher Charlson scores, but is still substantial in patients with low Charlson scores [12].

Charlson scores have been applied to a large cohort of American patients with non-metastatic prostate cancer in retrospective analysis [14]. At a median 6-year follow-up and a 3% prostate cancer mortality, patients with Charlson scores of 0, 1, 2, and 3+ had a 10-year non-prostate cancer mortality of 17%, 34%, 52%, and 74%, respectively [14]. This study highlighting the risk of overtreatment of low and intermediate risk localized prostate cancer in patients with significant competing co-morbidity. However, further studies are required to predict the accuracy of co-morbidity indices alone in predicting life expectancy in prostate cancer.

In view of the inaccuracies in life expectancy prediction highlighted above, a number of statistical nomograms have been developed to predict life expectancy in patients being treated for localized prostate cancer [15–18]. Of these, the nomogram developed by Walz is perhaps the simplest, using patient age and Charlson score as indices. It also has the highest reported accuracy of 84% in predicting 10-year life expectancy after either radical prostatectomy or external beam radiotherapy (EBRT) [10, 18]. Future studies are required to validate life expectancy nomograms prior to being accepted for use in routine clinical practice.

In addition to deciding whether a patient should have radical therapy for localized disease, patient age and co-morbidity have been shown as independent predictors of which mode of radical therapy patients should receive. It has been shown that younger patients more commonly opt to have surgical intervention, with older patients with increasing co-morbidity having radiation therapy [19].

## Patient beliefs, misconceptions, and reasons for treatment choice in localized disease

Patients select a specific therapy for localized prostate cancer due to a variety of beliefs. Patients often base a decision for surgery on the belief that it offers the best chance of cure with superiority over radiotherapy options [20]. This unproven belief about the superiority of surgery would seem to be still held by patients today as radical prostatectomy continues to be the most popular choice of radical treatment in localized disease [21–23]. The question remains as to whether improved patient counseling will alter the popularity of radical prostatectomy. The recent trend from Europe of an increase in popularity of active surveillance and radiotherapy may reflect indirectly that this is the case [23].

Surgery is often chosen by those patients motivated by the need for cancer eradication. Also, patients opting for surgery in localized disease have been shown to be commonly motivated by the need for physical removal of the cancer [21], providing knowledge about the tumor and giving the patient a psychological reassurance [20].

Some patients choosing EBRT do so due to fear of radical prostatectomy, seeing it as less invasive and with fewer side effects compared to surgery [20,21]. In one study, 39% of patients electing for brachytherapy did so for lifestyle convenience [21]. Brachytherapy is viewed as more convenient than EBRT in those who view EBRT as time-consuming [20].

Active surveillance is becoming an increasingly popular treatment choice in low-risk disease [22], likely reflecting a shift in clinician recommendation backed by clinical practice guidelines. The most popular reasons for electing active surveillance in one study of patients were those of urologists' opinion, age of patient, impact of treatment on urinary function, and impact of treatment on sexual function [24].

## Concern about potential treatment-induced morbidity

Treatment-induced morbidity from radical therapies for prostate cancer are well documented [25] and are a major factor in the treatment decision-making process. The most influential side effect is urinary dysfunction, closely followed by bowel and sexual dysfunction. Younger patients attribute more importance in the preservation of sexual function than older men [26]. Men considering radical prostatectomy are less likely to have concern over treatment-related side effect than those considering nonsurgical options, particularly active surveillance [21,27]. In one study, over two-thirds of men opting for nonsurgical options indicated that side-effects of treatment were the main factor in decision-making [27].

Patients with more aggressive tumors were less likely to consider side effects [27].

Although patients state the side effects of treatment as important, the influence of side effects in final decision-making may actually play a less-prominent role. For example, despite the perceived importance of sexual dysfunction one study has suggested that men without preexisting erectile dysfunction may discount the risks of side effects in the decision-making process [27]. In this study, patients who did not have sexual dysfunction prior to treatment were less likely to consider side effects prior to decision-making than those with preexisting sexual dysfunction [27]. The patient's spouse may also be less influenced by potential side effects in the decision-making process. In one study, only 6% of spouses of patients with localized disease viewed treatment side effects as the most important factor in decision–making, although 55% expressed it an important aspect of decision-making [28].

## Family and friends

As with other major illnesses, patients diagnosed with prostate cancer often turn to their spouse or partner for support in treatment decision-making. In addition, the patients' partner is increasingly being recognized as being affected by the cancer diagnosis and subsequent treatment received.

In a prospective study in the United States, a half of patients diagnosed with prostate cancer had their spouse/partner present when the diagnosis was given and nearly all were informed on the same day [29]. Thereafter, the majority of spouses/partners were actively involved in decision-making process; attending subsequent clinic appointments, reporting discussion of treatment options very often with their partner, providing emotional support, and indeed helping make the treatment decision itself [29]. Partners who were encouraged to participate in the decision-making process, as anticipated, were also shown to have increased reported satisfaction [29].

A retrospective study of localized prostate cancer in the United Kingdom demonstrated the partner's primary roles in emotional support and accumulation of information from both hospital visits and external sources [28]. The study again demonstrated that most partners believe they play an active role in the decision-making process. It indicated that the partner's conceptions for therapy of localized disease may influence decision-making, with younger partners favoring surgery and older partners preferring radiotherapy [28].

The partner's perceived prominent role in decision-making may not be that perceived by the patient however, with patients reporting only a minor influence from the spouse in studies [30, 31]. The discrepancy between patient's and partner's beliefs on impact in decision-making does require clarification in future studies.

It is generally accepted that clinicians, with the consent of the patient, should actively include the patient's partner at the initial diagnosis and subsequent consultation sessions for them to gain the necessary information to be able to facilitate in shared decision-making. This involvement may well enhance the couple's ability to cope with the diagnosis, improve satisfaction, and reduce decisional regret.

The role of friends in the decision-making process in prostate cancer is less documented. Anecdotal accounts of relatives or friends who have undergone treatment for prostate cancer, even if treatment is for different disease stage, have been reported as influencing factors [20]. One would hope that misconceptions from anecdotes could be minimized through patient education during the process of shared decision-making.

## Physician recommendation and bias

Patients continue to look to their physicians' clinical judgment in helping them make informed decisions and "what do you advise doctor?" is certainly a common question in consultations. A study of American patients electing for surgery or brachytherapy in localized disease has shown that urologists are seen as the most important source of information and the major influential factor [30]. Physician bias therefore is likely to play a role in influencing patient decision-making, particularly with the lack of level one evidence to support one treatment modality over another in localized disease. It is not surprising that studies have demonstrated that specialists (urologists vs. radiation oncologists) overwhelmingly prefer the therapy that they deliver [32]. In the United States, in men with localized prostate cancer diagnosed between 1994 and 2002, it has been demonstrated that 50% of men only saw a urologist and 44% saw both urologist and radiation oncologist [19]. Of those aged 65–69 years, 70% opted for surgery if they only saw a urologist, whereas 78% opted for radiation therapy if they consulted both urologist and radiation oncologist [19]. This study indirectly suggests that physician bias plays a role in the decision-making of patients with localized disease.

Methods of trying to overcome the potential for physician bias include patient decision aids, multidisciplinary team (MDT) review, and ensuring that all patients are offered consultations with all treatment specialists, including cancer specialist nurses, prior to decision-making.

The potential benefit of an MDT review prior to decision-making is highlighted by the fact that urologists have been shown to be unreliable in decision-making in early prostate cancer. A UK study of urologists has shown reliability of 56–79% in decision-making, with clinicians using few of the available cues when formulating decisions often ignoring cues of patient choice and co-morbidity [33]. If MDT case review of all patients were to take place, one would expect reliability of decision-making to increase. This hypothesis has not been formally tested for prostate cancer decision-making. MDT reviews have been shown to change treatment plans in 22% of prostate cancer referrals to a centre in the United States [34].

## Financial issues (patient and clinician)

Financial issues for both patient and healthcare provider are likely to influence treatment decisions. For the patient, loss of earnings due to time off work during and following treatment may strongly influence their decision. For the healthcare provider, the financial influences may be more complex.

The exponential increase in the number of robot-assisted laparoscopic prostatectomies performed in the past decade has occurred prior to the benefits of this surgery being documented despite the added cost [35]. The capital investments for equipment in robotic surgery are substantial and therefore once the investment has been made, there is obvious pressure for high patient caseloads to recoup this investment. The same could also be applied if the investment has been for intensity-modulated radiotherapy [35].

Novel therapies for castration-resistant prostate cancer come at a cost and cost–benefit analysis influences healthcare systems in approving their utilization where resources are finite [36]. In the United Kingdom, the National Institute for Health and Clinical Excellence (NICE) states that if a drug cost is between £20,000 and £30,000 per quality-adjusted life year (QALY) then it is not seen as cost-effective and not recommended.

In a private healthcare system, health insurance may influence decisions due to cost of treatment. For example, in the United States, marked differences in type of prostate cancer treatment received by men aged greater than 65 years have been demonstrated dependent on type of healthcare insurance [37].

Financial influences are likely to be not confined solely to private health-care systems. For example, in the Swedish national healthcare system, disparities have been demonstrated based on socioeconomic class in treatment received, and survival, in high-risk disease [38]. Patients from a higher socioeconomic group were more likely to receive radical therapy and radical prostatectomy with a lower prostate-cancer-specific mortality [38].

## Application and development of patient decision aids

Decision aids are evidence-based tools that are designed to prepare patients to participate in making specific healthcare treatment choices. They aim to supplement the clinicians' counseling about options. They can provide information about risks and benefits of treatment, help patients recognize the values they place on these risks and benefits, and can provide structured guidance in the steps of decision-making. Decision aids used in localized prostate cancer counseling often present individualized information in multiple formats such as written information, individual consultation, video, interactive CD-ROM, and internet-based tools [39].

Decision aids have been shown to improve knowledge, reduce decisional conflict and anxiety, reduce the number of patients who adopt a passive role in decision–making, and increase patient satisfaction [39, 40]. However, the overall impact of decision aids on the final treatment choice of patients in localized prostate cancer is less proven [39]. Therefore, decision aids are as yet not routine in clinical practice in prostate cancer counseling but may well gain popularity pending further research.

## Role of clinical nurse specialist and primary care physician

Patients diagnosed with prostate cancer in the United Kingdom are expected to have ongoing contact with clinical nurse specialists [41]. The primary role of clinical nurse specialists in prostate cancer is to provide patient support and information. Patients seen by a nurse specialist have been demonstrated in a study to be more likely to state that they have made the treatment decision themselves with more access to written information and support [42]. This positive impact on shared decision-making could be directly related to increased time spent discussing treatments and indirectly due to a reduction in physician bias.

The patient's primary care physician plays an important role prior to the initial diagnosis of prostate cancer in terms of investigation of symptoms or counseling prior to case detection through PSA screening. Following diagnosis, however, the role of the primary care physician in treatment decision-making is less prominent. This is demonstrated in a large cohort of American men diagnosed with prostate cancer between 1994 and 2002 where 79% of men were seen by a primary care physician within 12 months of diagnosis, however, only 22% saw a primary care physician between diagnosis and 9 months following treatment [19]. It would seem logical for the primary care physician to not to play a prominent role in treatment decision-making. Due to its complexities, counseling is likely to be best served by appropriate specialists who do it regularly and have the appropriate training. The role of the primary care physician during the decision-making process is likely to be more supportive, meeting the emotional needs of the patient.

## Clinical practice guidelines

Clinical practice guidelines provide a valuable resource for healthcare professionals and can aid evidence-based decision-making. A number of urological and oncological associations have published guidelines on the diagnosis and treatment of prostate cancer based on systematic review of the medical literature. They help to define established treatment options and guide future research.

Comprehensive guidelines reviewed in this section are those from the American Association of Urology (AUA; first published 1995, last update 2007) [43], European Association of Urology (EAU; first published 2001, last update 2012) [25], the National Comprehensive Cancer Network USA (NCCN; last update 2012) [44], the European Society of Medical Oncology (ESMO; 2010) [45], and the National Institute of Clinical Excellence, United Kingdom (NICE; 2008) [46]. In addition, guidelines from the American Society of Clinical Oncology (ASCO; 2007) [47, 48] and the Canadian Urological Association (CUA; 2010) [49] on metastatic disease were reviewed.

### Localized prostate cancer
Guidelines for the treatment of localized prostate cancer have been published by the AUA, EAU, NCCN, ESMO, and NICE.

### Risk stratification

Risk stratification is incorporated into all guidelines for treating localized prostate cancer. Most guidelines utilize the work by D'Amico and coworkers to define risk groupings, based on the risk of biochemical relapse and prostate cancer mortality following radical treatment [50]. Low-, intermediate-, and high-risk groups are derived from serum PSA, Gleason grade of prostate biopsy cores, and American Joint Committee on Cancer (AJCC) clinical stage [50]. Guidelines do differ slightly in their risk stratification of localized disease. These differences relate to clinical stage and are shown in the below table. NCCN guidelines in addition include a very low risk category using Epstein's criteria for clinically insignificant disease [51].

| | PSA | Gleason Score | Clinical stage by individual guideline | | | |
| | | | AUA | EAU/NCCN | NICE/ESMO | NCCN |
|---|---|---|---|---|---|---|
| Very low risk[a] (NCCN only) | <10 ng/mL | ≤6 | <3 cores +ve and <50% carcinoma in each core and PSAD <0.15 ng/mL/mL | | | T1c |
| Low risk[a] | <10 ng/mL | ≤6 | T1c-T2a | T1-T2a | T1-T2a | T1-T2a |
| Intermediate risk[b] | 10–20 ng/mL | 7 | T2b | T2b-T2c | T2b-T2c | T2b-T2c |
| High risk[b] | >20 ng/mL | 8–10 | T2c | T3a | T3-T4 | T3a |

PSAD, PSA density.
[a]Must fulfill all criteria.
[b]One or more criteria required.

### Treatment options of localized prostate cancer (AUA, NCCN, EAU, ESMO, NICE)

All guidelines recognize that no level one evidence is available comparing different treatment modalities other than the SPCG-4 study comparing watchful waiting and radical prostatectomy. The NCCN and EAU guidelines both recommend treatment options on a defined patient life expectancy.

### Very low risk disease

NCCN guidance recommends active surveillance for men with very low risk localized prostate cancer if the patient has a life expectancy of less than

20 years. In patients with greater than 20 year life expectancy, treatment options are as for low-risk disease.

### Low-risk disease

If the patient is not suitable for, or unwilling to have, radical treatment then watchful waiting with deferred hormonal therapy is the consensus recommendation of all guidelines reviewed. The NCCN and EAU state that radical treatment is not suitable if the patient's life expectancy is less than 10 years. Immediate hormonal therapy is not recommended.

In all guidelines, active surveillance, radical prostatectomy, radical EBRT (3D-conformal with or without intensity-modulated radiotherapy, IMRT), and transperineal interstitial brachytherapy with permanent implants are recognized treatment options in patients with low-risk disease and suitable for radical therapy (defined by NCCN and EAU as life expectancy of more than 10 years).

The NICE guidance is the only guideline to give a preferred option in low-risk disease of active surveillance. It goes further to state active surveillance is "particularly suitable" in men fulfilling Epstein's criteria for clinically insignificant disease identical to the NCCN's very low risk group. The EAU also recommend active surveillance as a treatment option if Epstein's criteria are fulfilled. The AUA and EAU both recognize that an ideal regimen of active surveillance has yet to be defined. All guidelines suggest follow-up based on regular digital rectal examination (DRE), PSA, and repeated prostate biopsies. The NCCN recommend repeat biopsies as often as annually, the EAU suggest annually or biannually.

The EAU and AUA are the only guidelines recommending cryosurgical ablation of the prostate as a treatment option in low-risk disease outside of a clinical trial. The EAU does state that long-term results of cryotherapy are lacking and that 5-year biochemical-free progression rates are inferior to radical prostatectomy. The AUA best practice statement (2008) also recognizes that long-term data are not currently available but differs in its conclusion stating that, because of lack of long-term data meaningful comparisons with other treatments are not possible.

High-intensity focused ultrasound is not a recommended treatment option unless in clinical trial.

### Intermediate-risk disease

As in low-risk disease, if the patient is not suitable for radical treatment (life expectancy less than 10 years in NCCN and EAU guidelines) then watchful waiting with deferred hormonal therapy is the consensus recommendation.

All guidelines reviewed recognize radical prostatectomy, EBRT (3D-conformal with or without IMRT), and permanent seed brachytherapy as treatment options. Extended lymph node dissection at the time of radical prostatectomy is recommended by the NCCN and EAU if the risks of metastases are 2% and 5%, for each respective guideline. Except for NICE, all guidelines suggest that neoadjuvant, concurrent, and adjuvant hormonal therapy should be considered for 6 months post-radiotherapy based on level one evidence [52].

Brachytherapy is not a "preferred" option according to NICE, and EAU restricts recommendation to only Gleason 3 + 4 disease with PSA <10 ng/mL and cT1c-T2. The NCCN recommends that permanent seed brachytherapy should be combined with 45 Gy EBRT (with or without neoadjuvant hormones) in intermediate-risk disease.

Active surveillance is not a recommended option for intermediate-risk disease by the EAU, ESMO, and NCCN if the patient is suitable for radical treatment. However, the AUA and NICE guidelines express that active surveillance is a treatment option in this group of patients.

Cryotherapy is recognized as an option in intermediate-risk disease by both the AUA and EAU.

**High-risk disease**

In patients with high-risk disease who are not candidates or those who are unwilling to have radical therapy, watchful waiting with deferred hormonal therapy is recommended by all guidelines. Immediate hormonal therapy is recognized by the AUA, EAU, and NCCN guidelines. The EAU and NCCN suggest that immediate hormonal therapy may be appropriate in selected men with high PSA levels (>50 ng/mL) and short PSA doubling time (<12 months). Evidence from this guidance mainly comes from the EORTC 30891 study [53]. Oral bicalutamide is recognized by the EAU and ESMO, but not by the NCCN, as an alternative to androgen deprivation therapy (ADT) in this setting citing evidence from the Early Prostate Cancer Programme study [54].

Radical prostatectomy and EBRT are recognized by all guidelines as the standard treatment option in high-risk disease. The NCCN guidelines state that patients with a life expectancy of over 5 years will benefit from radical treatment. The EAU acknowledges that radical prostatectomy in high-risk disease is often a part of multimodal therapy. Both NCCN and EAU give guidance on lymph node dissection at the time of prostatectomy and both recommend extended pelvic lymph node dissection. There is concordance within the guidelines reviewed that neoadjuvant, concomitant, and 2–3 years ADT offers survival advantage in patients having EBRT. This guidance is based on a number of randomized control trials. The EAU and NCCN give guidance on dose of radiotherapy, starting at 78 Gy and going up to 81 Gy. The NCCN recommends pelvic node irradiation in high-risk disease, whereas the EAU states that this requires further investigation in clinical trial.

The AUA is the only guideline to offer active surveillance as a treatment option in high-risk disease. However, this guideline does also state that "a high risk of disease progression and death from disease may make active treatment a preferred option."

Brachytherapy is a recognized treatment option in high-risk disease by the AUA, NCCN, and EAU but not by ESMO and NICE. The EAU and NCCN state that the role of brachytherapy in this setting is in combination with EBRT with or without short-term hormonal therapy.

Cryotherapy is recognized as an option in high-risk disease only by the AUA in its best practice statement in 2008. This statement does recognize that there is limited data for outcomes in T3 disease and the role of cryosurgery in this setting is undetermined. In addition, lymph node dissection is recommended prior to or concurrent with cryosurgery in men with greater than 25% risk of lymph node metastasis.

## Locally advanced disease
### Definition
Guidelines differ in defining locally advanced prostate cancer. Locally advanced disease is subcategorized by the NCCN and EAU into high-risk clinically localized disease (cT3 or Gleason score >7 or PSA > 20), as discussed above, and very high risk disease (cT3b-T4).

### Treatment of cT3b-T4 nonmetastatic prostate cancer
#### Hormonal treatment
Guidelines concur in recommending that primary hormonal therapy should be reserved for men who are not suitable for, or unwilling to have, radical treatment. The timing of hormonal therapy differs between guidelines. ESMO does not recommend immediate hormonal therapy in these patients. The EAU and NCCN recognize that the benefit of early hormonal therapy is unclear. However, both suggest that immediate rather than delayed hormonal therapy may be appropriate in selected men with

high PSA (>50 ng/mL) and short PSA doubling time (<12 months), citing evidence from the EORTC 30891 study [53].

The EAU is the only guideline to recommend bicalutamide as an alternative to castration for patients with locally advanced disease if progression-free survival is the treatment aim [53].

### Radical prostatectomy

According to NICE, the role of surgery and extended lymphadenectomy (eLND) as primary therapy for locally advanced disease should be studied in clinical trials. The EAU and NCCN recognize radical prostatectomy with eLND is an option in highly selected patients with cT3b-4 N0 disease. All guidelines agree in not recommending neoadjuvant hormonal therapy or adjuvant hormonal therapy post-radical prostatectomy except in node-positive disease.

Immediate adjuvant radiotherapy, rather than early salvage radiotherapy, post-prostatectomy is not routinely recommended by NICE or ESMO, even in margin positive disease. This recommendation is based on clinical trial data [55, 56]. However, the EAU guidelines review more mature data from the South West Oncology Group 8794 study and conclude that in T3 N0 M0 disease, immediate post-operative radiotherapy may improve overall survival, biochemical progression-free survival, and clinical disease-free survival [57]. The NCCN agrees with the EAU suggesting a likely benefit of immediate adjuvant radiotherapy in men with adverse prognostic features (margin positive, seminal vesical invasion, extracapsular extension).

### Radiotherapy

All the guidelines reviewed recommend radical EBRT as treatment of locally advanced prostate cancer. There is also consensus that radiotherapy should be accompanied with neoadjuvant (3–6 months), concomitant and adjuvant (2–3 years) ADT to improve overall survival. ESMO cites evidence from the Early Prostate Cancer Programme study to suggest that bicalutamide monotherapy is an alternative to gonadotrophin releasing hormone (GnRH) analogs in this setting [54]. The NCCN recommends that 3D-conformal IMRT and image-guided techniques using CT should be employed, giving up 81 Gy. The NCCN and NICE state that pelvic lymph node irradiation is an option in these patients, with the EAU recommending clinical trials of pelvic node irradiation.

The NCCN is the only guideline reviewed to recommend brachytherapy with EBRT boost (40–50 Gy) as an alternative treatment option in T3b-T4 disease. This treatment is recommended with 4–6 months of neoadjuvant, concomitant and adjuvant ADT.

## Metastatic prostate cancer
### Symptomatic disease
There is consensus in the reviewed guidelines that the standard of care in symptomatic metastatic prostate cancer is hormonal therapy. All guidelines state that bilateral orchidectomy is equivalent to GnRH agonists as first-line therapy. Bilateral orchidectomy is accepted as the most cost-effective therapy and should be offered as an alternative to GnRH agonists. No guidelines recommend diethylstilboestrol as first-line therapy due to its cardiovascular toxicity.

Maximal androgen blockade (MAB) with GnRH agonist plus bicalutamide has shown a potential small overall survival advantage with increased cost and toxicity [58]. Based on this level one evidence, MAB is not recommended as first-line therapy by ESMO, NICE; however, ASCO and NCCN state that it should be considered.

In one randomized study, nonsteroidal antiandrogen monotherapy has a 6-week adverse impact on overall survival as compared to androgen-deprivation therapy and it is not recommended by the NCCN [59]. The EAU, ESMO, and NICE, however, state that antiandrogen monotherapy is appropriate in the highly selected well-informed man who hopes to retain sexual function in the face of the potential adverse impact on overall survival.

GnRH antagonists are recognized by NCCN, EAU, and ESMO. The NCCN recommends GnRH antagonists as an option for first-line therapy due to equal efficacy [60], whereas the EAU states that the advantages of GnRH antagonists over GnRH agonists are far from proven and that further trials are required.

Intermittent androgen deprivation (IAD) is now not considered as investigational by the EAU and can be offered to patients. The NCCN are more cautious about IAD, suggesting that its long-term efficacy remains unproven. The NCCN guidance is in concordance with earlier guidelines from NICE and ASCO requesting further clinical trials of IAD.

### Asymptomatic disease
In asymptomatic metastatic prostate cancer, guidelines differ on when to commence hormonal therapy.

NCCN, ESMO, and NICE all recommend immediate ADT in asymptomatic metastases. The NCCN suggests immediate ADT to delay symptomatic progression but accepts that it is not clear whether earlier ADT will prolong survival. The EAU states that immediate castration is recommended to prevent symptoms and complications of disease and that "active clinical surveillance may be acceptable in clearly informed patients if survival is the main objective." ASCO states it "cannot give a strong recommendation for the early use of ADT" in asymptomatic metastatic prostate cancer.

## Conclusions

Treatment decision-making in prostate cancer is a difficult and complex process. The clinician requires knowledge of both clinical aspects of the disease and patient factors, which in many individuals can be very personal and influential. To optimize counseling and minimize decisional regret, counseling should be informed by clinical guidelines, delivered with equipoise within the framework of a MDT, and increasingly guided by evidence-based predictive nomograms, statistical tools, and decision aids.

## References

1  Salzburg Global Seminar. Salzburg statement on shared decision making. *BMJ*; 342:d1745.
2  Fischer M, Visser A, Voerman B, *et al.* Treatment decision making in prostate cancer: patients' participation in complex decisions. *Patient Educ Couns* 2006;63(3):308–313.
3  Denis L, Joniau S, Bossi A, *et al.* PCA: prostate cancer, patient-centred approach or both? *BJU Int* 2012;110(1):16.
4  Davison BJ, So AI, Goldenberg SL. Quality of life, sexual function and decisional regret at 1 year after surgical treatment for localized prostate cancer. *BJU Int* 2007;100(4):780–785.
5  Bill-Axelson A, Holmberg L, Ruutu M, *et al.* Radical prostatectomy versus watchful waiting in early prostate cancer. *N Engl J Med* 2011;364(18):1708–1717.
6  Wilt TJ, Brawer MK, Jones KM, *et al.* Radical prostatectomy versus observation for localized prostate cancer. *N Engl J Med* 2012;367(3):203–213.
7  Partin AW, Kattan MW, Subong EN, *et al.* Combination of prostate-specific antigen, clinical stage, and Gleason score to predict pathological stage of localized prostate cancer: a multi-institutional update. *J Am Med Assoc* 1997;277(18):1445.
8  Shariat SF, Kattan MW, Vickers AJ, *et al.* Critical review of prostate cancer predictive tools. *Future Oncol* 2009;5(10):1555.
9  Tamblyn DJ, Chopra S, Yu C, *et al.* Comparative analysis of three risk assessment tools in Australian patients with prostate cancer. *BJU Int* 2011;108:51.
10 Jeldres C, Latouff J-B, Saad F. Predicting life expectancy in prostate cancer patients. *Curr Opin Support Palliat Care* 2009;3(3):166–169.

11 Walz J, Gallina A, Perrotte P, *et al.* Clinicians are poor raters of life-expectancy before radical prostatectomy or definitive radiotherapy for localized prostate cancer. *BJU Int* 2007;100(6):1254.

12 Walz J, Suardi N, Shariat SF, *et al.* Accuracy of life tables in predicting overall survival in patients after radical prostatectomy. *BJU Int* 2008;102(1):33.

13 Charlson ME, Pompei P, Ales KL, MacKenzie CR. A new method of classifying prognostic comorbidity in longitudinal studies: development and validation. *J Chronic Dis* 1987;40(5):373–383.

14 Daskivich TJ, Chamie K, Kwan L, *et al.* Comorbidity and competing risks for mortality in men with prostate cancer. *Cancer* 2011;117(20):4642–4650.

15 Albertsen PC, Fryback DG, Storer BE, *et al.* The impact of co-morbidity on life expectancy among men with localized prostate cancer. *J Urol* 1996;156(1):127–132.

16 Cowen ME, Halasyamani LK, Kattan MW. Predicting life expectancy in men with clinically localized prostate cancer. *J Urol* 2006;175(1):99–103.

17 Tewari A, Johnson CC, Divine G, *et al.* Long-term survival probability in men with clinically localized prostate cancer: a case–control, propensity modeling study stratified by race, age, treatment and comorbidities. *J Urol* 2004;171(4):1513–1519.

18 Walz J, Gallina A, Saad F, *et al.* A nomogram predicting 10-year life expectancy in candidates for radical prostatectomy or radiotherapy for prostate cancer. *J Clin Oncol* 2007;25(24):3576–3581.

19 Jang TL, Bekelman JE, Liu Y, *et al.* Physician visits prior to treatment for clinically localized prostate cancer. *Arch Intern Med* 2010;170(5):440–450.

20 Denberg TD, Melhado TV, Steiner JF. Patient treatment preferences in localized prostate carcinoma: the influence of emotion, misconception, and anecdote. *Cancer* 2006;107(3):620–630.

21 Anandadas CN, Clarke NW, Davidson SE, *et al.* Early prostate cancer–which treatment do men prefer and why? *BJU Int* 2011;107(11):1762–1768.

22 McVey GP, McPhail S, Fowler S, *et al.* Initial management of low-risk localized prostate cancer in the UK: analysis of the British Association of Urological Surgeons Cancer Registry. *BJU Int* 2010;106(8):1161–1164.

23 Boevee SJ, Venderbos LD, Tammela TL, *et al.* Change of tumour characteristics and treatment over time in both arms of the European randomized study of screening for prostate cancer. *Eur J Cancer* 2010;46(17):3082–3089.

24 Davison BJ, Goldenberg SL. Patient acceptance of active surveillance as a treatment option for low-risk prostate cancer. *BJU Int* 2011;108(11):1787.

25 Heidenreich A, Bastian PJ, Bellmunt J, *et al.* EAU: Guidelines on Prostate Cancer, 2012.

26 Crawford ED, Bennett CL, Stone NN, *et al.* Comparison of perspectives on prostate cancer: analyses of survey data. *Urology* 1997;50(3):366–372.

27 Zeliadt SB, Ramsey SD, Potosky AL, *et al.* Association of preexisting symptoms with treatment decisions among newly diagnosed prostate cancer patients. *Patient* 2008;1(3):189.

28 Srirangam SJ, Pearson E, Grose C, *et al.* Partner's influence on patient preference for treatment in early prostate cancer. *BJU Int* 2003;92(4):365–369.

29 Zeliadt SB, Penson DF, Moinpour CM, *et al.* Provider and partner interactions in the treatment decision-making process for newly diagnosed localized prostate cancer. *BJU Int* 2011;108(6):851–856; discussion 856–857.

30  Hall JD, Boyd JC, Lippert MC, Theodorescu D. Why patients choose prostatectomy or brachytherapy for localized prostate cancer: results of a descriptive survey. *Urology* 2003;61(2):402–407.

31  Diefenbach MA, Dorsey J, Uzzo RG, *et al.* Decision-making strategies for patients with localized prostate cancer. *Semin Urol Oncol* 2002;20(1):55–62.

32  Fowler FJ, Jr., McNaughton Collins M, Albertsen PC, *et al.* Comparison of recommendations by urologists and radiaation oncologists for treatment of clinically localized prostate cancer. *J Am Med Assoc* 2000;283(24):3217–3222.

33  Wilson J, Kennedy K, Ewings P, Macdonagh R. Analysis of consultant decision-making in the management of prostate cancer. *Prostate Cancer Prostatic Dis* 2008; 11(3):288–293.

34  Kurpad R, Kim W, Rathmell WK, *et al.* A multidisciplinary approach to the management of urologic malignancies: does it influence diagnostic and treatment decisions? *Urol Oncol* 2011;29(4):378.

35  Nguyen PL, Gu X, Lipsitz SR, *et al.* Cost implications of the rapid adoption of newer technologies for treating prostate cancer. *J Clin Oncol* 2011;29(12):1517–1524.

36  Kmietowicz Z. NICE recommends abiraterone for prostate cancer after manufacturer reduces price. *BMJ* 2012;344:e3520.

37  Sadetsky N, Elkin EP, Latini DM, *et al.* Prostate cancer outcomes among older men: insurance status comparisons results from CaPSURE database. *Prostate Cancer Prostatic Dis* 2008;11(3):280–287.

38  Berglund A, Garmo H, Robinson D, *et al.* Differences according to socioeconomic status in the management and mortality in men with high risk prostate cancer. *Eur J Cancer* 2012;48(1):75–84.

39  Lin GA, Aaronson DS, Knight SJ, *et al.* Patient decision aids for prostate cancer treatment: a systematic review of the literature. *CA Cancer J Clin* 2009;59(6): 379–390.

40  Stacey D, Bennett CL, Barry MJ, *et al.* Decision aids for people facing health treatment or screening decisions. *Cochrane Database Syst Rev* 2011;(10):CD001431.

41  NICE. Guidance on Cancer Services: improving outcomes in urological cancers – The Manual. 2002.

42  Tarrant C, Sinfield P, Agarwal S, Baker R. Is seeing a specialist nurse associated with positive experiences of care? The role and value of specialist nurses in prostate cancer care. *BMC Health Serv Res* 2008;8:65.

43  Thompson I, Thrasher JB, Aus G, *et al.* Guideline for the management of clinically localized prostate cancer: 2007 update. *J Urol* 2007;177(6):2106.

44  NCCN. Clinical Practice Guidelines in Oncology. Prostate cancer, version 3.2012. 2012.

45  Horwich A, Parker C, Bangma C, Kataja V. Prostate cancer: ESMO Clinical Practice Guidelines for diagnosis, treatment and follow-up. *Ann Oncol* 2010;21(Suppl. 5):v129–v133.

46  National Collaborating Centre for Cancer. NICE Clinical Guideline 58. Prostate cancer: diagnosis and treatment. 2008.

47  Basch EM, Somerfield MR, Beer TM, *et al.* American Society of Clinical Oncology endorsement of the Cancer Care Ontario Practice Guideline on nonhormonal therapy for men with metastatic hormone-refractory (castration-resistant) prostate cancer. *J Clin Oncol* 2007;25(33):5313–5318.

48 Loblaw DA, Virgo KS, Nam R, *et al.* Initial hormonal management of androgen-sensitive metastatic, recurrent, or progressive prostate cancer: 2006 update of an American Society of Clinical Oncology practice guideline. *J Clin Oncol* 2007;25(12): 1596–1605.

49 Saad F, Hotte SJ. Guidelines for the management of castrate-resistant prostate cancer. *Can Urol Assoc J* 2010;4(6):380–384.

50 D'Amico AV, Whittington R, Malkowicz SB, *et al.* Biochemical outcome after radical prostatectomy, external beam radiation therapy, or interstitial radiation therapy for clinically localized prostate cancer. *J Am Med Assoc* 1998;280(11):969–974.

51 Epstein JI, Walsh PC, Carmichael M, Brendler CB. Pathologic and clinical findings to predict tumor extent of nonpalpable (stage T1c) prostate cancer. *J Am Med Assoc* 1994;271(5):368–374.

52 D'Amico AV, Manola J, Loffredo M, *et al.* 6-month androgen suppression plus radiation therapy vs radiation therapy alone for patients with clinically localized prostate cancer: a randomized controlled trial. *J Am Med Assoc* 2004;292(7):821–827.

53 Studer UE, Collette L, Whelan P, *et al.* Using PSA to guide timing of androgen deprivation in patients with T0-4 N0-2 M0 prostate cancer not suitable for local curative treatment (EORTC 30891). *Eur Urol* 2008;53(5):941–949.

54 Iversen P, McLeod DG, See WA, *et al.* Antiandrogen monotherapy in patients with localized or locally advanced prostate cancer: final results from the bicalutamide Early Prostate Cancer Programme at a median follow-up of 9.7 years. *BJU Int* 2010;105(8):1074–1081.

55 Thompson IM, Tangen CM, Paradelo J, *et al.* Adjuvant radiotherapy for pathologically advanced prostate cancer: a randomized clinical trial. *J Am Med Assoc* 2006;296(19):2329.

56 Bolla M, van Poppel H, Collette L, *et al.* Postoperative radiotherapy after radical prostatectomy: a randomised controlled trial (EORTC trial 22911). *Lancet* 2005;366(9485):572–578.

57 Thompson IM, Tangen CM, Paradelo J, *et al.* Adjuvant radiotherapy for pathological T3N0M0 prostate cancer significantly reduces risk of metastases and improves survival: long-term followup of a randomized clinical trial. *J Urol* 2009;181(3):956–962.

58 Samson DJ, Seidenfeld J, Schmitt B, *et al.* Systematic review and meta-analysis of monotherapy compared with combined androgen blockade for patients with advanced prostate carcinoma. *Cancer* 2002;95(2):361.

59 Tyrrell CJ, Kaisary AV, Iversen P, *et al.* A randomised comparison of 'Casodex' (bicalutamide) 150 mg monotherapy versus castration in the treatment of metastatic and locally advanced prostate cancer. *Eur Urol* 1998;33(5):447–456.

60 Klotz L, Boccon-Gibod L, Shore ND, *et al.* The efficacy and safety of degarelix: a 12-month, comparative, randomized, open-label, parallel-group phase III study in patients with prostate cancer. *BJU Int* 2008;102(11):1531–1538.

## CHAPTER 7

# Active Surveillance in the Management of Low-Risk Prostate Cancer

*L. Boccon-Gibod*

Department of Urology, CHU Bichat, Paris, France

## Introduction

The incidence of low-risk prostate cancer, defined with clinical stage T1-T2a, prostate-specific antigen (PSA) $< 10$ ng/mL, and Gleason score 6 or less, has dramatically risen recently due to the increase in PSA testing, and extensive prostate biopsy techniques triggered at low PSA levels (2.5 ng/mL); in parallel, extensive clinical research has demonstrated that the great majority of patients with low-risk prostate cancer die with, rather than from, the disease; in this setting, the limited benefits of radical therapy are offset by significant side effects [1, 2].

The concept of active surveillance (AS) with delayed treatment stems from these observations. It is completely different from the concept of watchful waiting which implies basically waiting for symptoms, essentially of clinical metastatic disease, to occur before treatment is offered. AS implies close monitoring of the patient so that progression from low- to high-risk disease can be detected in time to switch to active treatment at a time when it will keep its efficacy.

The major issues associated with AS are those of eligibility criteria both to start and to maintain AS, to avoid missing high-risk disease at onset, and further progression of low- to high-risk cancer during surveillance.

*Prostate Cancer: Diagnosis and Clinical Management*, First Edition.
Edited by Ashutosh K. Tewari, Peter Whelan and John D. Graham.
© 2014 John Wiley & Sons, Ltd. Published 2014 by John Wiley & Sons, Ltd.

## Patient selection

The ideal candidates for AS are patients with low-risk prostate cancer and potentially "insignificant/indolent" tumors: PT2, organ confined, Gleason score 6, no secondary or tertiary Gleason score 4 or 5, index tumor volume $<1.3$ cm$^3$, total tumor volume $<2.5$ cm$^3$ [3]. Although age of over 65 years may be considered, there is no obvious reason to deny AS to younger men, bearing in mind that the younger the patient, the higher the likelihood of delayed therapy.

Interestingly, there are as many sets of selection criteria as there are studies in the literature (Table 7.1): ranging from stringent such as the Hopkins criteria: T1, PSA $<$ 10 ng/mL, 2 positive cores or less, Gleason score 6 on $<50\%$ of the cores and a PSA density (PSAD) of $<0.15$, to more lax criteria such as those from Toronto: PSA up to 15 ng/mL, T2a, Gleason score $3 + 4 \ldots$ [4].

Iremashvili [5], after an extensive study of a PSA era series of radical prostatectomies, has recently shown that among the five different sets of criteria currently published, the most efficient in the prediction of indolent tumors were those of the Miami group: PSA $<$ 15 ng/mL, 2 positive cores or less, Gleason score 6, $<20\%$ cancer in cores; and those of the Prostate Cancer Research International Active Surveillance (PRIAS): clinical stage T1c-T2a; PSA $<$ 10 ng/mL, PSAD $<$ 0.20, 1 or 2 positive cores with Gleason score 6 adenocarcinoma [6].

It should be stressed that whatever the stringency of these criteria, they are based on suboptimal tools: the sensitivity and specificity of digital rectal examination (DRE) is limited, PSA is not a tumor marker, and transrectal ultrasound (TRUS)–guided biopsy remains a blind procedure targeting the gland but unable to visualize the tumor and failing to reach areas where significant tumors can develop such as the anterior zone. The limitations of the diagnostic tools explain the partially suboptimal results of the currently published series.

## Patient monitoring

Once the patient has been considered eligible for AS, there arises the critical issue of monitoring: when and how to monitor the patient in order to ascertain that he remains eligible for AS or requires active treatment because of tumor progression. Once again, there are as many monitoring protocols and triggers for intervention as there are published studies: the

**Table 7.1** Summary of surveillance studies in Reference 4

| Institution | Principal investigator | Most recent reports | Total no.[a] | Strict no.[b] | Median age (years) | Inclusion criteria |
|---|---|---|---|---|---|---|
| Royal Marsden | Parker | 2007 | 326 | 326 | 67 | Gleason $\leq$ 3 + 4; PSA $\leq$ 15 ng/mL; cT stage $\leq$ 2a; $\leq$50% of cores positive |
| University of Miami | Soloway | 2010 | 230 | 230 | 64 | Gleason $\leq$ 6; PSA $\leq$ 10 ng/mL; cT stage $\leq$ 2; $\leq$two cores; $\leq$20% of any core positive |
| Johns Hopkins | Carter | 2011 | 769 | 633 | 66 | Gleason $\leq$ 3 + 3; PSAD $\leq$ 0.15 ng/mL/mL; cT stage 1; $\leq$ two cores positive; $\leq$50% of any core positive |
| University of California San Francisco | Carroll | 2011 | 640 | 376 | 62 | Gleason $\leq$ 3 + 3; PSA $\leq$ 10 ng/mL; cT stage $\leq$ 2; $\leq$33% of cores positive; $\leq$50% of any core positive |
| University of Toronto | Klotz | 2010 | 453 | 453 | 70 | Gleason $\leq$6; PSA $\leq$ 10 ng/mL (until January 2000, for men age > 70 years: Gleason $\leq$3 + 4; PSA $\leq$ 15 ng/mL) |
| European Randomized Study of Screening for Prostate Cancer Sites | Schröder | 2009 | 988 | 616 | 66 | Gleason $\leq$3 + 3; PSA $\leq$ 10 ng/mL; PSAD $\leq$ 0.2 ng/mL/mL; cT stage 1c to 2; $\leq$ two cores positive |
| Memorial-Sloan Kettering | Eastham | 2011 | 238 | 238 | 64 | Gleason $\leq$3 + 3; PSA $\leq$ 10 ng/mL; cT stage $\leq$ 2a; $\leq$ three cores positive; $\leq$50% of any core positive |
| Total | | | 3644 | 2872 | 67 | |

*Source:* Reproduced from Reference 4 with permission from American Society of Clinical Oncology.

cT, clinical tumor; PSA, prostate-specific antigen; PSAD, prostate-specific antigen density.

[a]Total no. indicates total number of men undergoing surveillance.

[b]Strict no. is number reported who met institutional criteria for surveillance. In all cases, outcomes reported are based on Strict no.

Toronto group [7] and the PROTecT study rely only on PSA kinetics such as PSA doubling time (PSADT) or PSA velocity (PSAV). Other groups such as Hopkins [8], Miami [9], and PRIAS [6] require routine repeat biopsies at different intervals. The monitoring tools have the same pitfalls as the ones used for initial selection: PSA kinetics has been shown not to correlate with subsequent biopsy results, the limitations of which have been alluded to above.

## Current results of AS with delayed treatment

In spite of all the drawbacks associated with patient selection and monitoring, there is no doubt that AS has gained a prominent place in the management of low-risk prostate cancer as demonstrated by the consistency of the results of the different published studies: in May 2012, over 2800 patients had been reported [4] with a median follow-up, ranging from 2 to 7 years. The results observed are shown in Table 7.2.

The conversion to active therapy occurs in 15–30% of the patients, 80% of the conversions are due to progression in PSA kinetics or biopsy features: upgrading to Gleason grade 4 (mostly 3 + 4) or upstaging: increase of positive cores or percent of invaded tissue. It is worth noting that 25–30% of pathologic progressions occur at the first or second repeat biopsy suggesting that undergrading/understaging in fact occurred at the time of the initial biopsy. The remaining 20% of conversions relate to patient's wish [4, 6, 8–10], often motivated by anxiety related to the knowledge of harboring an untreated malignancy, or to the repeat biopsies and associated discomfort, as well as potentially significant side effects [11].

The percentage of PT3 at surgery ranges from 14% to 50% (the latter figure due to initially lax selection criteria from the Toronto group) [7]. Several groups have shown that there was no difference in PSA relapse at 1 year whether patients were operated on at diagnosis or at progression after AS [8, 12]:

The PSADT is superior to 10 years in 45% of the patients.

Metastases occur in 0–0.5% of the patients.

The overall survival ranges from 78.5% to 100%.

The prostate-cancer-specific survival ranges from 98% to 100%.

A decision model analysis performed by the Hopkins group [13] has shown that AS offered a significant benefit for men aged 74 years in excellent health, 65 years in medium health, and 54 years in poor health, regarding overall, cancer-specific survival and quality of life (QOL).

**Table 7.2** Results of surveillance studies in Reference 4

| Institution | Median follow-up (months) | Progress by grade/volume (%) | Progress by PSA/PSA kinetics (%) | Treatment without progression (%) | OS | CSS | PFS |
|---|---|---|---|---|---|---|---|
| Royal Marsden | 22 | 13 | 18 | 2 | 98 | 100 | 73 |
| University of Miami | 32 | 10 | NR | NR | 100 | 100 | 86 |
| Johns Hopkins | 32 | 14 | NR[a] | 9 | 98 | 100 | 54 |
| University of California San Francisco | 47 | 35 | 5 of 11[b] | 8 | 97 | 100 | 54 |
| University of Toronto | 82 | 9[c] | 14[c] | 3 | 68 | 97 | 70 |
| European Randomized Study of Screening for Prostate Cancer Sites | 52 | NR[d] | 13 | 18 | 91 | 99 | 68 |
| Memorial-Sloan Kettering | 22 | 13 | 14 | 11 | NA | NA | NA |

Source: Reproduced from Reference 4 with permission from American Society of Clinical Oncology.

Outcomes given reflect those for men meeting criteria for surveillance at each institution. University of California San Francisco and Johns Hopkins have reported outcomes for men with higher-risk disease (i.e., those not meeting criteria); these are not included in the table but are discussed in text. All progression/survival figures are raw, not actuarial.

CSS, prostate cancer-specific survival; NA, not applicable; NR, not reported; OS, overall survival; PFS, progression-free survival; PSA, prostate-specific antigen.

[a]Johns Hopkins studies do not use PSA-based definition of progression, but PSA outcomes for cohort have been reported in detail.

[b]Progression based on PSA doubling time <24 months/<36 months.

[c]Figures for University of Toronto do not include those who progressed but continued undergoing surveillance.

[d]Repeat biopsy information reported for only subset (23%) of European Randomized Study of Screening for Prostate Cancer cohort.

Finally, two issues remain to be considered: health-related quality of life (HRQOL) and costs induced by the adoption of AS.

As far as HRQOL is concerned, several studies did not show any deterioration with AS, and psychological distress within the time frame of the published studies does not appear to be significant. However, this may change with prolonged follow-up [4, 14].

Regarding costs, observational as well as modeling studies show that the estimated cost of AS over the long term was the lowest compared to the costs of immediate active treatment, be it surgery, radiation, or brachy therapy. Furthermore, AS is associated with more quality-adjusted life years than immediate treatment with similar or lower lifetime costs [15].

Undoubtedly, these results prove the validity of the concept of AS in the setting of low-risk prostate cancer; however, they definitely leave ample room for improvement which will come from the reevaluation of biological data previously collected, and more importantly from the dramatic progress in imaging techniques and molecular markers.

## Future improvements in selection and monitoring of patients offered AS

There is increasing evidence that the 25–30% progression rate at repeat biopsy implies that the tools currently used to characterize a prostate cancer as low risk are at best suboptimal.

The reevaluation of previously collected data can help to adjust the selection criteria:

The number of positive cores: 1 versus 2 appears to be a strong predictor of progression/reclassification in the PRIAS study [6].

PSAD is also a strong determinant: the currently accepted threshold value of 0.15 should probably be lowered to 0.08 as shown by the Hopkins group [16].

New molecular markers such as PCa.3 or the ratio pro-PSA/%free PSA may in the future yield promising results. Much is awaited in the future of molecular studies performed on the material collected and centrally analyzed from large cohorts of patients prospectively studied [4].

An improvement in ultrasound-guided biopsy techniques is undoubtedly necessary:

A confirmation TRUS-guided biopsy is considered by several authors as necessary [3]: even if a standard adequate 12 cores protocol has been used initially, a significant number of patients will then be reclassified as intermediate or high risk and proceed to active treatment. Nevertheless, the limitations of the current TRUS-guided biopsy, even the most extensive saturation ones, are well known: what is visible is the gland rather than the tumor, the precise determination of the biopsy sites to compare with future biopsies is not easy; the sampling of the anterior zone may be awkward in the presence of significant prostate enlargement.

Several groups have underlined the inadequacy of the traditional 12 cores protocol when compared to three-dimensional trans-perineal mapping (3D-TPM) [17].

Performed under general anesthesia, 3D-TPM will increase the number of cores up to 60. Such a wide systematic template-based sampling can lead to upgrading/staging of the tumor in 30–50% of the cases in relation to more accurate evaluation and sampling of the entire gland and particularly the anterior zone. However, the invasiveness and side effects, and not to mention the cost of the procedure, should not be underestimated [3].

The recent and ongoing dramatic improvements in imaging may in fact give an answer to these difficulties: multiparametric magnetic resonance imaging (MP-MRI) [18, 19] using a 3 T magnet and an endorectal coil; combined T1- and T2-weighted MRI and functional sequences the latter mostly useful to detect suspicious areas in the prostate (as well as extraprostatic extension); diffusion-weighted MRI (DW-MRI) with determination of the apparent diffusion coefficient (ADC); dynamic contrast-enhanced (DCE) MRI using gadolinium; and eventually MRI choline spectroscopy. The combination of these different techniques has a very high yield of cancer detection and can be used, alone or in combination with ultrasound, to guide targeted biopsies [20] with greater accuracy. MP-MRI is not only useful for diagnostic purposes, there is an increasing body of evidence demonstrating that based on the careful analysis of the various sequences of DW-MRI and DCE-MRI, it may predict the degree of aggressiveness of the tumor detected [19].

Consequently the future developments of modern MRI may hopefully lead to the preferential use of targeted biopsies to select the patients for AS, with further follow-up based on MP-MRI [21].

## Conclusions

AS represents a valuable option in the management of low-risk prostate cancer, however several key points cannot be underestimated:

1 The long-term results of AS remain, at this point in time, unknown as the longest available follow-up is less than 10 years, which considering the natural history of localized prostate cancer is undoubtedly short.

2 Consequently, the decision to offer and implement AS cannot be considered outside a structured program requiring the collaboration of a significant number of dedicated healthcare professionals: not only urologists but also uro-radiologists, uro-pathologists, and nurse specialists as well as a strong secretarial support to keep track of the patients; outside such a setting the adoption of AS may be fraught with many problems such as suboptimal patient selection and follow-up, potentially detrimental to the patients and leading to the eventual discredit of AS.

3 The selection criteria must be strict and characteristic of low-risk prostate cancer. Eventually elderly, frail patients with intermediate-risk disease may be offered AS but only after a full explanation of the issues related to the method.

4 The patient and the urologist must adhere to the rigorous monitoring which should be very clearly explained.

With these caveats AS should, at least, be offered to every patient with low-risk prostate cancer. Currently, although low-risk disease accounts for roughly 45% of the cases, only 15–20% of the patients are offered AS in the United States; in Europe through the use of a multidisciplinary approach this figure can be as high as 60–70% [6, 22], underlining once again the importance of the "team approach" in the management of this disease.

## References

1 Lu-Yao GL, Albertsen PC, Moore DF, *et al*. Outcomes of localized prostate cancer following conservative management. *J Am Med Assoc* 2009;302:1202–1209.

2 Wilt TJ, Brawer MK, Jones KM, *et al*. Radical prostatectomy versus observation. *N Eng J Med* 2012;367:203–213.

3 Lees K, Durve M, Parker C. Active surveillance in prostate cancer: patient selection and triggers for intervention. *Curr Opin Urol* 2012;22:210–2315.

4 Cooperberg MR, Carroll PR, Klotz L. Active surveillance for prostate cancer: progress and promises. *J Clin Oncol* 2011;29:3669–3676.

5 Iremashvili V, Pelaez l, Manoharan M, *et al*. Pathologic prostate cancer characteristicsin patients eligible for active surveillance: a head to head comparison of cotemporary protocols. *Eur Urol* 2012;62:462–468.

6 Bangma CH, Bul M, Roobol M. The prostate cancer research international: active surveillance study. *Curr Opin Urol* 2012;22:216-221.

7 Klotz L. Active surveillance: the canadian experience. *Curr Opin Urol* 2012;22:222–230.

8 Tosoian JJ, Trock BJ, Landis P, *et al.* Active surveillance program for prostate cancer: an update of the Johns Hopkins experience. *J Clin Oncol* 2011;29:2185–2190.

9 Iremashvili V, Soloway MS, Rosenberg DL. Clinical and demographic characteristics associated with prostate cancer progression in patients on active surveillance. *J Urol* 2012;187:1594–1600.

10 Porten SP, Whitson JM, Cowan Je, *et al.* changes in prostate cancer grade on serial biopsy in men undergoing active surveillance. *J Clin Oncol* 2011;29:2795–2800.

11 Carignan A, Roussy JF, Lapointe V, *et al.* Increasing risk of infectious complications after trans-rectal ultrasound-guided prostate biopsies: time to reassess anti microbial prophylaxis? *Eur Urol* 2012;62:453–459.

12 Bul M, Zhu X, Ranniko A, *et al.* Radical prostatectomy for low risk prostate cancer following active surveillance: results from a prospective observational study. *Eur Urol* 2012;62:195–200.

13 Liu D, Lehmann HP, Frick KD, *et al.* Active surveillance versus surgery for low risk prostate cancer: a clinical decision analysis. *J Urol* 2012;187:1241–1246.

14 Van den Bergh RCN, Korfage IJ, Bangma CH. Psychological aspects of active surveillance. *Curr Opin Urol* 2012;22:237–242.

15 Kim SI, Dall'Era MA, Evans CP. Economic analysis of active surveillance for localized prostate cancer. *Curr Opin Urol* 2012;22:247–253.

16 Tseng K, Landis P, Epstein J, *et al.* Risk stratification of men choosing surveillance for low risk prostate cancer. *J Urol* 2010;189:1779–1785.

17 Barzell WE, Melamed MR, Cathcart P, *et al.* Identifying candidates for active surveillance: an evaluation of the repeat biopsy strategy for men with favorable risk prostate cancer. *J Urol* 2012;188:762–768.

18 Ouzzane A, Puech P, Villers A. MRI and surveillance. *Curr Opin Urol* 2012;22:231–236.

19 Turkbey B, Choyke PL. Multiparametric MRI and prostate cancer diagnosis and risk stratification. *Curr Opin Urol* 2012;22:310–315.

20 Futterer JG, Barentsz JO. MRI guided and robotic – assisted prostate biopsy. *Curr Opin Urol* 2012;22:316–331.

21 Margel D, Yap SA, Lawrentschuk N, *et al.* Impact of multiparametric endorectal coil prostate magnetic resonance imaging on disease reclassification among active surveillance candidates: a prospective cohort study. *J Urol* 2012;187:1247–1252.

22 Aizer AA, Paly JJ, Zietman AL, *et al.* Multidisciplinary care and pursuit of active surveillance in low risk prostate cancer. *J Clil Oncol* 2012;30:3071–3076.

# CHAPTER 8

# Radical Surgery*

*Adnan Ali and Ashutosh Tewari*

Center for Prostate Cancer, Weill Cornell Medical College, New York Presbyterian Hospital, New York, NY

## Introduction

Radical surgery for clinically localized prostate cancer has come a long way since the first radical perinial prostatectomy was performed by H. Young in 1905 [1]. In 1947, Millin described the retropubic approach for radical prostatectomy (RP) which allowed access to pelvic lymph nodes for tumor staging [2]. Around 1980s, careful anatomical studies led to the development of modified radical retropubic prostatectomy (RRP) with better understanding of dorsal venous complex (DVC) [3], neurovascular bundles (NVBs) [4], and striated urinary sphincter [5]. This anatomical approach decreased intraoperative blood loss, preserved potency, and decreased urinary incontinence [6, 7]. In 1997, Schuessler performed the first laparoscopic radical prostatectomy (LRP) [8]. Over the next decade, advancement in optics, digital video, and computers and robotics led to further refinement of laparoscopic technique by Abbou and Guillonneau and Vallancien in 2000 [9, 10]. In May 2000, Binder and Kramer performed the first robot-assisted laparoscopic prostatectomy (RALP) using da Vinci Surgical System (Intuitive Surgical, Mountain View, CA) [11].

---

*Dr. Ashutosh Tewari discloses that he is the principal investigator on research grants from Intuitive Surgical, Inc. (Sunnyvale, CA) and Boston Scientific Corporation; he is a noncompensated director of Prostate Cancer Institute (Pune, India) and Global Prostate Cancer Research Foundation; he has received research funding from the LeFrak Family Foundation Prostate Cancer Foundation, Mr and Mrs Paul Kanavos, Craig Effron and Company, Charles Evans Foundation, and Christian and Heidi Lange Family Foundation.

---

The first-generation da Vinci Surgical System had three robotic arms, two for instruments and one for endoscope. Using this master–slave surgical system, surgeons were able to view the surgical field three-dimensionally in 10× magnification using stereo-endoscope lens and camera, and surgical instrument tips had a 360° range of movement. Later in 2002, Menon *et al.* described the surgical technique and reported outcomes following RALP [12, 13]. By 2008, greater than 60% of RPs in the United States were RALP [14].

The primary goal of RP is cancer extirpation, while the secondary goals are preservation of urinary continence and potency. The periprostatic space contains nerves, vessels, lymphatics, fat loose areolar and connective tissue in 3–5 mm condensed as fascial layers. Over the last few decades, better anatomic understanding of the periprostatic space and due to improved magnification of the surgical field, the previously binary decision of nerve sparing (NS) and non-nerve sparing can now be an incremental process [4, 15–19]. This risk-stratified approach allows an appropriate balance between NS and oncological efficacy of the procedure. The key developments that led to this are as follows: (a) preoperative risk stratification allowing us to group patients into four (rather than two) groups with incremental risk in incidence of extraprostatic extension (EPE) [20]; (b) anatomic studies clarified the periprostatic space anatomy and also established that these nerves are organized as a hammock of interconnected nerves, ganglions, arteries, and veins [21]; (c) the anatomic studies also clarified that nerves are mostly lateral to the veins and capsular arteries which can serve as landmark during surgery [19, 22]; (d) the use of high-resolution, 3 T multiparametric endorectal magnetic resonance imaging (eMRI) for risk stratification and study of periprostatic space and surgical planning in patients not contraindicated for multiparametric MRI using endorectal coil [23].

## Types of surgery

Radical prostatectomy (RP) is the removal of prostate gland and seminal vesicles. Prostatectomy is a common treatment for patients having clinically localized cancer or in patients who have failed to respond to radiation therapy (salvage prostatectomy). Depending on the approach chosen and the type of technique, following are the types of surgeries:
1 Open approaches
   a Radical retropubic prostatectomy—This is done using an infraumbilical midline or transverse incision usually 8–10 cm in length.

**b** Radical perineal prostatectomy—This is done using a curvilinear incision in the perineum between the scrotum and the anus starting and ending just medial to ischial tuberosities on either side. This approach is used less often.

**2** Minimally invasive approaches

   **a** Laparoscopic radical prostatectomy—Access to the abdomen is gained through creation of laparoscopic ports and pneumoperitoneum is created. The surgery is carried out using laparoscopic instruments inserted through these ports while visualizing the surgical field using a laparoscope.

   **b** Robot-assisted laparoscopic radical prostatectomy—It is similar to the laparoscopic approach with the addition of a robotic interface. The surgeon sits on the surgical console and controls robotic arms with robotic instruments to perform the surgery. This provides the surgeon with greater maneuverability and enhanced vision of the surgical field in three dimension and magnification. The transperitoneal anterior approach is described in detail in this chapter.

## Patient selection

The indications for RALP are similar to that for open RP, that is, patients with clinical stage T2 or less with no evidence of metastasis either clinically or radiographically (computed tomography (CT) and bone scan). Severe cardiopulmonary disease and uncorrectable bleeding diatheses are absolute contraindications for RALP.

## Preoperative workup

A complete history and physical examination including a digital rectal examination (DRE) is done. Serum PSA is drawn. Transrectal-ultrasound-guided prostate needle biopsy is used for diagnosis of prostate cancer. Additionally, a targeted fusion biopsy may also be done in selected cases. The 3 T multiparametric eMRI findings are used in patients when eMRI is not contraindicated. These findings help in better surgical planning and tuning the procedure to each individual patient's unique requirement based on preoperative disease characteristics and MRI findings. These findings are reviewed before the procedure starts and are kept handy during the procedure to make informed surgical decisions.

## Instrumentation

### Port access

1 Versaport Plus bladeless (5–12 mm) (Covidien, Dublin, Ireland)
2 Versaport bladeless (5 mm) (Covidien)
3 Endopath® dilating tip trocar and housing (10/12 mm) (Ethicon, Somerville, NJ)
4 Dilating tip (Cardinal Health, Dublin, OH)

### Robotic instruments

1 da Vinci Surgical System (Intuitive Surgical, Sunnyvale, CA)
2 InSite Vision System da Vinci robotic 0-degree and 30-degree scopes (Intuitive Surgical, Sunnyvale, CA)
3 Endowrist Maryland bipolar forceps (Intuitive Surgical, Sunnyvale, CA)
4 Endowrist curved monopolar scissors (Intuitive Surgical, Sunnyvale, CA)
5 Endowrist ProGrasp forceps (Intuitive Surgical, Sunnyvale, CA)
6 Endowrist needle drivers (Intuitive Surgical, Sunnyvale, CA)
7 New robotic fourth arm and accessories
8 Karl Storz robotic urology instrument tray (Karl Storz GmbH, Tuttlingen, Germany)

### Conventional instruments (disposable)

1 Hydroline trumpet valve with pulsewave cassette (Cardinal Health)
2 Weck Hem-o-lok clips (Teleflex Medical, Research Triangle Park, NC)
3 Endoscopic needles—Polysorb (Covidien)
4 Biosyn sutures (Cardinal Health)
5 Endo Catch Gold (10 mm) (Covidien)
6 Endo Shears (5 mm) (Covidien)
7 V-Loc 26 mm sutures (Covidien)
8 Chromic Gut V-20 (26 mm) (Covidien)
9 Sofsilk cutting (26 mm) (Covidien)
10 Maxon sutures (40 mm) (Covidien)

## Positioning

After induction of general anesthesia the patient is placed in steep Trendelenberg position. The patient's arms are tucked and padded at the sides.

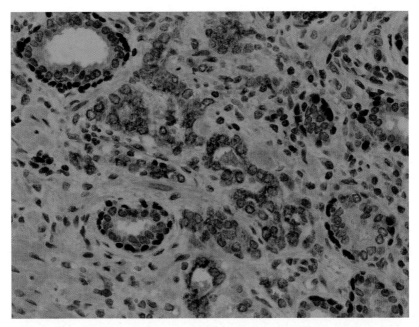

**Plate 3.1** Immunohistochemistry for AMACR and p63: The benign glands around the edge have basal cells that show nuclear staining for p63 (brown), the cancer glands centrally lack these basal cells but show positive staining for AMACR (red).

*Prostate Cancer: Diagnosis and Clinical Management*, First Edition.
Edited by Ashutosh K. Tewari, Peter Whelan and John D. Graham.
© 2014 John Wiley & Sons, Ltd. Published 2014 by John Wiley & Sons, Ltd.

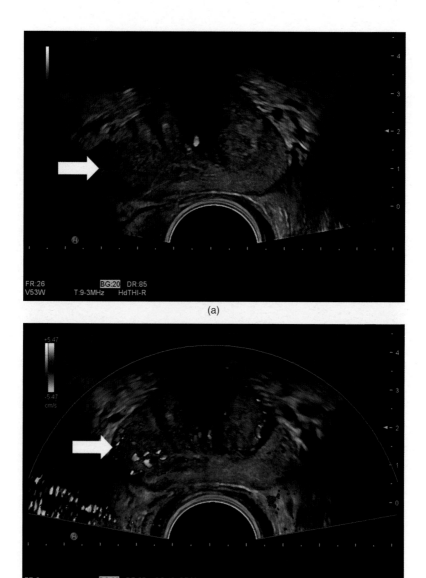

(a)

(b)

**Plate 5.3** Prostate cancer (arrows) Gleason 7 (3 + 4) biopsy confirmed on (a) grayscale, (b) color Doppler.

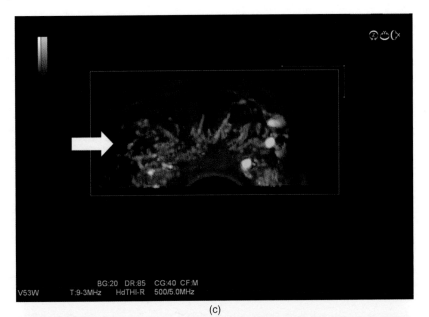

(c)

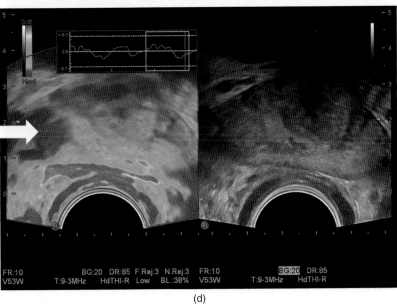

(d)

**Plate 5.3** (*Continued*) (c) 3D color Doppler, (d) seen as an area of increased stiffness on elastography.

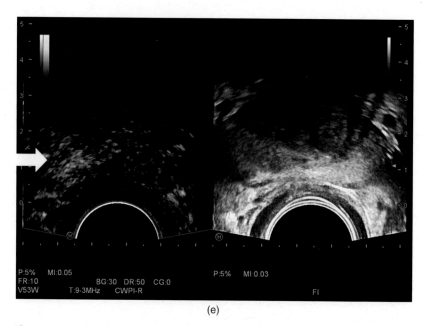

**Plate 5.3** (*Continued*) (e) as a focal enhancing lesion following intravenous Sonovue (Bracco, Italy) microbubbles using microbubble-specific imaging. Prostate cancer right mid zone shown as a focal enhancing lesion following intravenous Sonovue (Bracco, Italy) microbubbles using microbubble-specific imaging. Biopsy confirmed a Gleason 7 (3 + 4) prostate cancer.

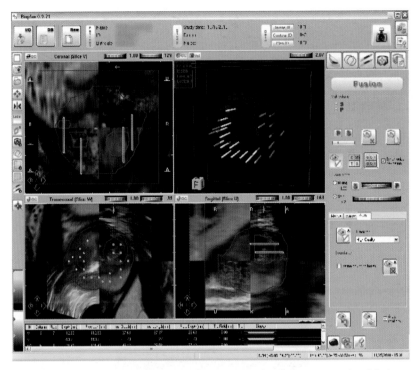

**Plate 5.5** Fusion of mpMRI dataset on TRUS as part of real-time transperineal fusion biopsy of focal lesions of the prostate gland detected on mpMRI.

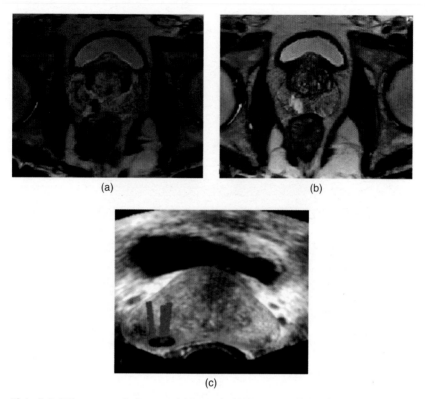

(a)    (b)

(c)

**Plate 5.6** MR transrectal ultrasound (TRUS) fusion image. (a, b) Multiparametric axial MR images with functional information (related to diffusion-weighted MRI) identifying a cancer (arrowheads) not visible on TRUS (study not shown). (c) Fused dataset, superimposing after coregistering the MR images that identify the tumor based on its reduced diffusion onto the real-time TRUS images. The red bars represent biopsy trajectories. Biopsy directed by the TRUS revealed a Gleason 7 cancer. Courtesy of Dr Erik Rud, Oslo University Hospital, Oslo, Norway.

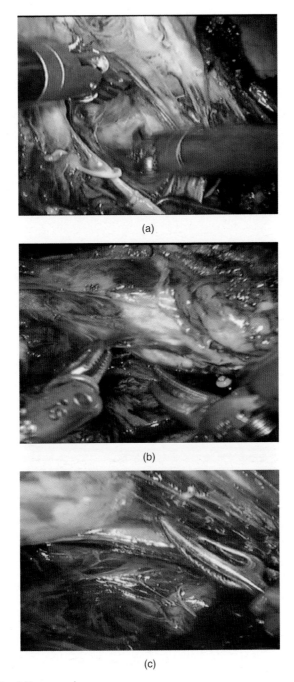

(a)

(b)

(c)

**Plate 8.1** (a–c) Nerve sparing.

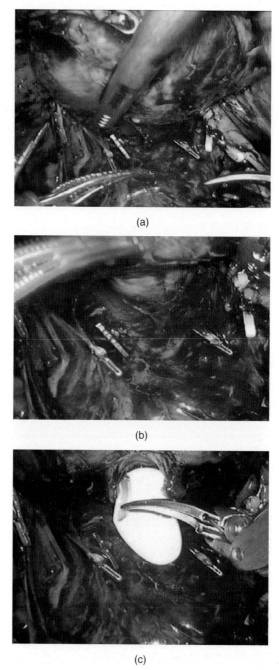

**Plate 8.2** Circumapical dissection. (a) Posterior aspect of the prostate gland. (b) Clearly visible urethra. (c) Foley catheter tip being pulled posterior to the urethra.

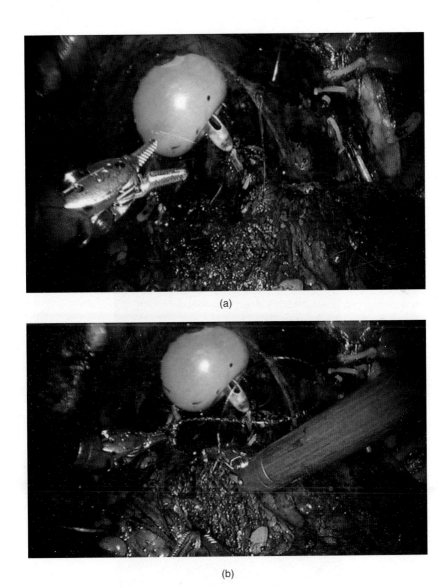

(a)

(b)

**Plate 8.3** (a,b) Dynamic detrusor cuff trigonoplasty.

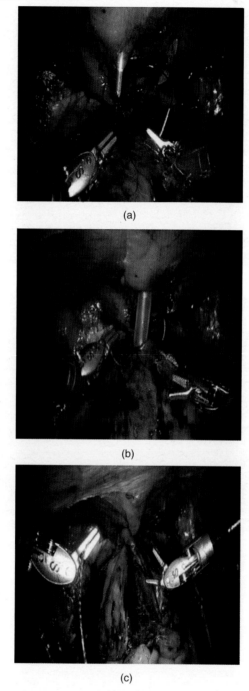

(a)

(b)

(c)

**Plate 8.4** (a–c) Suprapubic catheter placement.

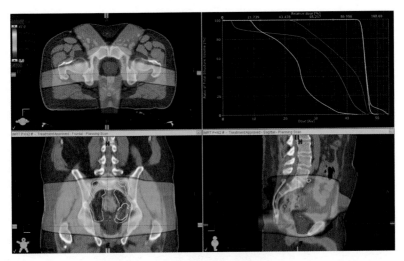

**Plate 9.2** The top left and bottom two images represent the color wash dose distributions from an IMRT prostate and pelvic lymph node radiotherapy plan. The top right image shows the corresponding dose–volume histogram for the plan. Note the increased number of beams which has allowed a higher level of conformity around the prostate gland.

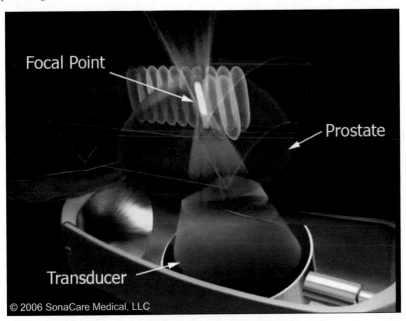

Focal Point

Prostate

Transducer

© 2006 SonaCare Medical, LLC

**Plate 10.3** Ultrasonic waves generated with transducer are focused onto a target area with focal lengths of either 3.0 or 4.0 cm. The intervening tissue and surrounding areas remain undamaged as the secondary intensity is low. Used with permission from Sonacare Medical.

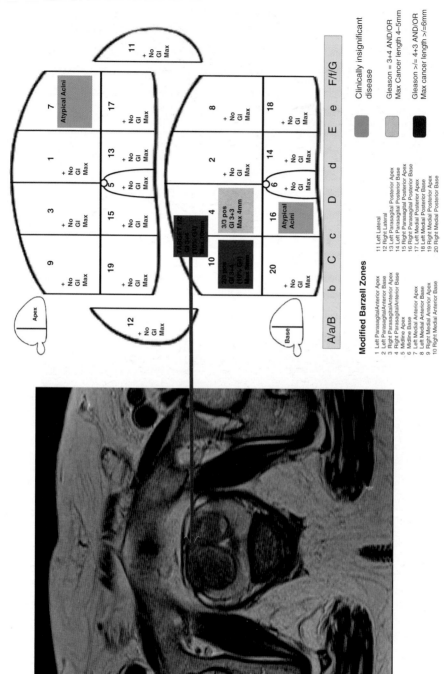

**Modified Barzell Zones**

1 Left ParasagitalAnterior Apex
2 Left ParasagitalAnterior Base
3 Right ParasagitalAnterior Apex
4 Right ParasagitalAnterior Base
5 Midline Apex
6 Midline Base
7 Left Medial Anterior Apex
8 Left Medial Anterior Base
9 Right Medial Anterior Apex
10 Right Medial Anterior Base

11 Left Lateral
12 Right Lateral
13 Left Parasagital Posterior Apex
14 Left Parasagital Posterior Base
15 Right Parasagital Posterior Apex
16 Right Parasagital Posterior Base
17 Left Medial Posterior Apex
18 Left Medial Posterior Base
19 Right Medial Posterior Apex
20 Right Medial Posterior Base

Clinically insignificant disease

Gleason = 3+4 AND/OR
Max Cancer length 4–5mm

Gleason >/= 4+3 AND/OR
Max cancer length >/=6mm

**Plate 10.4** Right anterior location of a tumor (*red arrow*) on multiparametric MRI and TPM biopsy in a man who subsequently underwent focal HIFU.

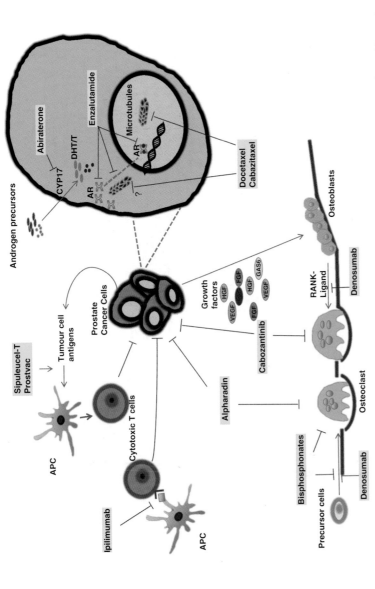

**Plate 14.1** Targets of current/emerging treatments for advanced prostate cancer. Abiraterone, CYP17 inhibitor; enzalutamide, antiandrogen, blocks AR shuttling into the nucleus, blocks interaction of activated AR with DNA; denosumab, RANK-ligand inhibitor; bisphosphonates, microtubule inhibitors, potentially also block AR shuttling into the nucleus; denosumab, RANK-ligand inhibitor; bisphosphonates, antiresorptive activity by osteoclast inhibition; alpharadin, α-radiation emitting radioisotope; cabozantinib, c-MET and VEGFR2 inhibitor; sipuleucel-T and PROSTVAC, vaccine therapies; ipilimumab, anti-CTLA-4 antibody. APC, antigen-presenting cell; DHT, dihydrotestosterone; T, testosterone; HGF, hepatocyte growth factor; FGF, fibroblast growth factor; IGF-1, insulin-like growth factor; VEGF, vascular endothelial growth factor; GAS6, growth arrest-specific 6.

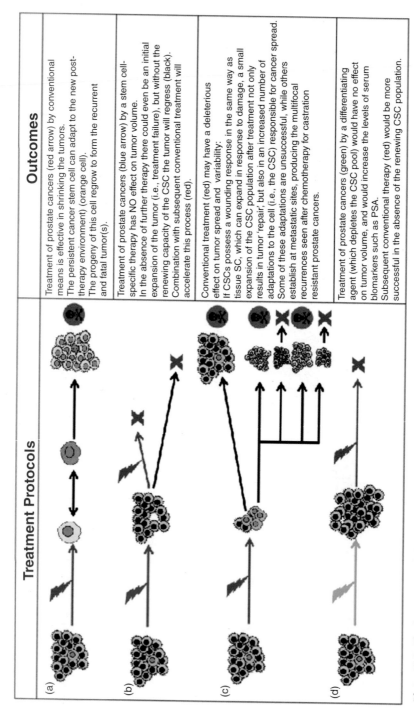

**Plate 17.2** The importance of the timing of treatments to account for the existence of cancer stem cells.

The patient's legs are abducted and secured on a split leg table. Orogastric tube and urethral catheter are placed using aseptic precautions to decompress the stomach and bladder, respectively.

## Port placement

A Veress needle inserted infraumbilicaly is used for creating a pneumoperitoneum. After adequate insufflation, trocar placement is done, beginning with a 12 mm trocar placed supraumbilically or at umbilicus for the placement of stereoscopic endoscope. Five trocars, three for robotic arms and two for assistants are placed. First, two 8 mm pararectus trocars for the robotic arms are placed on the right and the left side for the second and third robotic arms. Another 8 mm trocar is placed in the left lumbar region for the fourth arm of the robot. Additionally, 12 mm and 5 mm assistant ports are placed on the patient's right side, used to provide retraction, suction, irrigation, and passing clips and sutures. Following the placement of trocars, the da Vinci robot is placed between the patient's legs and the robotic arms are brought above the patient and docked.

## Surgical technique

Herein transperitoneal anterior approach for RALP is described.
1  Dropping the bladder.
   After gaining abdominal access of peritoneum, inspection is carried out, urachus and medial umbilical ligaments are identified, and adhesions are lysed, if present. Using monopolar cautery, a wide inverted U-shaped peritoneal incision is made. The incision starts lateral to the left medial umbilical ligament and extended anteromedially dividing the urachus in the midline to the right medial umbilical ligament. This U-shaped incision is then extended bilaterally to the vas deferns.

   Blunt and dissection are carried along the avascular plane within the space of Retzius to develop retropubic space. This exposes pubis, endopelvic fascia, bladder, prostate, and puboprostatic ligaments. Athermal dissection of the periprostatic space is carried out between the endopelvic fascia and lateral prostatic fascia. During development of the retropubic space and incision of the endopelvic fascia, we proceed distally and medially. Meticulous dissection is performed to minimize disruption of the puboprostatic ligaments and arcus tendineus until the urethra is exposed and there is a clear space for the placement of the dorsal venous stitch. The arcus tendineus and puboprostatic ligaments are used later in the anterior reconstruction.

2  Bladder neck dissection

A 30° downward angle lens is used for this part. The prostatovesical junction (PVJ) is identified by "bimanual bladder neck pinch" [24]. The prostate is trapped using blunt robotic instruments and pulled proximally until there is a sudden feeling of "giving way" at the junction with collapsed bladder. At this point, the PVJ can be easily identified. The surface is scored to precisely mark the PVJ anteriorly. The bladder neck is incised in the midline using Maryland bipolar forceps and hot shears with 1:1 scaling for adequate coagulation of any bleeders. Dissection proceeds until the Foley catheter is seen. The Foley balloon is deflated and the left-side assistant grasps the tip of the catheter with firm anterior traction. The dissection then proceeds laterally. Care is taken to maintain the appropriate plane of dissection. With traction on the shaft of the catheter, the exact location for the posterior incision becomes visible and the mucosa of the posterior bladder neck is now incised precisely. After dissection through the mucosa, the retrotrigonal fibromuscular layer is identified [25]. Beyond this plane, athermal dissection is carried out to preserve the neural hammock surrounding the prostate and the trigonal nerves until the shiny white surface of the vas deferens is seen.

3  Athermal dissection of seminal vesicles and vas deferens

After the bladder neck dissection, the seminal vesicles and vas deferens are identified and dissected one at a time using athermal technique, the ends are clipped and cut. The cut ends are lifted by the fourth arm of the robot. A plane is developed between the seminal vesicles and the surrounding fascia, arteries entering into the seminal vesicles are identified. These are cut using clips and sharp dissection. Lateral to the seminal vesicles, it is important to be aware of the proximity to the NVBs. Every attempt is made to preserve them. Both the seminal vesicles and vas deferens are then pulled upward. In patients who are appropriate candidates for NS, an intracompartmental seminal vesicle dissection is performed [26].

4  Nerve sparing (Figure 8.1, Plate 8.1)

Anatomic grades of nerve sparing (NS) technique strive to achieve the competing goals of cancer clearance and preservation of potency based on the patient's probability of ipsilateral EPE [20]. It is based on neurosurgical principles. The patient's PSA level, biopsy Gleason score, clinical

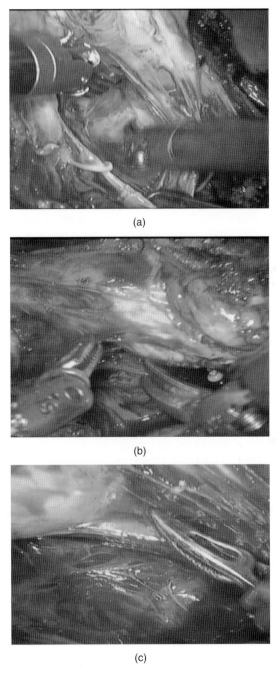

(a)

(b)

(c)

**Figure 8.1** (a–c) Nerve sparing. (See also Plate 8.1.)

stage, and findings on the eMRI parameters were used for risk stratification. Approach to athermal and traction-free NS during RALP involves varying degrees of preservation of the nerve fibers in the various fascial planes. They are described as follows:

- Grade 1 NS: The Denonvilliers' fascia and the later pelvic fascia (LPF) are incised just outside the prostatic capsule to preserve the neural hammock. We also describe this as medial venous plane for complete hammock preservation. This is the greatest degree of NS possible, and we perform this procedure for patients with no to minimal risk of EPE.
- Grade 2 NS: The Denonvilliers' fascia (leaving deeper layers on the rectum) and LPF are incised just outside the layer of veins of the prostate capsule. This allows the preservation of most large neural trunks and ganglia and is used for patients at low risk of EPE.
- Grade 3 NS (partial/incremental): Incision is made through the outer compartment of the LPF (leaving some yellow adipose and neural tissue on the specimen), excising all layers of Denonvilliers' fascia. This is performed for patients with moderate risk of EPE because some of the medial trunks are sacrificed, whereas the lateral trunks are preserved.
- Grade 4 NS (non-NS): These patients have high risk of EPE and are not candidates for NS. In such cases, we perform a wide excision of the LPF and Denonvilliers' fascia containing most of the periprostatic neurovascular tissue. In selected patients, we attempt nerve advancement of the identifiable ends of the NVBs.

These planes are developed athermally by sharp and blunt dissection, proceeding distally toward the apex and laterally on both sides. At the lateral attachments, the perforating arteries enter into the prostatic capsule. They are sharply cut after being secured by clips and the plane is created between the capsule and the medial aspect of the pedicular vessels [19, 27, 28].

5 Circumapical dissection of the urethra (Figure 8.2, Plate 8.2)
Prostatic apex is a frequent site of positive surgical margin (PSM). Therefore, extra care has to be taken during apical dissection. After the prostate is mobilized, it is lifted anteriorly and a plane is developed along the posterior surface of the prostate. At this time, the posterior prostatic apex is covered by a few layers of Denonvilliers' fascia and the rectourethralis muscle.

The prostate is lifted to develop a distinct plane between the prostatic apex and the urethra using blunt dissection. The apex is swept

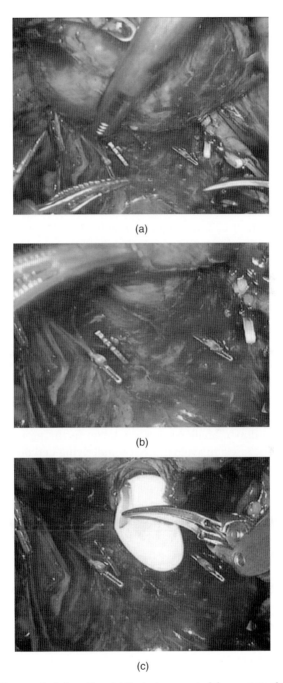

(a)

(b)

(c)

**Figure 8.2** Circumapical dissection. (a) Posterior aspect of the prostate gland. (b) Clearly visible urethra. (c) Foley catheter tip being pulled posterior to the urethra. (See also Plate 8.2.)

away from the urethra to gain 1–2 mm of ventral membranous urethral length prior to transection. The posterior hemicircumference of
the urethra is sharply incised and the Foley catheter tip is exposed.
The transection of the urethra is completed circumferentially via the
retro-apical approach [29]. After completing transection of the membranous urethra, the prostate is loosely attached by the DVC anteriorly
as the urethra has been cut posteriorly. After securing the prostate with
suture, we then use both blunt and sharp dissection to find the distinct
plane between the anterior prostatic apex and the membranous urethra.
The DVC is ligated using CT-1 needle and 0-polyglactin suture. Once
the prostate is free, lymph node dissection is done and the specimen is
bagged.

6  Dynamic detrusor cuff trigonoplasty (Figure 8.3, Plate 8.3)

The fourth arm of the robot is used to held anterior bladder and the
bladder opening, mucosa and uretric orifices are identified. A 4–0 Biosin
suture is used to close the posterior extent of the bladder opening using
a "tennis racquet" stitch. The mucosa is everted using the same suture
and the posterior gap is covered using a flap of detrusor muscle and
approximated in the midline using a 3–0 V-Lock suture to support the
bladder neck creating a dynamic detrusor cuff. This posterior reinforce-
ment is based on the principles of Pagano [30].

7  Posterior reconstruction

Few shallow bites are passed into the posterior aspect of Denonvilliers'
fascia and the same suture is passed through the retrotrigonal layer
and cinched down. Shallow bites are taken in the posterior aspect of
Denonvilliers' fascia to avoid injury to underlying nervous tissue.

8  Anastomosis and anterior repair

A two-layer anastomosis is completed by synchronized pull and push
technique to cinche the retrotrigonal layer close to rectourethralis using
a V-lock suture [31]. By proper mucosal approximation, tension-free
approximation and avoidance of NVBs, a secure water-tight anastomosis is created. The anterior reconstruction is done by suturing previously
preserved arcus tendinius to detrusor muscle using a single-knotted
suture [32]. This helps in positioning and stabilizing the vesico-urethral
junction.

9  Suprapubic catheter placement (Figure 8.4, Plate 8.4)

A suprapubic catheter is inserted into the bladder after it has been filled
with 180 mL of water. This helps in elevation of the bladder to its normal
preoperative position and also serves as a urinary diversion route in
cases in which we do not use a catheter [33]. Finally, reperitonization
is done to restore preoperative anatomy.

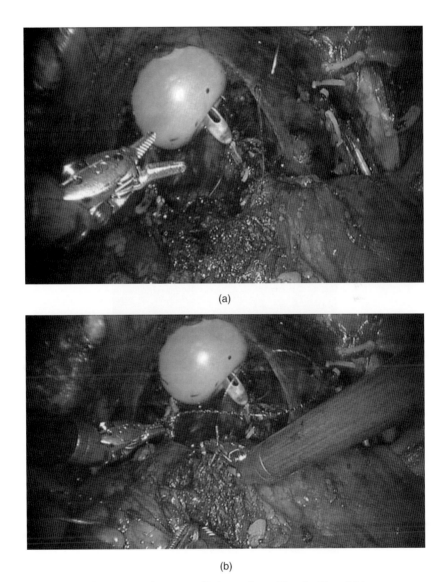

(a)

(b)

**Figure 8.3** (a,b) Dynamic detrusor cuff trigonoplasty. (See also Plate 8.3.)

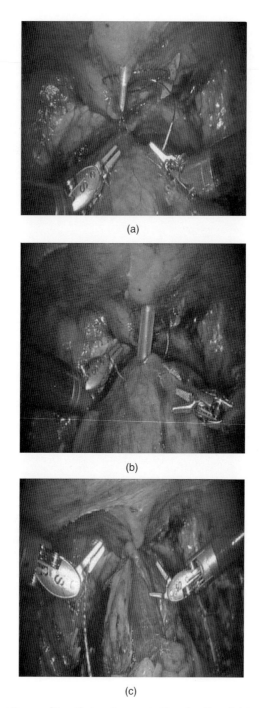

(a)

(b)

(c)

**Figure 8.4** (a–c) Suprapubic catheter placement. (See also Plate 8.4.)

## Postoperative management

Following surgery, the suprapubic catheter, bulb drain, and occasionally a Foley catheter are left in place. Postoperative pain is managed with parenteral narcotics. Early ambulation is encouraged to prevent deep venous thrombosis (DVT). The patient is started on a clear liquid diet and advanced as tolerated. Once the patient has been taught catheter care, is ambulatory, and tolerating oral pain medication, he is discharged. Patient returns 1 week after surgery for catheter removal. Patients then begin Kegel exercises.

## Complications

The perioperative complication rate for RALP ranges from 2.5% to 26%. [34].

The complications of radical surgery include

1 Hemorrhage

Hemorrhage had been a major concern for open surgery, but most studies show that for RALP and LRP, blood loss was about 50–200 mL during the procedure and the blood transfusion rate of 2% or less are commonly reported [35]. This decrease in blood loss is due to the tamponade effect of the pneumoperitoneum and improved visualization. The excessive bleeding generally is often due to the injury to DVC. Sometimes the superior epigastric artery can also be injured during trocar insertion. Increasing the pneumoperitoneum pressure could minimize minor bleeding [36].

2 Rectal injury

The incidence of rectal injury during LRP and RALP varies from 0.7% to 2.4% and can be managed successfully without open conversion [37, 38]. Rectal injuries may occur with large prostates, with inflammation and scarred tissue between the anterior rectal wall and the Denonvilliers' fascia. The injuries may occure during dissection of the posterior prostatitc plane or the seminal vesicles, and some cases could occur at the apex of prostate when dissecting the NVBs or separation of prostatic apex.

3 Ureter injury

Ureteral injuries occur very rarely in <0.5% of cases, most of cases are detected postoperatively because of intra or retro peritoneal urinary leakage [39]. The urinary leakage can be diagnosed contrast enhanced pelvis CT scan. Ureteral injuries might happen during extended lymphadenectomy or bladder neck dissection. Large prostates or median lobes, and history of prostatitis, are known risk factors of ureter injury, especially ureteral orifices injury during dissection of the posterior bladder neck [40].

4 Anastomotic strictures and urethrovesical anastomotic urinary leakage
  Anastomotic stricture incidence ranges from <2% to 14.0%, which is likely to be dependent on the surgical technique [41, 42]. Age, obesity, smoking, diabetes mellitus, hypertension, coronary artery disease, postoperative bleeding, low surgeon experience, and trans urethral resection of prostateTURP history are all the risk factors of postoperative anastomotic stricture [43]. Surgeon experience is the most important factor related to the anastomotic strictures, especially the postoperative bleeding, which causes formation of a hematoma, and induce the local inflammation to disrupt the anastomosis. Some studies demonstrated that the patients with postoperative bleeding will have a higher risk of anastomotic strictures. Some surgical techniques can decrease the postoperative anastomotic stricture incidence, including the closure of the bladder neck with mucosal eversion to prevent stricture, although it would increase the risk of extravasation of enteric contents [44]. For the patients with anastomotic strictures, the treatment options include chronic catheter drainage, intermittent self-dilation, repeating endoscopic incision or dilation, placement of a urethral stent, and open bladder neck reconstruction.

  The definition of anastomotic urinary leakage depends on the postoperative days [45]. The current literature defines anastomotic urinary leakage as persistent contrast extravasation on cystography between postoperative days 3 and 14 [46]. Urinary leakage can be diagnosed by using cystogaphy, CT cystography, or creatinine level measurement in pelvis. Patients with anastomotic urinary leakage can present with abdominal distention, pain, and fever. Urinary leakage is divided into three grades according to the extent of extravasation [18]. Surgical suturing technique is important predictive factor of anastomotic urinary leakage. Some studies have shown that a double layer suture is much better than the single layer. When anastomotic urinary leakage occurs, conservative treatment choices include catheter insertion and placement of a pelvic drain. The other choice is reoperation: mono-J stent inserted to drain the urine and help the anastomotic stoma healing.

5 Other complications: infection, rectourethral fistula, urinary retention, thrombosis, lymphocele

Rectourethral fistula is a rare complication, with incidence of <2% [47]. Usually the clinical signs occur about 10–14 days after the surgery. Although few publications described that fistula with minimal symptoms can spontaneously close with prolonged urethral catheter drainage alone [48], most of cases require surgical intervention. Fecal diversion and diverting colostomy, which prevent rectal distention and pressure during healing, are recommended before tenuous repair.

Systematic review have shown that DVT incidence ranges approximately from 0.3% in the robotic prostatectomy to 1.0% in the open prostatectomy [49]. One of the possible reasons is that the robotic procedure is minimally invasive, and early ambulation could benefit to prevent thrombosis formation. For the patients with risk of thrombosis, preoperative heparin injection can be administered. The symptoms of DVT of lower extremity include tenderness and swelling in the lower extremity. Doppler ultrasound can identify the thrombosis and its location. If the pulmonary embolism is identified, inferior vena cava (IVC) filter can be placed.

A lymphocele is a postoperative complication induced by lymph node dissection and inadequate closure in the RP. Lymphocele can be detected by CT or ultrasound, but urinary cyst and pelvic infection should be excluded. The management depends on multiple factors including size, position, infection, and risk. Management choices include percutaneous aspiration drainage, sclerotherapy, and open surgical methods. Studies have reported that the success rate is about 50–70% for aspiration drainage, whereas the open surgical success rate for peritoneal marsupialization is more than 90% [50].

## Outcomes

1 Perioperative outcomes
  a Operative times
    Operative times are typically longer with LRP and RALP compared with open surgery, especially earlier during the learning curve. Once experience is gained, operative times of 3 hours and less are reported.
  b Blood loss
    The tamponade effect from the pneumoperitoneum during RALP and laparoscopic procedures considerably decrease the intraoperative blood loss. As for homologous blood transfusion, most studies have shown significant decrease in blood transfusion requirements in patients undergoing LRP and RALP [21, 51].

**Table 8.1** Summary of pathologic-stage-specific positive surgical margin rates

| Study (References) | *n* | Positive margins (%) | | |
| --- | --- | --- | --- | --- |
| | | pT2 | pT3 | Overall |
| RALP | | | | |
| Ahlering [51] | 109 | | | 13 |
| Badani [52] | 2766 | 13 | 35 | 12.3 |
| Patel [53] | 1500 | 4 | 34 | |
| Menon [18] | 1142 | | | 13 |
| Tewari [54] | 1335 | | | 8.5 |
| Lavery [55] | 1436 | | | 18 |
| Laparoscopic | | | | |
| Guillonneau [56] | 1000 | 15.5 | 31.1 | 19.2 |
| Rassweiler [57] | 500 | 7.4 | 31.8 | 19 |
| Rozet [58] | 600 | 14.6 | 25.6 | 17.7 |
| Lein [59] | 1000 | 14.8 | 21.1 | |
| Stolzenburg [60] | 2000 | 9.7 | 33.9 | |
| Open | | | | |
| Grossfeld [61] | 1383 | | | 19.9 |
| Hsu [62] | 1024 | | | 20.6 |
| Roehl [63] | 3478 | | 18.1 | 19 |
| Ward [64] | 7268 | 28 | 58 | 38 |
| Saranchuk [65] | 1133 | 18.3 | 38.9 | 23.5 |

**2** Oncological outcomes

**a** Surgical margins (Table 8.1)

The 2009 International Society of Urological Pathology Consensus Conference in Boston recommended the standardization of pathology reporting of RP specimens. Issues related to surgical margin assessment were coordinated by working group 5 [66]. Pathologists agreed that tumor extending close to the "capsular"' margin, yet not to it, should be reported as a negative margin, and that locations of positive margins should be indicated as either posterior, posterolateral, lateral, anterior at the prostatic apex, mid-prostate or base.

Based on our experience, the key point is to create tumor map before the surgery, including the DRE, eMRI to determine the tumor location, volume, capsular extension. This will help the surgeon in making informed decision for cancer removal, urethral amputation, and neurovascular preservation. Intraoperative real-time transrectal ultrasound (US) and surgical loupes are new technical adjuncts that have been recently reported as a dissection guide to reduce margin positivity during RP [67].

**b** Biochemical recurrence

In 2009 Update, the AUA defined biochemical recurrence as an initial PSA value ≤0.2 ng/mL followed by a subsequent confirmatory test [68]. Biochemical recurrence is found to be associated with the PSM, tumor stage, and Gleason grade. PSA elevations developed within the first 2 years following surgery are more often associated with distant recurrences. For the management of patients with biochemical recurrence, there is still no long-term result of prospective randomized study. Radiation therapy and hormone therapy are the choices following biochemical recurrence.

**3** Functional outcomes

The adverse effects of urinary incontinence and sexual dysfunction following RP still persist and have a significant impact on health-related quality of life (HRQoL) [69]. Widespread usage of PSA as a screening test has resulted in earlier detection and diagnosis of prostate cancer in younger men and has further necessitated the importance of postoperative recovery of genitourinary functions. The primary goal of cancer extirpation has to be balanced with the functional outcomes. Potency outcomes are dependent on many factors such as patient's age, type and extent of NS, and preoperative erectile function [70, 71]. However, the return of urinary continence has been found to be dependent on factors such as patient demographics, presence of median lobe, degree of NS, and changes in surgical technique [72, 73].

**a** Urinary incontinence (Table 8.2)

Urinary incontinence is one of the most common postoperative complications following RP, with a current incidence ranging from 1% [81] to 47% [82]. The widely used definitions for urinary continence currently used are no pads, a pad for security or 0–1 pad per 24 hour. The urinary incontinence after RP is attributed to damage of urinary sphincter, alterations in the pelvic floor musculature. Apart from the aforementioned factors, unstable detrusor muscle, low-compliance bladders could induce urgency incontinence; while postoperative urethral stricture could induce the overflow incontinence. Various surgical techniques such as (a) optimizing preservation of urethral rhabdosphincter length, without affecting the PSM rate [29]; (b) total reconstruction of the

**Table 8.2** Summary of urinary continence outcomes

| Study (References) | n | Evaluated patients | Age | Follow-up period (months) | Continence rate (%) |
|---|---|---|---|---|---|
| RALP | | | | | |
| Ahlering [51] | 60 | 60 | 62.9 | 3 | 76 |
| Costello [74] | 89 | 89 | | 6 | 82 |
| Patel [75] | 1100 | 393 | 58 | 18 | 97.9 |
| Menon [18] | 2652 | 1142 | 60.2 | 12 | 95 |
| Tewari [54] | 2536 | 1100 | 58 | 12 | 96.07 |
| Lavery [55] | 1436 | 1436 | 59.4 | 12 | 93% |
| Laparoscopic | | | | | |
| Guillonneau [76] | 550 | 550 | | 12 | 82.3 |
| Rassweiler [77] | 500 | 500 | 64 | 12 | 83.6 |
| Rozet [58] | 600 | 498 | 62 | 12 | 98 |
| Lein [59] | 1000 | 952 | 62 | 18 | 76 |
| Stolzenburg [60] | 2000 | 1530 | 63.2 | 12 | 92 |
| Open | | | | | |
| Stanford [78] | 1291 | 1291 | 62.9 | 18 | 58 |
| Walsh [79] | 64 | 64 | 57 | 18 | 93 |
| Kundu [71] | 3477 | 2737 | 61 | 12 | 93 |
| Lepor [80] | 500 | 491 | 58.8 | 18 | 98.5 |

vesico-urethral junction [32]; (c) preservation of puboprostatic ligaments and arcus tendineus (Incising the puboprostatic ligaments just proximal to the prostate apex and careful dissection in that plane is used so as to avoid detaching the urethral rhabdosphincter from its anterolateral ligamentous attachments [83]); (d) periurethral retropubic suspension stitch [84]; and (e) NS [85] are known to improve urinary continence outcomes.

Other conservative and surgical treatments can be chosen for urinary incontinence. The conservative treatments include pelvic floor exercises, biofeedback, and transcutaneous electrical nerve stimulation. The surgical treatment methods include periurethral silicone implants and artificial urinary sphincter insertion.

**b** Erectile dysfunction (Table 8.3)

The published postoperative potency rates vary from 3.4% to 75.6% [86] following RP. After the NS technology was applied in the RP, the erectile function has been significantly improved. Some meta-analysis have shown that potency rates according the NS procedure were 47–80% for unilateral NS and 63.8–100% for bilateral

**Table 8.3** Summary of potency outcomes

| Study (References) | n | Evaluated patients | Age | Follow-up period (months) | % Receiving BNS (%) | Nerve sparing | Intercourse (%) |
|---|---|---|---|---|---|---|---|
| RALP | | | | | | | |
| Ahlering [86] | 110 | 59 | 62.9 | ≤12 | 40.9 | BNS | 24.4 |
| Zorn [87] | 300 | 258 | 59.4 | 12 | 59.7 | BNS | 80 |
| Patel [75] | 1100 | 387 | 58 | 18 | 36.7 | BNS | 96.6 |
| Menon [18] | 2652 | 1142 | 60.2 | 12 | 42 | BNS | 95 |
| Tewari [54] | 2536 | 659 | 58 | 12 | | Grade 1 NS | 92.4 |
| Lavery [55] | 1436 | 1436 | 59.4 | 12 | 89% | BNS | 84% |
| Laparoscopic | | | | | | | |
| Guillonneau [76] | 550 | 47 | | 12 | 100 | BNS | 66 |
| Rassweiler [77] | 562 | 562 | | | 61.2 | BNS | 76 |
| Rozet [58] | 600 | 89 | 62 | 12 | 63.7 | BNS | 43 |
| Gill [88] | 200 | 76 | NA | 12 | 38 | BNS | 88 |
| Stolzenburg [60] | 2000 | 730 | 63.2 | 12 | 65.3 | BNS | 67.7 |
| Open | | | | | | | |
| Stanford [78] | 1291 | 1042 | 62.9 | 18 | | | 44 |
| Walsh [79] | 64 | 64 | 57 | 18 | 89 | BNS | 86 |
| Kundu [71] | 3477 | 1834 | 61 | >18 | 91 | BNS | 76 |
| Saranchuk [65] | 1133 | 647 | 58 | 24 | 92.5 | BNS | 62 |

NS procedure after 18 months of robotic surgery. For the patients with erectile dysfunction postoperatively, the choices of treatment include PDE-5 inhibitors, vacuum erection devices, and intraurethral or intracavernosal vasodilators. The studies have testified that the sildenafil could help nearly 80% patients with bilateral NS to improve their sex function, and help 25% patients with unilateral NS to improve their sex function. Therefore, for the patients whose bilateral NVBs are destroyed in the surgery, penile implants could be considered.

# References

1 Young HH. The early diagnosis and radical cure of carcinoma of the prostate: being a study of 40 cases and presentation of a radical operation which was carried out in four cases. *Johns Hopkins Hosp Bull* 1905;16:315–321.
2 Millin T. *Retropubic Urinary Surgery*. Edinburgh, UK: E. & S. Livingstone; 1947.

3 Reiner WG, Walsh PC. An anatomical approach to the surgical management of the dorsal vein and Santorini's plexus during radical retropubic surgery. *J Urology* 1979;121:198.

4 Walsh PC, Donker PJ. Impotence following radical prostatectomy: insight into etiology and prevention. *J Urology* 1982;128:492.

5 Oelrich TM. The urethral sphincter muscle in the male. *Am J Anat* 1980;158:229–246.

6 Walsh PC. Radical prostatectomy for localized prostate cancer provides durable cancer control with excellent quality of life: a structured debate. *J Urology* 2000;163:1802.

7 Nielsen ME, Schaeffer EM, Marschke P, Walsh PC. High anterior release of the levator fascia improves sexual function following open radical retropubic prostatectomy. *J Urology* 2008;180:2557–2564.

8 Schuessler WW, Schulam PG, Clayman RV, Kavoussi LR. Laparoscopic radical prostatectomy: initial short-term experience. *Urology* 1997;50:854–857.

9 Abbou CC, Salomon L, Hoznek A, *et al.* Laparoscopic radical prostatectomy: preliminary results. *Urology* 2000;55:630–633.

10 Guillonneau B, Vallancien G. Laparoscopic radical prostatectomy: the Montsouris technique. *J Urology* 2000;163:1643–1649.

11 Binder J, Kramer W. Robotically-assisted laparoscopic radical prostatectomy. *BJU Int* 2001;87:408–410.

12 Menon M, Shrivastava A, Tewari A, *et al.* Laparoscopic and robot assisted radical prostatectomy: establishment of a structured program and preliminary analysis of outcomes. *J Urology* 2002;168:945–949.

13 Tewari A, Peabody J, Sarle R, *et al.* Technique of da vinci robot-assisted anatomic radical prostatectomy. *Urology* 2002;60:569–572.

14 Trinh QD, Sammon J, Sun M, *et al.* Perioperative outcomes of robot-assisted radical prostatectomy compared with open radical prostatectomy: results from the nationwide inpatient sample. *Eur Urol* 2012;61:679–685.

15 Ahlering TE, Skarecky D, Borin J. Impact of cautery versus cautery-free preservation of neurovascular bundles on early return of potency. *J Endourol* 2006;20: 586–589.

16 Kiyoshima K, Yokomizo A, Yoshida T, *et al.* Anatomical features of periprostatic tissue and its surroundings: a histological analysis of 79 radical retropubic prostatectomy specimens. *Jpn J Clin Oncol* 2004;34:463–468.

17 Eichelberg C, Erbersdobler A, Michl U, *et al.* Nerve distribution along the prostatic capsule. *Eur Urol* 2007: 51:105–111.

18 Menon M, Shrivastava A, Kaul S, *et al.* Vattikuti Institute prostatectomy: contemporary technique and analysis of results. *Eur Urol* 2007;51:648–658.

19 Tewari A, Takenaka A, Mtui E, *et al.* The proximal neurovascular plate and the tri zonal neural architecture around the prostate gland: importance in the athermal robotic technique of nerve sparing prostatectomy. *BJU Int* 2006;98:314–323.

20 Tewari AK, Srivastava A, Huang MW, *et al.* Anatomical grades of nerve sparing: a risk stratified approach to neural hammock sparing during robot assisted radical prostatectomy (RARP). *BJU Int* 2011;108:984–992.

21 Tewari A, Peabody JO, Fischer M, *et al*. An operative and anatomic study to help in nerve sparing during laparoscopic and robotic radical prostatectomy. *Eur Urol* 2003;43:444.

22 Rao S, Tu JJ, Jhaveri JK, *et al*. Distributions of peri-prostatic nerves in the fascial planes around the prostate–implications for technique of nerve sparing radical prostatectomy. *J Urology* 2008;179:228.

23 Ramanathan R, Shih G, Yang XJ, *et al*. MRI based classification of variations in neurovascular structures around the seminal vesicles: implication for a modified seminal vesicle dissection technique during robotic radical prostatectomy. *J Urology* 2008;179:611.

24 Tewari AK, Rao SR. Anatomical foundations and surgical manoeuvres for precise identification of the prostatovesical junction during robotic radical prostatectomy. *BJU Int* 2006;98:833–837.

25 Tewari A, El Hakim A, Rao S, Raman JD. Identification of the retrotrigonal layer as a key anatomical landmark during robotically assisted radical prostatectomy. *BJU Int* 2006;98:829–832.

26 Srivastava A, Grover S, Sooriakumaran P, *et al*. Neuroanatomic basis for traction-free preservation of the neural hammock during athermal robotic radical prostatectomy. *Curr Opin Urol* 2011;21:49.

27 Tewari A, Rao S, Martinez-Salamanca JI, *et al*. Cancer control and the preservation of neurovascular tissue: how to meet competing goals during robotic radical prostatectomy. *BJU Int* 2008;101:1013–1018.

28 Tewari A, Tan G, Dorsey P. Optimizing erectogenic outcomes during athermal robotic prostatectomy: a risk-stratified tri-zonal approach. *Urol Times Clin Edition* 2008;3:s4–s12.

29 Tewari AK, Srivastava A, Mudaliar K, *et al*. Anatomical retro apical technique of synchronous (posterior and anterior) urethral transection: a novel approach for ameliorating apical margin positivity during robotic radical prostatectomy. *BJU Int* 2010;106:1364–1373.

30 Pagano F, Prayer Galetti T, d'Arrigo L, *et al*. Radical surgery for clinically confined prostate cancer. *Ann NY Acad Sci* 1996;784:85–92.

31 Tewari AK, Srivastava A, Sooriakumaran P, *et al*. Use of a novel absorbable barbed plastic surgical suture enables a "self-cinching" technique of vesicourethral anastomosis during robot-assisted prostatectomy and improves anastomotic times. *J Endourol* 2010;24:1645–1650.

32 Tewari A, Jhaveri J, Rao S, *et al*. Total reconstruction of the vesico urethral junction. *BJU Int* 2008;101:871–877.

33 Tewari A, Rao S, Mandhani A. Catheter less robotic radical prostatectomy using a custom made synchronous anastomotic splint and vesical urinary diversion device: report of the initial series and perioperative outcomes. *BJU Int* 2008;102:1000–1004.

34 Sanchez-Salas R, Flamand V, Cathelineau X. Preventing complications in robotic prostatic surgery. *Eur Urol Suppl* 2010;9:388–393.

35 Ficarra V, Novara G, Artibani W, *et al*. Retropubic, laparoscopic, and robot-assisted radical prostatectomy: a systematic review and cumulative analysis of comparative studies. *Eur Urol* 2009;55:1037–1063.

36 Djavan B, Agalliu I, Laze J, *et al*. Blood loss during radical prostatectomy: impact on clinical, oncological and functional outcomes and complication rates. *BJU Int* 2012;110:69–75.

37 Guillonneau B, Gupta R, El Fettouh H, *et al*. Laparoscopic management of rectal injury during laparoscopic radical prostatectomy. *J Urology* 2003;169:1694–1696.

38 Yee DS, Ornstein DK. Repair of rectal injury during robotic-assisted laparoscopic prostatectomy. *Urology* 2008;72:428–431.

39 Carlsson S, Nilsson AE, Schumacher MC, *et al*. Surgery-related complications in 1253 robot-assisted and 485 open retropubic radical prostatectomies at the Karolinska University Hospital, Sweden. *Urology* 2010;75:1092–1097.

40 Crisci A, Young MD, Murphy BC, *et al*. Ureteral reimplantation for inadvertent ureteral injury during radical-perineal prostatectomy. *Urology* 2003;62:941.

41 Msezane LP, Reynolds WS, Gofrit ON, *et al*. Bladder neck contracture after robot-assisted laparoscopic radical prostatectomy: evaluation of incidence, risk factors, and impact on urinary function. *J Endourol* 2008;22:377–384.

42 Buckley JC. Complications after radical prostatectomy: anastomotic stricture and rectourethral fistula. *Curr Opin Urol* 2011;21:461.

43 Sandhu JS, Gotto GT, Herran LA, *et al*. Age, obesity, medical comorbidities and surgical technique are predictive of symptomatic anastomotic strictures after contemporary radical prostatectomy. *J Urology* 2011;185:2148–2152.

44 Schoeppler GM, Zaak D, Clevert DA, *et al*. The impact of bladder neck mucosal eversion during open radical prostatectomy on bladder neck stricture and urinary extravasation. *Int Urol Nephrol* 2012;44:1403–1410.

45 Tyritzis SI, Katafigiotis I, Constantinides CA. All you need to know about urethrovesical anastomotic urinary leakage following radical prostatectomy. *J Urology* 2012;188:369–376.

46 Mochtar CA, Kauer PC, Laguna MP, de la Rosette J. Urinary leakage after laparoscopic radical prostatectomy: a systematic review. *J Endourol* 2007;21:1371–1380.

47 Thomas C, Jones J, Jger W, *et al*. Incidence, clinical symptoms and management of rectourethral fistulas after radical prostatectomy. *J Urology* 2010;183:608–612.

48 Nyam DCNK, Pemberton JH. Management of iatrogenic rectourethral fistula. *Dis Colon Rectum* 1999;42:994–997.

49 Tewari A, Sooriakumaran P, Bloch DA, *et al*. Positive surgical margin and perioperative complication rates of primary surgical treatments for prostate cancer: a systematic review and meta-analysis comparing retropubic, laparoscopic, and robotic prostatectomy. *Eur Urol* 2012;62:1–15.

50 Pepper RJ, Pati J, Kaisary AV. The incidence and treatment of lymphoceles after radical retropubic prostatectomy. *BJU Int* 2005;95:772–775.

51 Ahlering TE, Woo D, Eichel L, *et al*. Robot-assisted versus open radical prostatectomy: a comparison of one surgeon's outcomes. *Urology* 2004;63:819–822.

52 Badani KK, Kaul S, Menon M. Evolution of robotic radical prostatectomy. *Cancer* 2007;110:1951–1958.

53 Patel VR, Palmer KJ, Coughlin G, Samavedi S. Robot-assisted laparoscopic radical prostatectomy: perioperative outcomes of 1500 cases. *J Endourol* 2008;22:2299–2306.

54 Tewari AK, Ali A, Metgud S, *et al*. Functional outcomes following robotic prostatectomy using athermal, traction free risk-stratified grades of nerve sparing. *World J Urol* 2013;31:471–480.

55 Lavery HJ, Levinson AW, Brajtbord JS, Samadi DB. Candidacy for active surveillance may be associated with improved functional outcomes after prostatectomy. Urologic Oncology: Seminars and Original Investigations; 2011: Elsevier, 2011

56 Guillonneau B, El-Fettouh H, Baumert H, *et al*. Laparoscopic radical prostatectomy: oncological evaluation after 1,000 cases at Montsouris Institute. *J Urology* 2003;169:1261–1266.

57 Rassweiler J, Schulze M, Teber D, *et al*. Laparoscopic radical prostatectomy with the Heilbronn technique: oncological results in the first 500 patients. *J Urology* 2005;173:761–764.

58 Rozet F, Galiano M, Cathelineau X, *et al*. Extraperitoneal laparoscopic radical prostatectomy: a prospective evaluation of 600 cases. *J Urology* 2005;174:908–911.

59 Lein M, Stibane I, Mansour R, *et al*. Complications, urinary continence, and oncologic outcome of 1000 laparoscopic transperitoneal radical prostatectomies— experience at the Charit Hospital Berlin, Campus Mitte. *Eur Urol* 2006;50:1278–1284.

60 Stolzenburg JU, Rabenalt R, Do M, *et al*. Endoscopic extraperitoneal radical prostatectomy: the University of Leipzig experience of 2000 cases. *J Endourol* 2008;22:2319–2326.

61 Grossfeld GD, Chang JJ, Broering JM, *et al*. Impact of positive surgical margins on prostate cancer recurrence and the use of secondary cancer treatment: data from the CaPSURE database. *J Urology* 2000;163:1171.

62 Hsu EI, Hong EK, Lepor H. Influence of body weight and prostate volume on intraoperative, perioperative, and postoperative outcomes after radical retropubic prostatectomy. *Urology* 2003;61:601–606.

63 Roehl KA, Han M, Ramos CG, *et al*. Cancer progression and survival rates following anatomical radical retropubic prostatectomy in 3,478 consecutive patients: long-term results. *J Urology* 2004;172:910–914.

64 Ward JF, Zincke H, Bergstralh EJ, *et al*. The impact of surgical approach (nerve bundle preservation versus wide local excision) on surgical margins and biochemical recurrence following radical prostatectomy. *J Urology* 2004;172:1328–1332.

65 Saranchuk JW, Kattan MW, Elkin E, *et al*. Achieving optimal outcomes after radical prostatectomy. *J Clin Oncol* 2005;23:4146–4151.

66 Tan PH, Cheng L, Srigley JR, *et al*. International Society of Urological Pathology (ISUP) consensus conference on handling and staging of radical prostatectomy specimens. Working group 5: surgical margins. *Modern Pathol* 2010;24:48–57.

67 Magera JS Jr., Inman BA, Slezak JM, *et al*. Increased optical magnification from 2.5 to 4.3 with technical modification lowers the positive margin rate in open radical retropubic prostatectomy. *J Urology* 2008;179:130–135.

68 Greene KL, Albertsen PC, Babaian RJ, *et al*. Prostate specific antigen best practice statement: 2009 update. *J Urology* 2009;182:2232.

69 Sanda MG, Dunn RL, Michalski J, *et al*. Quality of life and satisfaction with outcome among prostate-cancer survivors. *New Engl J Med* 2008;358:1250–1261.

70 Rabbani F, Stapleton AMF, Kattan MW, *et al*. Factors predicting recovery of erections after radical prostatectomy. *J Urology* 2000;164:1929–1934.

71 Kundu SD, Roehl KA, Eggener SE, *et al*. Potency, continence and complications in 3,477 consecutive radical retropubic prostatectomies. *J Urology* 2004;172:2227–2231.

72 Sandhu JS, Eastham JA. Factors predicting early return of continence after radical prostatectomy. *Curr Urol Rep* 2010;11:191–197.

73 Rocco F, Carmignani L, Acquati P, *et al*. Restoration of posterior aspect of rhabdosphincter shortens continence time after radical retropubic prostatectomy. *J Urology* 2006;175:2201–2206.

74 Costello AJ, Haxhimolla H, Crowe H, Peters JS. Installation of telerobotic surgery and initial experience with telerobotic radical prostatectomy. *BJU Int* 2005;96: 34–38.

75 Patel VR, Coelho RF, Chauhan S, *et al*. Continence, potency and oncological outcomes after robotic assisted radical prostatectomy: early trifecta results of a high volume surgeon. *BJU Int* 2010;106:696–702.

76 Guillonneau B, Cathelineau X, Doublet JD, *et al*. Laparoscopic radical prostatectomy: assessment after 550 procedures. *Crit Rev Oncol Hemat* 2002;34:33–321.

77 Rassweiler J, Schulze M, Teber D, *et al*. Laparoscopic radical prostatectomy: functional and oncological outcomes. *Curr Opin Urol* 2004;14:75–82.

78 Stanford JL, Feng Z, Hamilton AS, *et al*. Urinary and sexual function after radical prostatectomy for clinically localized prostate cancer. *J Am Med Assoc* 2000;283:354–360.

79 Walsh PC, Marschke P, Ricker D, Burnett AL. Patient-reported urinary continence and sexual function after anatomic radical prostatectomy. *Urology* 2000;55: 58–61.

80 Lepor H, Kaci L. The impact of open radical retropubic prostatectomy on continence and lower urinary tract symptoms: a prospective assessment using validated self-administered outcome instruments. *J Urology* 2004;171:1216–1219.

81 Kielb S, Dunn RL, Rashid MG, *et al*. Assessment of early continence recovery after radical prostatectomy: patient reported symptoms and impairment. *J Urology* 2001;166:958–961.

82 Fowler FJ, Barry MJ, Lu-Yao G, *et al*. Patient-reported complications and follow-up treatment after radical prostatectomy: the national medicare experience: 1988–1990 (updated June 1993). *Urology* 1993;42:622–628.

83 Tewari AK, Bigelow K, Rao S, *et al*. Anatomic restoration technique of continence mechanism and preservation of puboprostatic collar: a novel modification to achieve early urinary continence in men undergoing robotic prostatectomy. *Urology* 2007;69:726–731.

84 Patel VR, Coelho RF, Palmer KJ, Rocco B. Periurethral suspension stitch during robot-assisted laparoscopic radical prostatectomy: description of the technique and continence outcomes. *Eur Urol* 2009;56:472–478.

85 Srivastava A, Chopra S, Pham A, *et al*. Effect of a risk-stratified grade of nerve-sparing technique on early return of continence after robot-assisted laparoscopic radical prostatectomy. *Eur Urol* 2013;63:438–444.

86 Ahlering TE, Eichel L, Skarecky D. Rapid communication: early potency outcomes with cautery-free neurovascular bundle preservation with robotic laparoscopic radical prostatectomy. *J Endourol* 2005;19:715–718.

87 Zorn KC, Gofrit ON, Orvieto MA, *et al.* Robotic-assisted laparoscopic prostatectomy: functional and pathologic outcomes with interfascial nerve preservation. *Eur Urol* 2007;51:755.

88 Gill IS, Ukimura O. Thermal energy-free laparoscopic nerve-sparing radical prostatectomy: one-year potency outcomes. *Urology* 2007;70:309–314.

# CHAPTER 9

# Radiation Therapy in the Management of Prostate Cancer

*J. Conibear[1] and P.J. Hoskin[2]*
[1] Mount Vernon Cancer Centre, Middlesex, UK
[2] University College London, Mount Vernon Cancer Centre, Northwood, UK

## Introduction

Radiation is one of the principal treatment modalities for prostate cancer [1, 2]. Since the early twentieth century, radiation has been used to treat all stages of the disease. In 1904, Armand and Léon Imbert were the first clinicians to report on the successful use of X-ray therapy to treat an advanced prostate cancer [3]. In 1908, both Minet and Desnos used radium-containing catheters to deliver an early form of brachytherapy, and in 1923 Waters and Pierson used "deep" X-rays to treat a prostate cancer bony metastasis [4–7]. Over the past century, radiation therapy for prostate cancer has undergone dramatic changes as a result of advances in radiobiology, physics, and computer technology. Now in the twenty-first century, practitioners of prostate cancer radiation therapy can tailor their treatments to the stage and needs of the patient.

## External beam radiotherapy

The first attempts to use X-rays to treat prostate cancer relied upon low-energy beams. Compared to modern megavoltage X-rays, they lacked the comparative depth of penetrance and consequently led to high-radiation doses at the patient's skin surface. This meant early prostate cancer patients suffered significant acute skin toxicity and an increased risk of radiation-induced skin cancers. Due to these early drawbacks the use of low-energy beams to treat localized prostate cancer remained relatively low in the first half of the twentieth century.

*Prostate Cancer: Diagnosis and Clinical Management*, First Edition.
Edited by Ashutosh K. Tewari, Peter Whelan and John D. Graham.
© 2014 John Wiley & Sons, Ltd. Published 2014 by John Wiley & Sons, Ltd.

Prior to World War II important discoveries were made in radiation science that led to new developments in radiotherapy. The work of Leó Szilárd, Rolf Widerøe, and Gustav Ising during the 1920s led to subatomic particle acceleration theory and the creation of particle accelerators termed linear accelerators or "linacs" [8, 9]. These new machines were capable of producing megavoltage X-rays that offered deeper tissue penetrance and an important skin sparing effect. This effect allowed tumors lying beneath the skin surface to receive higher doses of radiation without the high levels of surface toxicity seen previously with lower-energy electron beams. In 1953, an 8-megavoltage (MV) linac was installed in the Hammersmith Hospital in London, which was the first to begin treating patients with various tumors [10]. This achievement was to herald a new age in external beam radiotherapy (EBRT).

Over the next 50 years EBRT underwent further refinement through the discovery of X-ray computed tomography (CT) and advances in linear accelerator design and technology. Up until the early 1990s, EBRT for prostate cancer was typically planned and delivered using a two-dimensional technique usually termed as "conventional radiotherapy." This technique meant that the patient's prostate gland and a significant portion of their surrounding pelvis were encompassed within a typically box-shaped radiation field. Due to the uncertainties of tumor location and organ movement, shielding of normal tissue was relatively minimal. This of course meant that the volume of normal tissue treated was great and that patients often developed significant acute gastrointestinal (GI) and genitourinary (GU) toxicities [11]. Because of these toxicities patients were often unable to tolerate radiotherapy doses in excess of 67–70 Gy when delivered using conventional radiotherapy.

The discovery of CT imaging and its integration into radiotherapy planning during the 1980s led to the creation of three-dimensional conformal radiotherapy (3D-CRT) [12, 13]. This term describes how the linear accelerator performs complex beam shaping to conform the X-rays to match the outline of the patient's tumor on the patient's treatment planning scan. Conforming the beams also helps minimize the dose of radiation delivered to the patient's normal pelvic organs (Figure 9.1) [14]. A phase III randomized controlled trial comparing this technique with conventional radiotherapy using a standard dose of 64 Gy has shown a significant reduction in the dose-limiting late side effect of proctitis with no impact on disease control when using 3D-CRT [15].

More recent advances in 3D planning and dosimetry have led to the creation of a more advanced form of 3D-CRT termed "intensity-modulated

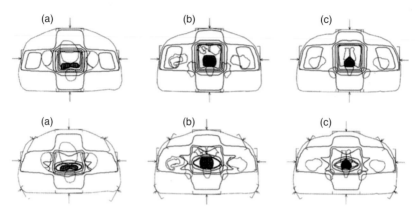

**Figure 9.1** Top three images represent the isodose distributions from a conventional radiotherapy plan and the bottom three images represent the isodose distribution from a 3D-CRT prostate plan. The *arrows* indicate beam direction. (a) CT-scan slice at the level of the seminal vesicles; (b) CT-scan slice through mid-prostate; (c) CT-scan slice through the prostate above the apex. The 78, 77, 70, 55, 45, and 25 Gy lines are shown [14]. Reproduced from Reference 14 with permission from Elsevier.

radiotherapy" (IMRT). With IMRT radiation, physicists are able to plan more complex treatments by utilizing an increased number of X-ray beams, sometimes as many as 9, which allows an even higher level of conformity to be achieved (Figure 9.2, Plate 9.2). The adoption of IMRT and inverse planning techniques has allowed clinicians to increase the dose delivered to the prostate gland while maintaining acceptably low doses of radiation to the patient's normal pelvic organs and GI tract [16, 17]. 3D-CRT and now IMRT have helped to reduce the incidence of GI and GU late toxicity commonly seen with early conventional radiotherapy. These new radiotherapy treatment techniques have permitted further studies to safely investigate the potential benefits of radiotherapy dose escalation to the prostate gland and pelvic lymph nodes.

## Dose escalation

Several phase III randomized clinical trials have investigated the potential benefits of dose escalation on tumor control. Each trial utilized 3D-CRT or IMRT and studied radiation doses ranging from the original conventional dose of 64 Gy up to a dose of 86 Gy. Studies from The Royal Marsden Hospital (RMH), MRC RT01, MD Anderson, and the Dutch multicenter trial reported improvements in overall PSA control of between 6% and

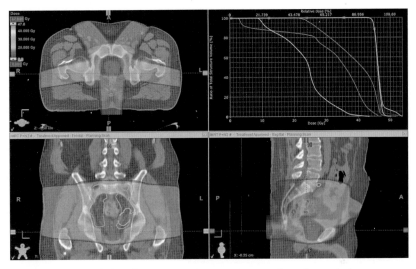

**Figure 9.2** The top left and bottom two images represent the color wash dose distributions from an IMRT prostate and pelvic lymph node radiotherapy plan. The top right image shows the corresponding dose–volume histogram for the plan. Note the increased number of beams which has allowed a higher level of conformity around the prostate gland. (See also Plate 9.2.)

12% using higher doses of radiation [18–21]. The RMH pilot study and MRC RT01 trial compared 64 Gy with 74 Gy, the MD Anderson compared 70 Gy with 78 Gy, and the Dutch trial compared 68 Gy with 78 Gy [18–21]. More recently, Kuban *et al.* has published an updated analysis on the long-term outcomes of the MD Anderson dose escalation trial; 301 patients with stage T1b to T3 prostate cancer [22]. They reported superior freedom from biochemical or clinical failure in the group randomized to 78 Gy compared with 70 Gy (78% vs. 59%, $p = .004$) after a median follow-up of 8.7 years. In light of these findings, the conventional dose of 64 Gy is no longer considered adequate and a dose of 74–78 Gy in conventional 2 Gy fractions to the prostate is appropriate for patients with low-risk cancers. Intermediate- and high-risk prostate cancer patients should receive doses up to 81 Gy [16, 23, 24].

Despite the advantages of dose escalation on disease control, it should be noted that dose escalation does come with the risk of increased GI and GU toxicity. The MRC RT01 trial showed that patients treated in the dose-escalated conformal arm had higher rates of late grade 2 or above GI toxicity (24%), reflecting a major increase in urethral stricture rate, and GU (11%) toxicity compared with those in the conventional arm (8% and 24%, respectively) [19]. Sexual function assessment in these patients is compounded by the use of androgen deprivation; however, at 2 years and beyond around 60% of patients had significant sexual dysfunction.

## Androgen deprivation therapy and nodal irradiation

Patients with locally advanced T3 prostate cancers have a high risk of pelvic lymph node involvement. As a consequence, in historical series they have relatively poor disease-free survival rates; only 22.5% (95% CI = 19–26) at 10 years [25]. In the United Kingdom, approximately one-third of newly diagnosed patients present with T3 disease and the majority of them are suitable for radiotherapy given with curative intent [26]. Normally these patients are now treated with a combination of EBRT and androgen deprivation therapy (ADT).

The largest study which has shown an advantage for adding ADT to radical radiotherapy in these patients is that undertaken by the EORTC in which patients received 70 Gy radiotherapy with a randomization to receive 3 years of ADT starting on the first day of radiotherapy [25]. The 10-year disease-free survival was 22.7% in the radiotherapy alone group and 47.7% in the radiotherapy plus ADT group. Even more compelling was a difference in overall survival at 10-years which was 39.8% in the radiotherapy alone group and 58.1% in the radiotherapy plus ADT group.

It is also clear that radiotherapy with ADT is superior to ADT alone. The SPCG-7 trial, reported in 2009, was the first to show an overall survival advantage for endocrine therapy in combination with radiotherapy in the treatment of locally advanced prostate cancer [27]. The trial showed a 12% improvement (23.9% vs. 11.9%) in the 10-year cumulative incidence for prostate-cancer-specific mortality [27]. More recently in 2011, the PR07 trial, a phase III trial investigating combined ADT and EBRT for locally advanced prostate cancer, reported that radiotherapy in combination with ADT improved not just local control but also overall survival for patients with high-risk localized or locally advanced prostate cancer [28]. Consequently, patients with high-risk disease, T1/T2 N+ M0 or T3/T4 N0/+ M0, should be advised to receive ADT for a total duration of 2–3 years with radiotherapy. Evidence has also shown that even patients with only one high-risk disease feature can benefit from 4–6 months of ADT in combination with EBRT [29].

With regard to pelvic nodal irradiation, international opinion is split on what should be considered the standard of care. In the SPCG-7 trial, patients randomized to the radiotherapy plus ADT arm received radiotherapy to the prostate and seminal vesicles alone which was considered the standard of care for UK centers. In the PR07 trial, patients randomized to radiotherapy plus ADT arm received radiotherapy to prostate, seminal vesicles, and the pelvic lymph nodes, which is considered the standard of care for patients in North America and some European countries [30, 31]. The Radiation Therapy Oncology Group (RTOG) 94-13 trial, which compared prostate-only radiotherapy against whole-pelvic radiotherapy, initially found a 7% improvement in progression-free survival for patients in the prostate and pelvis radiotherapy arm after a median follow-up of 5 years [32]. The initial results of this study changed clinical practice for intermediate- and high-risk prostate cancer patients in the United States where the addition of whole-pelvic radiotherapy to prostate radiotherapy became the new standard of care. An update in 2007 though found that there was no longer any statistical significance between the two groups and that the 5-year biochemical progression-free survival for both groups was now just under 50% [33]. A smaller French phase III trial conducted by the French Fédération Nationale des Centres de Lutte Contre le Cancer (FNLCC) group also failed to find a significant difference between whole-pelvic and prostate-only radiotherapy. The GETUG-01 trial recruited a total of 444 patients and randomized them between whole-pelvic and prostate-only radiotherapy. They found a nonsignificant 3% difference in 5-year progression-free survival, 63% vs. 60%, between the high-risk prostate-alone group and high-risk whole-pelvis group, respectively ($p = 0.20$) [34]. These results cast further doubt on the true benefits of whole-pelvic radiotherapy in high-risk prostate cancer patients.

A phase II trial (PIVOTAL) has been designed to determine the feasibility and toxicity of treating locally advanced prostate cancer with escalated doses of radiotherapy to the prostate and pelvic nodes using IMRT. By utilizing IMRT, the trial aims to deliver a higher dose of radiation to the pelvic lymph nodes in the hope that it will lead to a significant improvement in biochemical progression-free and overall survival. Both the RTOG and GETUG-01 trials relied upon CRT and consequently the dose delivered to the pelvic lymph nodes was 50.4 Gy in 1.8 Gy per fraction and 46 Gy in 2 Gy per fraction, respectively. By utilizing IMRT, the PIVOTAL trial aims to escalate the dose to the pelvic nodes to 60 Gy in 1.62 Gy per fraction (55.4 Gy in 2 Gy per fraction dose equivalent), which is a significant increase over the doses used in the older trials. The trial is currently open and in the early stages of recruitment so any definitive conclusions will be some time yet.

## Adjuvant or salvage radiotherapy following radical surgery

Following radical prostatectomy, there are a significant number of patients who on postoperative histology are found to have high-risk features and/or a positive surgical margin that places them at increased risk of tumor recurrence. The results of the SWOG 8794 trial has allowed clinicians to counsel patients more clearly on the potential benefits of adjuvant radiotherapy. The SWOG 8794 trial has randomized 425 patients, who had been found to have extra-prostatic disease extension following radical prostatectomy to either adjuvant radiotherapy or routine care and follow-up. When the trial was initially reported they found that the rates of disease and biochemical relapse were significantly lower in the adjuvant radiotherapy arm compared with the routine follow-up arm [35]. In 2009, updated results from the trial showed that adjuvant radiotherapy improved the rates of metastasis-free survival and overall survival [36]. Two further trials have also reported statistically significant improvements in the 5-year biochemical progression-free survival in patients receiving adjuvant radiotherapy rather than observation alone [37, 38]. Based on these trial results, it would seem that adjuvant radiotherapy offers a potential benefit to post-prostatectomy patients.

To help clarify the situation further, the RADICALS trial has been designed to answer two important questions: what is the best way to use radiotherapy after surgery? and what is the best way to use hormone treatment with any radiotherapy given after surgery? The RADICALS trial is a randomized phase III international trial that hopes to recruit 3000 post radical prostatectomy patients. As of March 2012, the trial had managed to recruit just over 1200 patients. Based on their target patient population, it will be a few years yet before the answers to these questions will be ready.

## Hypofractionation

The application of radiobiology to radiotherapy has led to the fractionation of radiotherapy. Generally speaking, radiation fractionation provides an increased therapeutic benefit that balances tumor control and late treatment side effects. By fractionating radiotherapy, that is, dividing the total dose into 1.8–2 Gy daily doses over a course of 6–8 weeks, normal tissues sustain less late toxicity while still maintaining tumor control. Hypofractionation in radiotherapy describes schedules in which the total dose of radiation is divided into larger doses given over a shorter period of time. Current radiobiological concepts suggest that prostate cancer has radiation response characteristics which are closer to those of late reactions than acute reactions, which means that it is much more sensitive to fraction size and that large doses per fraction cause relatively more radiation damage.

This sensitivity to differing radiation fractionation regimens can be expressed mathematically using the linear quadratic equation which describes two phases of cell kill, the initial alpha phase followed by an exponential beta phase. The ratio of these two is termed the alpha:beta ratio. The radiobiology of prostate cancer has been of particular interest recently following the proposal that the alpha:beta ratio of the prostate cancer cells seem to be more in keeping with late responding tissues rather than early ones. Radiobiological modeling initially using low dose rate brachytherapy data suggested the alpha:beta ratio for prostate cancer could be in the region of only 0.8–2.2 Gy [39, 40]. Further modeling using high dose rate brachytherapy data placed the alpha:beta ratio in the region of 0.03–4.1 Gy [41]. If these alpha:beta ratio estimates were correct, then it would support the idea that prostate cancer radiotherapy might be better suited to hypofractionated radiotherapy regimens. This would mean that patients would no longer need to be treated over a 6–8-week period. To investigate this further, the CHHIP trial was designed to randomize patients between three different radiotherapy schedules: 74 Gy over 7.5 weeks, 60 Gy over 4 weeks, and 57 Gy over just under 2 weeks. The trial closed to recruitment in June 2011 after recruiting 3216 patients. Its full results are currently awaited, although an analysis of toxicity in those patients taking part found no significant differences in toxicity after a median follow-up of 50.5 months. So far, it would seem based on this initial data that treating patients with hypofractionated radiotherapy is safe and does not cause more side effects than standard fractionated treatments [42].

## Stereotactic body radiotherapy

The interest in the potentially low alpha:beta ratio of prostate cancer has also led to the introduction of extreme hypofractionated radiotherapy regimens for the disease. Stereotactic body radiotherapy (SBRT) utilizes state-of-the-art radiotherapy technology to deliver a highly CRT treatment in five fractions or less [43]. Currently though there is a paucity of randomized evidence to support its use, and much of the data surrounding SBRT for prostate cancer treatment comes from single-center series. It is hoped though that the newly launched international, multicenter, randomized trial, PACE, which plans to compare Cyberknife SBRT with IMRT, will confirm its therapeutic benefits in prostate cancer.

## Proton therapy

Protons are charged sub-atomic particles that cause ionization in cells similar to the effect of X-rays and photons. However, because they are particulate they travel for a finite range in tissue, related to their accelerating energy, unlike X-ray beams. Due to their relatively large mass, they suffer little lateral scatter and deposit the majority of their energy in the final few millimeters of their path. This deposition of energy is termed as "Bragg peak" and when exploited in the treatment of cancer means that the normal tissue surrounding the tumor receives little of the ionizing radiation. This in turn translates to reduced acute and late toxicity for the patient. The benefit of proton therapy over modern linear-accelerator-based IMRT in treating prostate cancer is yet to be proven in clinical trials, although a proof of principal study has demonstrated their efficacy in achieving dose escalation [44]. One factor that restricts the more widespread use of proton therapy is its huge cost in terms of equipment and consequently at present only a few centers internationally have installed high-energy proton accelerators for clinical use.

## Brachytherapy

An alternative means of delivering radiation to the prostate is by direct insertion of a radiation source into the prostate. The transperineal transrectal ultrasound-guided approach is now widely established and undertaken as a routine procedure to achieve this with high accuracy. The advantage of brachytherapy is that it delivers dose intensely around the radiation source with a rapid fall off obeying the inverse square law. This means that high doses can be concentrated in the prostate with low doses to surrounding normal tissue in particular the rectum and bladder. Thus, for low-risk prostate cancer, where the risk of significant extracapsular extension, seminal vesicle, or lymph node involvement is small, brachytherapy alone offers an excellent choice for radiotherapy; in intermediate- and higher-risk disease, localized cancer carrying a higher risk of extraprostatic spread then in combination with EBRT treatment it offers an excellent means of dose escalation within the prostate gland itself.

There are two forms of brachytherapy:

- Low dose rate (LDR) permanent seed brachytherapy with which radioactive sources are implanted as tiny 5 mm seeds containing the radioisotope, either iodine-125, caesium-131, or palladium-103.
- Temporary afterloading brachytherapy that uses a temporary implant with needles or plastic catheters that are then used to guide a single radiation source using a computer-controlled afterloader through the implant at a calculated rate to deliver the required dose. The usual form of this approach is high dose rate (HDR) brachytherapy using iridium-192 delivering the dose in minutes; less common is the use of a low-activity source which is pulsed hourly (pulsed dose rate; PDR) over several days. At the end of treatment, with both HDR and PDR the implant is removed.

## Patient selection for brachytherapy

Patients must have localized disease on routine staging and be able to undergo a general or spinal anesthetic for the procedure. Other specific criteria have been defined below.

## LDR seed brachytherapy alone

Patients should have disease with a low risk of extracapsular extension or regional spread based on:

- PSA $\leq$ 10 ng/mL
- Gleason score $\leq$ 6 or 7 (3 + 4)
- Stage <T2c

Staging with a multifunctional MRI is also recommended to provide maximum information on disease extent and distribution.

Patients should also have no features which may predispose to significant post-brachytherapy complications including

- Prostate volume should be approximately <50 mL
- Pubic arch obstruction should be assessed
- Obstructive urinary symptoms should be minimal; as a guide an IPSS score > 15 and maximum flow rate <15 mL/min predict for a higher risk of catheterization and long-term urinary symptoms
- Recent transurethral resection (TURP) (within the previous 6–12 months) also predicts for a higher risk of urinary complications.

## Brachytherapy in combination with EBRT

This is appropriate for all patients having radical radiotherapy for prostate cancer. Low-risk patients as defined above will be better served by brachytherapy alone provided they are prepared to undergo the procedure; in doing so they will avoid the additional potential side effects of EBRT.

For the remainder then dose escalation using additional brachytherapy should be considered. LDR brachytherapy boosts may be less appropriate for those with T3 disease as retention of seeds outside the gland is less reliable. This is not an issue for temporary implants using HDR or PDR.

### HDR (PDR) brachytherapy alone

Although there is an emerging literature on the role and efficacy of HDR brachytherapy used alone in the same way as LDR seed implants, this remains at present investigational but with considerable promise for the future being able to offer radical brachytherapy treatment to low-, intermediate-, and high-risk localized prostate cancer patients.

## Procedure

Brachytherapy may be undertaken as a day case or ward-based inpatient. It should always be performed by an experienced team undertaking the procedure on a regular basis which may comprise input from urologists, radiologists, brachytherapy physicists, specialist radiographers, and nurses alongside the oncologist.

*LDR permanent seed brachytherapy* is undertaken as a one- or two-step procedure. The requirements are a transrectal ultrasound series of images to be acquired in the position in which implantation will be undertaken. This may be done as a separate procedure following which the implantation of sources occurs some days or even weeks later. Increasingly, the procedure is undertaken as a single-step procedure with the volume study and implantation performed in one episode. Once the volume study has been acquired, the target volume is defined and using a sophisticated computer algorithm the position of sources within that volume is defined. Seeds are then placed in the prostate under direct ultrasound vision to reproduce the dosimetric plan. Modern systems will track each source as it is deposited and build up the dose contribution so that fine adjustments can be made during the implant procedure. Typically 80–100 seeds will be used for each patient.

*HDR or PDR temporary implantation*s use a similar approach but instead of live radioactive sources being placed in the gland, inactive afterloading needles or catheters are placed within the gland using the transrectal ultrasound transperineal-guided approach. Once in position, imaging with the transrectal ultrasound will be used to define the volume to be treated or alternatively the patient will be transferred for CT or MR imaging which will be used for volume definition. Once defined, the rate of passage for the source within each catheter or needle is calculated using 2–5 mm "dwell times" at which it may rest for several seconds. Treatment is then delivered by connecting the implant tubes to the afterloader, which contains the source and will reproduce the dosimetric plan as it passes the source through each tube.

Organs at risk will be carefully defined alongside the target volume for both techniques, in particular the urethra and anterior rectal wall. Dose constraints will be used for these structures to ensure the dose they receive is kept within acceptable limits.

Patients can be discharged from hospital the same or the following day after completion of seed implantation and HDR treatment delivery. An alpha-blocker to enhance the urine flow and a week of prophylactic antibiotics are often recommended.

Following HDR brachytherapy there are no radioprotection issues however after seed brachytherapy, while the dose outside the patient is very low and within radiation safety limits, it is usual to recommend that for the first 2 months after implant children do not sit on the lap of the patient. For men who resume sexual activity, condom use is recommended for the first 2 months although loss of seeds following implantation is now a rare event. Cremation can cause contamination of the crematorium and liberate radioactive material into the atmosphere and current UK recommendations are that cremation should not be undertaken in the first 2 years after seed implantation.

## Results

In all cases the probability of biochemical disease-free survival is closely related to the prognostic factors and risk category at presentation. For patients with PSA < 10 ng/mL, Gleason score <7, and stage T2A or less, little impact is seen on natural life expectancy; even for those with high-risk disease, 70% or more will be alive 10 years after treatment.

### LDR permanent seed brachytherapy

There is now an extensive literature reporting the results of LDR seed brachytherapy with mature results out to 15 years and beyond. A selection of the larger series is shown in Table 9.1. The largest cohort is that of

**Table 9.1** Selected published series of LDR I125 seed brachytherapy with >10 years follow-up

| | | | Biochemical relapse-free survival (%) | | |
| | | | Risk group | | |
| Author | Number | Follow-up (years) | Low | Intermediate | High |
|---|---|---|---|---|---|
| Grimm [45] | 125 | 10 | 87 | 78 | – |
| Potters [46] | 1449 | 12 | 89 | 78 | 63 |
| Henry [47] | 1298 | 10 | 86 | 77 | 61 |
| Hinnen [48] | 921 | 10 | 88 | 61 | 30 |
| Stone [49] | 1171 | 12 | 88 | 79 | 67 |
| Taira [50] | 463 | 12 | 97 | 96 | 91 |
| Crook[a] [51] | 1111 | 10 | – | 95 | |

[a]Seven-year disease-free survival reported.

2693 patients pooled from 11 US institutes [52] of which 1831 received LDR I125 brachytherapy (median dose 144 Gy) and 893 received Pd103 implants (median dose 130 Gy). The 8-year PSA relapse-free survival was 82%, 70%, and 48%, respectively, for low-, intermediate-, and high-risk patients using the ASTRO definition of three successive PSA rises and 74%, 61%, and 39%, respectively, using the nadir $+ 2$ ng/mL definition. No significant difference between the two isotopes was found on multivariate analysis. Using the same risk groups, the 15-year outcome data from Seattle report PSA relapse-free survivals of 85.8%, 80.3%, and 67.8% for low-, intermediate-, and high-risk groups, respectively.

Two important features of the response after LDR seed brachytherapy are the time taken to reach PSA nadir and the phenomenon of a PSA "bounce." For many patients, the PSA nadir is not reached until around 3 years from implant. In the large US collaborative cohort, nadir PSA at 3 years was a prognostic factor, the 8-year PSA relapse-free survival being 88%, 69%, 57%, and 41% after nadir counts of 0–0.49, 0.5–0.99, 1.0–1.99, and ≥2.0, respectively.

The PSA bounce is seen in approximately 15% of patients. This occurs when after an initial fall there is a rise in PSA before settling to the nadir. This is usually seen between 12 and 24 months after implant with average rises of around 3 ng/mL being seen during this period in those who demonstrate the bounce. It is important to recognize this phenomenon and continue PSA monitoring rather than proceeding to unnecessary salvage treatment.

Most series demonstrate a relationship between implant quality as measured by the $D_{90}$ and PSA response based on a standard prescription of 145 Gy to the minimum peripheral isodose. In the US series, when the $D_{90}$ for I125 implants was $\geq 130$ Gy the PSA relapse-free survival was 92% compared with 76% in those patients whose implant had a lower $D_{90}$ value. Another large series of 1377 patients having LDR seed brachytherapy reported that when the $D_{90}$ was $<154$ Gy the 10-year PSA relapse-free survival was 69% compared with 91% when the $D_{90}$ was $>150$ Gy [53].

## HDR temporary brachytherapy alone

The first experience with HDR monotherapy was reported from Osaka using a schedule of 48–54 Gy in 8–9 fractions in a population of predominantly high-risk patients [54]. The 5-year PSA failure-free rate was 70%. A series of 298 patients treated at Oakland and Michigan reports a 94% biochemical control rate at 5 years [55]. This was a relatively good prognosis group having a median presenting PSA of 5.4, stage IC, and Gleason score 6; and the two centers used two different schedules, 42 Gy in six fractions in Oakland and 36 Gy in four fractions in Michigan. No statistically significant difference between the two schedules was seen. A dose escalation study reporting three cohorts receiving 34 Gy in four fractions, 36 Gy in four fractions, and 31.5Gy in three fractions from Mount Vernon has a 100% biochemical control rate with median follow-ups of 30, 18, and 11.8 months, respectively [56].

## Brachytherapy in combination with EBRT
### HDR boost with external beam

One randomized controlled trial has been reported from Mount Vernon that compared external beam treatment delivering 55 Gy in 20 daily fractions with a combined schedule of external beam 35.7 Gy in 13 fractions and an HDR boost of 17 Gy in 2 fractions [57]. The relative doses of the two schedules in 2 Gy equivalents are 62.5 Gy and 77.7 Gy with an alpha:beta ratio of 3.5; and 66.9 Gy and 92.1 Gy with an alpha:beta ratio of 1.5. The results show an advantage in biochemical control for the combined HDR group at 7 years with lower acute rectal morbidity and equivalent late morbidity demonstrating that using an HDR boost is a highly effective means of achieving biological dose escalation.

**Table 9.2** Selected published series of HRD brachytherapy with external beam with ≥5 years follow-up

| Author | Number | Follow-up (months) | Biochemical relapse-free survival (%) Risk group | | |
| --- | --- | --- | --- | --- | --- |
| | | | Low | Intermediate | High |
| Pellizzon [59] | 209 | 64 | 91 | 90 | 89 |
| Phan [60] | 309 | 64 | 98 | 90 | 78 |
| Kalkner [61] | 154 | 73 | 97 | 83 | 51 |
| Sato [62] | 53 | 61 | 100 | 43 | |
| Demanes [63] | 209 | 84 | 90 | 87 | 69 |
| Zwahlen [64] | 196 | 65 | 94 | 83 | 76 |
| Wilder [65] | 284 | 66 | 100 | 100 | 93 |
| Kaprealian [66] | 165 | 105 | 92 | 79 | 89 |

A case–control series comparing external beam 50.4 Gy followed by 21 Gy in three fractions HDR brachytherapy with external beam IMRT delivering 86.4 Gy showed an advantage for the brachytherapy group for all risk groups, most marked in the intermediate-risk group of patients [58].

There are in addition a number of mature single-center and co-operative group studies using HDR brachytherapy in combination with external beam, all of which demonstrate high rates of biochemical and local control as shown in Table 9.2.

### LDR seed boost with external beam

Similarly LDR brachytherapy using either I125 in a dose of 110 Gy or Pd103 in a dose of 90—100 Gy has been reported from a number of single centers showing that it is effective in achieving durable biochemical control. No comparative data with external beam alone or between LDR and HDR brachytherapy as a boost have been reported.

### PDR boost with external beam

Few centers choose to use PDR in this setting and published results are few; in principle however there is no reason to think that they will be different to those achieved with HDR or LDR.

# Side effects of brachytherapy

## Acute toxicity

Urethritis is the most common problem and very variable. Most patients also will notice frequency, urgency, and mild dysuria with reduced flow in more severe cases. It usually follows one of two patterns:

- After LDR seed brachytherapy symptoms start 5 or 6 days after implantation and may persist reaching a peak in the first month or two and persisting at decreasing levels for 6–9 months.

- In contrast, after HDR brachytherapy, there is an acute phase of urethritis developing in the first 2 weeks after implantation, which resolves much more rapidly, usually within 6 weeks from the implant.

Urinary retention requiring catheterization occurs in around 10% of patients after LDR seed brachytherapy. The majority resume normal micturition after 10–14 days but some need a catheter for a few months. Surgical intervention should be delayed for as long as possible but if there are still obstructive symptoms after 12 months, a bladder neck incision or channel TURP can be performed. This is safer than a full TURP, which carries a significant risk of incontinence. Further delay to longer periods after implantation may also be associated with a higher risk of incontinence due to fibrosis.

Predictive factors for obstruction include a high urinary symptom score, prostate volume >50 mL at implant, and the use of initial hormone therapy to downsize the volume. Other factors that have been proposed include number of needles used and number of needle passes.

## Late effects

Urethral strictures occur in 5–10% of patients requiring dilatation or self-catheterization.

Urinary incontinence is rare and usually only seen in patients who have had prostate surgery within 6–12 months of the implants.

Erectile dysfunction (ED) occurs in 15–40% of patients. Comparative nonrandomized studies demonstrate that as a primary treatment modality LDR brachytherapy has a lower rate of ED compared with prostatectomy or EBRT. When LDR or HDR brachytherapy is used with external beam, then comparable rates to external beam alone are reported. Predictive factors for ED after LDR brachytherapy include age, premorbid erectile function score, prior use of androgen blockade, smoking, diabetes, and hypertension. It remains unclear whether the dose to the neurovascular bundle or to the penile bulb is can predict ED [67, 68].

Phosphodiesterase inhibitors such as sildenafil and tadalafil are effective in this setting with response rates of over 60%.

Radiation proctitis occurs in between 2% and 12% following permanent brachytherapy, but is usually mild with intermittent rectal bleeding. HDR brachytherapy when used as a boost after external beam treatment has been shown to reduce acute radiation proctitis compared with EBRT alone.

Ulceration and fistula formation is reported in <1% of cases and usually reflects misplaced seeds with the result of a higher dose to the rectum.

Inappropriate biopsy and cauterization of the rectal mucosa to stop bleeding can also result in ulceration and fistula and should be avoided unless clearly indicated to confirm an alternative diagnosis for rectal symptoms [69].

## Summary

Modern radiotherapy offers effective, durable treatment for all stages of prostate cancer with low levels of clinically significant toxicity. For the patient with low-risk disease, LDR seed brachytherapy offers an attractive alternative to prostatectomy with low rates of long-term urinary and sexual toxicity. For intermediate- and high-risk prostate cancer, dose-escalated radiotherapy using state-of-the-art approaches with IMRT, HDR brachytherapy, or protons in combination with a period of androgen deprivation has dramatically improved the long-term outlook for these patients with the expectation of 10-year relapse-free survival rates of greater than 70%.

## References

1 The Royal College of Radiologists' Clinical Oncology Information Network. British Association of Urological Surgeons. Guidelines on the management of prostate cancer. *Clin Oncol* 1999;11(2):S53–S88.

2 Consensus conference. The management of clinically localized prostate cancer. *J Am Med Assoc* 1987;258(19):2727–2730.

3 Imbert, A, Imbert L. Carcinome prostatopelvienne diffuse à marche aiguë, guérie par la radiothérapie. *Bull Acad Med* 1904;52:139–142.

4 Minet H. Applications du radium aux tumeurs vésicales, à l'hypertrophie et au cancer de la prostate. *Assoc Franc Urol* 1909;13:629–633.

5 Murphy LJT. *History of Urology.* Springfield: Charles C. Thomas; 1972.

6 Waters CA, Pierson JW. Deep X-ray therapy in the treatment of metastatic pain in carcinoma of the prostate. *South Med J* 1923;16:620–624.

7 Desnos E. Action du radium sur la prostate hypertrophiée. *Proc Verb Mem Assoc Franc Urol.* 1909;13:646–656.

8 Widerøe R. Ueber ein neues prinzip zur herstellung hoher spannungen. *Archiv fuer Elektronik und Uebertragungstechnik* 1928;21(4):387.

9 Ising G. Prinzip einer methode zur herstellung von kanalstrahlen hoher voltzahl. *Arkiv Fuer Matematik, Astronomi Och Fysik* 1928;18: 1–4.

10 Thwaites DI, Tuohy JB. Back to the future: the history and development of the clinical linear accelerator. *Phys Med Biol* 2006;51(13):R343–R362.

11 Morris DE, Emami B, Mauch PM, *et al.* Evidence-based review of three-dimensional conformal radiotherapy for localized prostate cancer: an ASTRO outcomes initiative. *Int J Radiat Oncol Biol Phys* 2005;62(1):3–19.

12 Fuks Z, Leibel SA, Kutcher GJ, *et al.* Three-dimensional conformal treatment: a new frontier in radiation therapy. *Important Adv Oncol* 1991:151–172.

13 Fuks Z, Horwich A. Clinical and technical aspects of conformal therapy. *Radiother Oncol* 1993;29(2):219–220.

14 Pollack A, Zagars GK, Starkschall G, *et al.* Conventional vs. conformal radiotherapy for prostate cancer: preliminary results of dosimetry and acute toxicity. *Int J Radiat Oncol Biol Phys* 1996;34(3):555–564.

15 Dearnaley DP, Khoo VS, Norman AR, *et al.* Comparison of radiation side-effects of conformal and conventional radiotherapy in prostate cancer: a randomised trial. *Lancet* 1999;353(9149):267–272.

16 Zelefsky MJ, Levin EJ, Hunt M, *et al.* Incidence of late rectal and urinary toxicities after three-dimensional conformal radiotherapy and intensity-modulated radiotherapy for localized prostate cancer. *Int J Radiat Oncol Biol Phys* 2008;70(4):1124–1129.

17 Jani AB, Su A, Correa D, Gratzle J. Comparison of late gastrointestinal and genitourinary toxicity of prostate cancer patients undergoing intensity-modulated versus conventional radiotherapy using localized fields. *Prostate Cancer Prostatic Dis* 2007;10(1):82–86.

18 Dearnaley DP, Hall E, Lawrence D, *et al.* Phase III pilot study of dose escalation using conformal radiotherapy in prostate cancer: PSA control and side effects. *Br J Cancer* 2005;92(3):488–498.

19 Dearnaley DP, Sydes MR, Graham JD, *et al.* Escalated-dose versus standard-dose conformal radiotherapy in prostate cancer: first results from the MRC RT01 randomised controlled trial. *Lancet Oncol* 2007;8(6):475–487.

20 Pollack A, Zagars GK, Starkschall G, *et al.* Prostate cancer radiation dose response: results of the M. D. Anderson phase III randomized trial. *Int J Radiat Oncol Biol Phys* 2002;53(5):1097–1105.

21 Peeters ST, Heemsbergen WD, Koper PC, *et al.* Dose-response in radiotherapy for localized prostate cancer: results of the Dutch multicenter randomized phase III trial comparing 68 Gy of radiotherapy with 78 Gy. *J Clin Oncol* 2006;24(13):1990–1996.

22 Kuban DA, Tucker SL, Dong L, *et al.* Long-term results of the M. D. Anderson randomized dose-escalation trial for prostate cancer. *Int J Radiat Oncol Biol Phys* 2008;70(1):67–74.

23 Xu N, Rossi PJ, Jani AB. Toxicity analysis of dose escalation from 75.6 gy to 81.0 gy in prostate cancer. *Am J Clin Oncol* 2011;34(1):11–15.

24 Eade TN, Hanlon AL, Horwitz EM, *et al.* What dose of external-beam radiation is high enough for prostate cancer? *Int J Radiat Oncol Biol Phys* 2007;68(3):682–689.

25  Horwitz EM, Bae K, Hanks GE, *et al*. Ten-year follow-up of radiation therapy oncology group protocol 92-02: a phase III trial of the duration of elective androgen deprivation in locally advanced prostate cancer. *J Clin Oncol* 2008;26(15):2497–2504.

26  British Uro-oncology Group, British Association of Urological Surgeons: Section of Oncology, and British Prostate Group. *MDT (Multi-disciplinary Team) Guidance for Managing Prostate Cancer*; 2009.

27  Widmark A, Klepp O, Solberg A, *et al*. Endocrine treatment, with or without radiotherapy, in locally advanced prostate cancer (SPCG-7/SFUO-3): an open randomised phase III trial. *Lancet* 2009;373(9660):301–308.

28  Warde P, Mason M, Ding K, *et al*. Combined androgen deprivation therapy and radiation therapy for locally advanced prostate cancer: a randomised, phase 3 trial. *Lancet* 2011;378(9809):2104–2111.

29  D'Amico AV, Manola J, Loffredo M, *et al*. 6-month androgen suppression plus radiation therapy vs radiation therapy alone for patients with clinically localized prostate cancer: a randomized controlled trial. *J Am Med Assoc* 2004;292(7):821–827.

30  Pilepich MV, Winter K, Lawton CA, *et al*. Androgen suppression adjuvant to definitive radiotherapy in prostate carcinoma–long-term results of phase III RTOG 85-31. *Int J Radiat Oncol Biol Phys* 2005;61(5):1285–1290.

31  Bolla M, Collette L, Blank L, *et al*. Long-term results with immediate androgen suppression and external irradiation in patients with locally advanced prostate cancer (an EORTC study): a phase III randomised trial. *Lancet* 2002;360(9327):103–106.

32  Roach M 3rd, DeSilvio M, Lawton C, *et al*. Phase III trial comparing whole-pelvic versus prostate-only radiotherapy and neoadjuvant versus adjuvant combined androgen suppression: Radiation Therapy Oncology Group 9413. *J Clin Oncol* 2003;21(10):1904–1911.

33  Lawton CA, DeSilvio M, Roach, M 3rd, *et al*. An update of the phase III trial comparing whole pelvic to prostate only radiotherapy and neoadjuvant to adjuvant total androgen suppression: updated analysis of RTOG 94-13, with emphasis on unexpected hormone/radiation interactions. *Int J Radiat Oncol Biol Phys* 2007;69(3):646–655.

34  Pommier P, Chabaud S, Lagrange JL, *et al*. Is there a role for pelvic irradiation in localized prostate adenocarcinoma? Preliminary results of GETUG-01. *J Clin Oncol* 2007;25(34):5366–5373.

35  Thompson IM Jr., Tangen CM, Paradelo J, *et al*. Adjuvant radiotherapy for pathologically advanced prostate cancer: a randomized clinical trial. *J Am Med Assoc* 2006;296(19):2329–2335.

36  Thompson IM, Tangen CM, Paradelo J, *et al*. Adjuvant radiotherapy for pathological T3N0M0 prostate cancer significantly reduces risk of metastases and improves survival: long-term followup of a randomized clinical trial. *J Urol* 2009;181(3):956–962.

37  Van der Kwast TH, Bolla M, Poppel HVan, *et al*. Identification of patients with prostate cancer who benefit from immediate postoperative radiotherapy: EORTC 22911. *J Clin Oncol* 2007;25(27):4178–4186.

38  Wiegel T, Bottke D, Steiner U, *et al*. Phase III postoperative adjuvant radiotherapy after radical prostatectomy compared with radical prostatectomy alone in pT3 prostate cancer with postoperative undetectable prostate-specific antigen: ARO 96-02/AUO AP 09/95. *J Clin Oncol* 2009;27(18):2924–2930.

39  Brenner DJ, Hall EJ. Fractionation and protraction for radiotherapy of prostate carcinoma. *Int J Radiat Oncol Biol Phys* 1999;43(5):1095–1101.

40  D'Souza WD, Thames HD. Is the alpha/beta ratio for prostate cancer low? *Int J Radiat Oncol Biol Phys* 2001;51(1):1–3.

41  Brenner DJ, Martinez AA, Edmundson GK, *et al.* Direct evidence that prostate tumors show high sensitivity to fractionation (low alpha/beta ratio), similar to late-responding normal tissue. *Int J Radiat Oncol Biol Phys* 2002;52(1):6–13.

42  Dearnaley D, Syndikus I, Sumo G, *et al.* Conventional versus hypofractionated high-dose intensity-modulated radiotherapy for prostate cancer: preliminary safety results from the CHHiP randomised controlled trial. *Lancet Oncol* 2012;13(1):43–54.

43  Buyyounouski MK, Price RA, Jr., Harris EE, *et al.* Stereotactic body radiotherapy for primary management of early-stage, low- to intermediate-risk prostate cancer: report of the American Society for Therapeutic Radiology and Oncology Emerging Technology Committee. *Int J Radiat Oncol Biol Phys* 2010;76(5):1297–1304.

44  Zietman AL, Bae K, Slater JD, *et al.* Randomized trial comparing conventional-dose with high-dose conformal radiation therapy in early-stage adenocarcinoma of the prostate: long-term results from Proton Radiation Oncology Group/American College of Radiology 95-09. *J Clin Oncol* 2010;28(7):1106–1111.

45  Grimm PD, Blasko JC, Sylvester JE, *et al.* 10-year biochemical (prostate-specific antigen) control of prostate cancer with (125)I brachytherapy. *Int J Radiat Oncol Biol Phys* 2001;51(1):31–40.

46  Potters L, Morgenstern C, Calugaru E, *et al.* 12-year outcomes following permanent prostate brachytherapy in patients with clinically localized prostate cancer. *J Urol* 2008;179(Suppl. 5):S20–S24.

47  Henry AM, Al-Qaisieh B, Gould K, *et al.* Outcomes following iodine-125 monotherapy for localized prostate cancer: the results of Leeds 10-year single-center brachytherapy experience. *Int J Radiat Oncol Biol Phys* 2010;76(1):50–56.

48  Hinnen KA, Battermann JJ, Roermund JGVan, *et al.* Long-term biochemical and survival outcome of 921 patients treated with I-125 permanent prostate brachytherapy. *Int J Radiat Oncol Biol Phys* 2010;76(5):1433–1438.

49  Stone NN, Stone MM, Rosenstein BS, *et al.* Influence of pretreatment and treatment factors on intermediate to long-term outcome after prostate brachytherapy. *J Urol* 2011;185(2):495–500.

50  Taira AV, Merrick GS, Butler WM, *et al.* Long-term outcome for clinically localized prostate cancer treated with permanent interstitial brachytherapy. *Int J Radiat Oncol Biol Phys* 2011;79(5):1336–1342.

51  Crook J, Borg J, Evans A, *et al.* 10-year experience with I-125 prostate brachytherapy at the Princess Margaret Hospital: results for 1,100 patients. *Int J Radiat Oncol Biol Phys* 2011;80(5):1323–1329.

52  Zelefsky MJ, Kuban DA, Levy LB, *et al.* Multi-institutional analysis of long-term outcome for stages T1-T2 prostate cancer treated with permanent seed implantation. *Int J Radiat Oncol Biol Phys* 2007;67(2):327–333.

53  Stock RG, Stone NN, Cesaretti JA, Rosenstein BS. Biologically effective dose values for prostate brachytherapy: effects on PSA failure and posttreatment biopsy results. *Int J Radiat Oncol Biol Phys* 2006;64(2):527–533.

54  Yoshioka Y, Konishi K, Sumida I, *et al.* Monotherapeutic high-dose-rate brachytherapy for prostate cancer: five-year results of an extreme hypofractionation regimen with 54 Gy in nine fractions. *Int J Radiat Oncol Biol Phys* 2011;80(2):469–475.

55  Demanes DJ, Martinez AA, Ghilezan M, *et al.* High-dose-rate monotherapy: safe and effective brachytherapy for patients with localized prostate cancer. *Int J Radiat Oncol Biol Phys* 2011;81(5):1286–1292.

56  Corner C, Rojas AM, Bryant L, *et al.* A phase II study of high-dose-rate afterloading brachytherapy as monotherapy for the treatment of localized prostate cancer. *Int J Radiat Oncol Biol Phys* 2008;72(2):441–446.

57  Hoskin PJ, Rojas AM, Bownes PJ, *et al.* Randomised trial of external beam radiotherapy alone or combined with high-dose-rate brachytherapy boost for localised prostate cancer. *Radiother Oncol* 2012;103(2):217–222.

58  Deutsch I, Zelefsky MJ, Zhang Z, *et al.* Comparison of PSA relapse-free survival in patients treated with ultra-high-dose IMRT versus combination HDR brachytherapy and IMRT. *Brachytherapy* 2010;9(4):313–318.

59  Pellizzon AC, Nadalin W, Salvajoli JV, *et al.* Results of high dose rate afterloading brachytherapy boost to conventional external beam radiation therapy for initial and locally advanced prostate cancer. *Radiother Oncol* 2003;66(2):167–172.

60  Phan TP, Syed AM, Puthawala A, *et al.* High dose rate brachytherapy as a boost for the treatment of localized prostate cancer. *J Urol* 2007;177(1):123–127; discussion 127.

61  Kalkner KM, Wahlgren T, Ryberg M, *et al.* Clinical outcome in patients with prostate cancer treated with external beam radiotherapy and high dose-rate iridium 192 brachytherapy boost: a 6-year follow-up. *Acta Oncol* 2007;46(7):909–917.

62  Sato M, Mori T, Shirai S, *et al.* High-dose-rate brachytherapy of a single implant with two fractions combined with external beam radiotherapy for hormone-naive prostate cancer. *Int J Radiat Oncol Biol Phys* 2008;72(4):1002–1009.

63  Demanes DJ, Brandt D, Schour L, Hill DR. Excellent results from high dose rate brachytherapy and external beam for prostate cancer are not improved by androgen deprivation. *Am J Clin Oncol* 2009;32(4):342–347.

64  Zwahlen DR, Andrianopoulos N, Matheson B, *et al.* High-dose-rate brachytherapy in combination with conformal external beam radiotherapy in the treatment of prostate cancer. *Brachytherapy* 2010;9(1):27–35.

65  Wilder RB, Barme GA, Gilbert RF, *et al.* Preliminary results in prostate cancer patients treated with high-dose-rate brachytherapy and intensity modulated radiation therapy (IMRT) vs. IMRT alone. *Brachytherapy* 2010;9(4):341–348.

66  Kaprealian T, Weinberg V, Speight JL, *et al.* High-dose-rate brachytherapy boost for prostate cancer: comparison of two different fractionation schemes. *Int J Radiat Oncol Biol Phys* 2012;82(1):222–227.

67  Merrick GS, Butler WM, Wallner KE, *et al.* The importance of radiation doses to the penile bulb vs. crura in the development of postbrachytherapy erectile dysfunction. *Int J Radiat Oncol Biol Phys* 2002;54(4):1055–1062.

68  Stock RG, Kao J, Stone NN. Penile erectile function after permanent radioactive seed implantation for treatment of prostate cancer. *J Urol* 2001;165(2):436–439.

69  Gelblum DY, Potters L. Rectal complications associated with transperineal interstitial brachytherapy for prostate cancer. *Int J Radiat Oncol Biol Phys* 2000;48(1):119–124.

## CHAPTER 10

# Novel Therapies for Localized Prostate Cancer

*Massimo Valerio[1,2,3], Mark Emberton[1,2], Manit Arya[2,4], and Hashim U. Ahmed[1,2]*

[1] Division of Surgery and Interventional Science, University College London, London, UK
[2] Department of Urology, University College London Hospitals NHS Foundation Trust, London, UK
[3] Centre Hospitalier Universitaire Vaudois, Lausanne, Switzerland
[4] Barts Cancer Institute, Queen Mary University, London, UK

## Introduction

Traditionally the management of organ-confined prostate cancer has been focused on radical treatments and more recently in expectant management as watchful waiting and active surveillance protocols. Standard radical therapies include radical prostatectomy, external beam radiotherapy (EBRT), and brachytherapy. Despite recent innovations in these respective procedures and excellent medium- to long-term oncological outcomes, the morbidity of each therapy remains significant. Further, the task to determine the superiority of one treatment over another with respect to their toxicity and efficacy profiles has not been possible as no randomized controlled trial comparing these procedures with each other has been successfully completed to date. As a result, the American Urological Association clinical guidelines panel on prostate cancer stated that given the selection biases, the heterogeneity in reporting complications after treatment and various other forms of bias and variability, it was unfeasible to determine whether one therapy had more overall toxicity than others [1]. Although differences do exist in the type and rate of complications expected after every treatment, the morbidity is significant for each of these therapies. On an average, 10–20% will experience urinary incontinence and 50% erectile dysfunction. Rectal toxicity after radiotherapy and surgery occurs in 10–20%.

*Prostate Cancer: Diagnosis and Clinical Management*, First Edition.
Edited by Ashutosh K. Tewari, Peter Whelan and John D. Graham.
© 2014 John Wiley & Sons, Ltd. Published 2014 by John Wiley & Sons, Ltd.

Two randomized controlled trials have completed comparing surgery with watchful waiting. The first trial, the Scandinavian Prostate Cancer Group-4 trial (SPCG-4), showed that after a median follow-up of 12.8 years there was an absolute risk reduction of 6.1% in prostate-cancer-specific mortality in patients undergoing surgery [2]. This pivotal study was the first level I evidence showing superiority of treatment over no treatment. However, the findings of this study cannot be applied to patients currently diagnosed with prostate cancer in Western countries. Indeed, the recruitment of this trial began in 1989 when the formal and informal screening practices in Europe and particularly in the Scandinavian countries where the trial was carried out were significantly different than the current strategy used. For instance, only 12% of the patients had prostate-specific antigen (PSA)-detected disease and a majority of patients had palpable disease on digital rectal examination. In effect, this mortality reduction is likely to represent the best possible we can achieve in high-risk prostate cancer.

Recently, the PIVOT trial has reported on outcomes from a randomized controlled trial in which men were randomized between surgery and watchful waiting. These 731 men were diagnosed with prostate cancer in the early PSA screening era in the United States. The headline results showed that among men randomized to radical prostatectomy, 21 (5.8%) died from prostate cancer or treatment, as compared with 31 men (8.4%) assigned to observation (hazard ratio = 0.63; 95% CI = 0.36–1.09; $p$ = .09; absolute risk reduction = 2.6%) [3]. This sobering finding has found additional weight alongside the publication of two large screening studies on prostate cancer which showed conflicting outcomes with significant concerns about overdiagnosis, overtreatment, and the harms of prostate-cancer-related therapy [4, 5].

The initial response has been to look for an intermediate solution between radical treatment and watchful waiting, namely active surveillance. This active strategy, better discussed elsewhere in this book, is growing fast and the initial results are very encouraging with high rates of disease-specific survival in the medium term. In the largest cohort, reported overall and disease-specific survival at 10 years were 78.6% and 97.2%, respectively [6]. However, these findings need to be tempered for several reasons. First, the prostate-cancer-specific mortality is extremely low and this follow-up in a highly selected group of low-risk patients is insufficient to draw completely valid conclusions. Second, although active surveillance is considered a type of strict expectant management aiming to delay or avoid active treatment in prostate cancer when not needed, the burden for patients and healthcare services costs can be significant. Indeed, clinical examinations, numerous biopsies (every 1–2 years), and 3 monthly serum PSA measurements may not make this strategy so appealing to some men and physicians. There is also a very small risk of prostate cancer progression. Further, the absence of reliable biological markers of prostate cancer progression and the random and systematic error associated with standard transrectal ultrasound (TRUS) biopsy may make this approach lead to potentially under-treatment. Indeed, on average one-third of patients in active surveillance usually require active treatment after 2–3 years. To underline the fact that the current active surveillance protocol may be inadequate, a recent study reclassified 80% of patients in an active surveillance cohort from low-risk to intermediate- or high-risk disease not suited to monitoring, using transperineal template mapping biopsy (TPM) instead of standard TRUS biopsy [7].

Given the shortcomings of each of the current strategies, there has been increasing interest among physicians and patients in other active minimally invasive treatments which could reduce treatment-related morbidity and at the same time maintain good disease control rates.

## Minimally invasive treatment

The primary objective for the use of minimally invasive treatment has been to reduce the side effects of standard treatment by minimizing damage to surrounding structures of the prostate—such as the bladder, seminal vesicles, rhabdo-sphincter, neurovascular bundles, Denonvilliers' fascia, and rectum. Initially, this was through a whole-gland approach in which cryosurgery or high-intensity focused ultrasound (HIFU) attempted to mimic conventional whole-gland surgery or radiotherapy. More recently, there has been a tremendous amount of interest and work on tissue-preserving focal therapy in which the tumor alone is targeted with a margin of normal tissue [8]. Of course, conventional therapies find this difficult since radiation therapy (even intensity-modulated or radiosurgical techniques) does not allow a precise preservation of contiguous structures to the target and because surgical approaches have traditionally been unable to dissect into the prostate due to lack of a natural tissue plane. Research in other ablative technologies has thus been necessary. Cryotherapy, HIFU, photodynamic therapy (PDT), irreversible electroporation, and photothermal therapy have all been investigated in prospective trials to determine their feasibility, toxicity, and ablative efficacy in prostate cancer.

A common ability of these technologies has been the possibility to deliver the treatment in an outpatient setting or with a less than 24 hours hospital stay. In addition, because of the ability to precisely ablate with the capacity to spare tissue adjacent to prostate cancer, it was postulated that such modalities could be used when other treatments had failed or re-applied in more than one session. With these premises, the initial experience with the majority of these treatments has been in salvage cases, mostly after local EBRT failure. The application of these treatments in primary disease has been forthcoming particularly over the past 5–10 years.

## Focal therapy

After the first trials investigating whole-gland therapies and given the good results in a high-risk population represented by salvage patients, an appealing strategy has been to not only preserve surrounding tissue, but prostatic tissue unaffected by significant cancer as well. This strategy has been deemed "focal therapy." Focal therapy aims to maximize the preservation of tissue by targeting the cancer and not the organ. This approach has been increasingly used in other solid tumors such as breast, thyroid, kidney, liver, and even pancreas.

The application of organ-preserving therapy in prostate cancer has come from a better understanding of the natural history of prostate cancer and from new technologies which are able to accurately identify, localize, and sample single foci of prostate cancer within the gland. Prostate cancer has traditionally been considered as a multifocal disease; the use of organ-sparing approaches was thereby deemed ineffective. However, given the shift to diagnosing prostate cancer earlier in its natural history driven by formal and informal PSA screening, recent series of patients undergoing surgery for instance show that nearly half of the patients have unifocal or unilateral disease [9]. In addition, new evidence from basic research have pointed out that the natural history of prostate cancer is mediated and driven by index tumors which have histological characteristics of aggressiveness—such as Gleason pattern 4 or greater or large lesion volumes of 0.5 cm$^3$ or greater. Indeed, a recent study has demonstrated that progression of prostate cancer to metastasis could be mediated by only one single precursor cell [10, 11]. Thus, destroying the index lesion in the case of multifocal prostate cancer with clinically insignificant satellite lesions may also be a reasonable strategy to investigate, especially as some are now questioning, if these small low-grade lesions should even be called "cancer" [12, 13].

Thus, efforts have particularly focused around tools to precisely localize cancer lesions and particularly the index lesion within the prostate. Two complementary tools have been explored with the aim to increase the diagnostic ability to define the exact location of the index lesion: template transperineal prostate mapping biopsies and MRI. As in the majority of other solid organ cancers, imaging is likely to play an essential role in the detection of significant prostate cancer. Continuous development of the MRI technique using a multiparametric approach is ongoing. The initial results seem to confirm the role of multiparametric MRI in detecting the index lesion. In the setting of focal therapy, in which tissue is preserved, the negative predictive value of multiparametric MRI of 95% is particularly pertinent [14–17]. Template prostate mapping biopsy is performed under TRUS guidance using a brachytherapy stepper and grid with biopsies taken every 5 mm through the perineum and not through the rectum (Figure 10.1). Systematic TPM has undergone wide evaluation in the last years and currently must be considered as the gold standard prior to thinking of a focal approach in treating prostate cancer. A 5 mm distance sampling allows an accuracy of 95% for detection of significant prostate cancer lesions and allows one to accurately risk stratify disease based on volume and grade of cancer [18–24].

Once the spatial location of the index lesion has been established, the next objective is to determine which ablative technology is best suited to destroy cancerous cells and avoid damage to adjacent structures and tissue and to determine the margin of normal tissue that will be applied. No classification exists at the moment defining the boundaries of focal therapy and its margins. The terms subtotal ablation, hemi-ablation, quadrant ablation, and true focal ablation or wide local ablation of a single or multiple foci of prostate cancer are all equally defined as focal therapy (Figure 10.2). Such distinctions seem not to be that important at the moment. As in the history of other novel tissue-preserving surgical paradigm shifts, adjacent tissue to disease is at the beginning treated widely; with subsequent experience, limiting the margin of destruction to a few millimeters has been possible with further refinement in technology and techniques.

## Defining success and failure after minimally invasive therapy

Major concerns in the field of minimally invasive treatment for prostate cancer remain the follow-up of patients after therapy, and defining success and failure. The use of disease-specific mortality with the purpose to

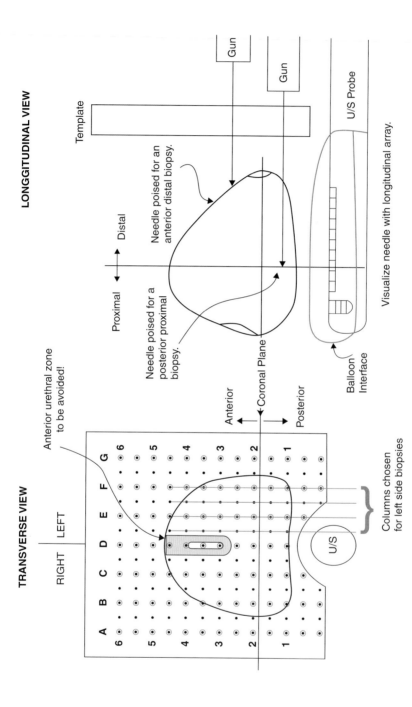

**Figure 10.1** Three-dimensional template prostate mapping (TPM) using a brachytherapy-like grid to insert needles under TRUS guidance. From Reference [7], used with permission from Elsevier.

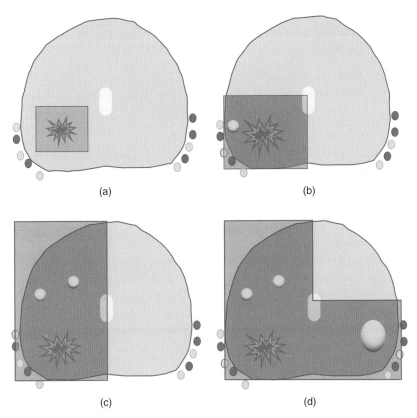

**Figure 10.2** Several types of organ-sparing approaches may be used to deliver treatment according to the number and the location of prostate cancer lesions. (a) True focal, (b) quadrant, (c) hemi-, or (d) subtotal ablations are illustrated.

evaluate an active treatment may not be feasible, practical, or cost-efficient in prostate cancer as the rate is very low and a study of 15–20 years duration would likely be needed. As a surrogate, PSA level is used as a marker of efficacy in radical therapies. However, in the setting of treatment which leaves the majority of the prostate untreated and which continues to secrete PSA, biochemical outcomes are less effective.

There is a need for an international consensus about benchmarks of success and failure after minimally invasive treatment to allow comparison between different groups using the same kind of energy and different kinds of energy. Until such consensus or validated biochemical parameters, the most reliable method to evaluate each technology seems to be the same used for diagnosis, namely biopsy and imaging (Table 10.1).

**Table 10.1** Overall disease control and functional outcomes using focal therapy

| Technology | Tissue damage | Approach | Phase development | Positive biopsy | Erectile dysfunction | Incontinence |
|---|---|---|---|---|---|---|
| Cryotherapy | Thermal | Transperineal | Approved | 4–45.5% | 14–42% | 0–4% |
| HIFU | Thermal | Transrectal | Phase III | 8–23.5% | 5–46% | 0–5% |
| PDT | Oxidative | Transperineal | Phase III | – | – | – |
| IRE | Electric | Transperineal | Phase II | – | – | – |
| Photothermal | Thermal | Transperineal | Phase II | – | – | – |

## Cryotherapy

### Technology

This form of thermal ablation aims to destroy prostate cancer cells by extreme cold temperatures—under $-40°C$. This is the only form of minimally invasive treatment considered as an established alternative to conventional treatment for whole-gland therapy. Indeed, the American Urology Association developed a Best Practice Statement in 2008 on the use of cryotherapy in localized prostate cancer [25]. The use of this technology in prostate cancer was first introduced in 1964 with both application of energy transurethrally and through a direct approach via the perineum. The technique was abandoned because of its extreme toxicity with rectourethral fistulae and urinary incontinence representing frequent complications [26]. The development of the technology with smaller probes inserted under image guidance has led to fourth-generation devices able to significantly reduce the morbidity. Several innovations were necessary to accomplish this task. First, TRUS guidance of cryoneedle placement via the perineum. Second, the use of safety measures such as urethral warmers and thermocouples to increase the preservation of adjacent structures. Next, a determinant innovation was the replacement of liquid with gas. With this advancement, cryosurgeons were able to take advantage of the Joule–Thomson effect by using argon and helium gas instead of liquid in the same time with the goal of both freeze and thaw with greater speed. In addition, the introduction of multiprobe cryogenic systems allowed the achievement of a better ablative efficacy and avoided the use of tract dilators to gain access to the prostate.

The first series using cryoablation in prostate cancer showed a survival comparable to surgical and radiation patients; with these innovations, cryotherapy became the first energy source approved by the Food and Drug Administration for the treatment of prostate cancer. Nowadays cryotherapy is delivered as an outpatient procedure in most of the cases, using general or spinal anesthesia. The cryoprobes are positioned transcutaneously under TRUS guidance with patients lying in a lithotomy position. A warming transurethral catheter is put in place during the procedure and then removed; thermocouples can be positioned to monitor the temperature within the rhabdo-sphincter, the Denonvilliers' fascia, and the neurovascular bundles. Sometimes a suprapubic catheter is left in place but often now a urethral catheter is commonly used to avoid urinary retention due to prostate inflammation and swelling after treatment.

The extreme cold temperatures destroy tissue through a series of mechanisms such as induction of apoptosis, vascular injury, osmotic damage, pH changes, ice crystal formation, and finally direct cytolysis through the extracellular or intracellular route. To maximize the ablative effect of cryosurgery and to safely perform the treatment, the Best Practice Statement from the AUA stated a number of procedures to follow during treatment. Temperature surveillance, nadir temperature of $-40°C$, rapid tissue freeze rate, slow thaw rate, and the use of two freeze–thaw cycles were all considered basic requirements for best practice [25].

## Whole-gland results

Nowadays patients having organ-confined prostate cancer or focal extracapsular extension and any Gleason grade with a negative metastatic assessment are considered good candidates for this approach. Indeed cryoablation is known to be effective against poorly differentiated cancer cells including those resistant to radiation and hormonal therapy [26]. It is known that it is difficult to achieve effective and uniform ablation in glands over 50 cm$^3$, so preoperative cytoreduction is considered in these cases. Traditionally, ideal patients have been considered, those not potent or disinterested in maintaining erections since many series showed an extremely high impotence rate [27]. The Cryo On-Line Database (COLD) including cases from various institutions allowed the most recent analysis on primary cryotherapy in patients affected by localized prostate cancer. The results in this population included 1198 consecutive patients with a mean age of 69.8 years, pretreatment PSA of 9.6 ng/mL, median Gleason score of 7, and median clinical stage of T2a [28]. The 5-year biochemical disease-free survival (bDFS) was 84.7%, 73.4%, and 75.3% for low-, moderate-, and high-risk patients using the ASTRO criteria. When the latest ASTRO-Phoenix criteria were applied, the 5-year bDFS was 91.1%, 78.5%, and 62.2%, respectively. When biopsy was performed in the absence of biochemical failure, the positive biopsy rate was 14.5%, compared with 38% when the biopsy was performed "for cause" due to a rising PSA. The urinary toxicity was low with 3.6% rate of urinary retention and incontinence at 2.9%. Impotence in the subgroup of potent patients was at 74.8% and rectal fistula was rare (0.4%). These results are comparable to previous reported series [29, 30]. Interestingly, one randomized controlled trial was performed in Canada comparing cryotherapy with EBRT in patients with localized prostate cancer [31, 32]. In both arms, all patients received neoadjuvant androgen deprivation therapy (ADT) since hormonal treatment prior to EBRT was included in the local protocol as standard of care. The primary endpoint in the 244 patients randomized control trial was failure at 36 months, defined according to ASTRO criteria. The failure rate in the cryotherapy group was 17.1% compared with 13.2% in the EBRT group. However, these results were not statistically significant and the failure trend between the two groups was reversed in further follow-up. The survival was not different in the two groups, whereas there were significantly more positive biopsies in the radiation group ($p < .01$). Overall toxicity was similar with gastrointestinal toxicity being more significant in the EBRT group and erectile dysfunction being more significant in the cryotherapy group ($P < .001$). Since this trial was underpowered with recruitment closing before reaching the sample size, the authors were unable to draw any definitive conclusions.

## Focal therapy results

The use of cryotherapy in a focal manner has widely increased in the last decade. An analysis of the COLD registry found that in the period between 1997 and 2007 there was an increase in this approach of over 1000-fold [33]. Compared with the group managed by whole-gland cryotherapy, this population is younger, has a lower Gleason score and stage. Apart from this registry, other series of patients treated in this manner have been reported [34–38]. In the first study by Onik *et al.* published in 2007, 55 patients underwent focal cryotherapy with a mean follow-up of 3.6 years [34]. With respect to cancer control, 13% of patients undergoing follow-up biopsy had residual disease in a previously untreated area, 95% had stable PSA, and 85% were potent at follow-up. In 2011, a series of 73 patients reported on hemi-cryoablation for unilateral, low–intermediate-risk prostate cancer which was biopsy proven by TRUS and target sampling based on Doppler signal [38]. Residual cancer in the treated side was found in only 1 patient out of 48 undergoing posttreatment biopsy. In regard of genitourinary toxicity, all patients were fully continent and potency was preserved in 86% of patients. In a matched analysis with surgical patients from the same institution, the relative risk for need of salvage therapy was similar in the population of radical prostatectomy and cryotherapy patients.

The results of these first series of patients demonstrate the feasibility of focal cryotherapy with promising functional and oncological outcomes. However, these findings must be confirmed in prospective development studies according to the IDEAL recommendations on evaluating new surgical and interventional techniques [39].

## HIFU

### Technology

High-intensity focused ultrasound (HIFU) is a thermal energy technique that aims to destroy cancer cells by heating with ultrasound frequencies of 0.8–3.5 MHz delivered in a focused manner to raise temperature in the target tissue above 56°C while sparing intervening tissue (Figure 10.3, Plate 10.3). Tissue is destroyed by two complementary mechanisms:

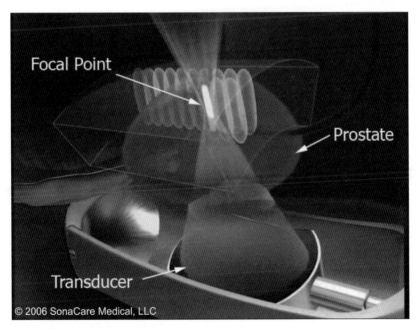

**Figure 10.3** Ultrasonic waves generated with transducer are focused onto a target area with focal lengths of either 3.0 or 4.0 cm. The intervening tissue and surrounding areas remain undamaged as the secondary intensity is low. Used with permission from Sonacare Medical. (See also Plate 10.3.)

thermal effect and internal cavitation due to the interaction between ultrasound waves and water microbubbles. In the application of HIFU in prostate cancer, two TRUS-guided devices have been developed since 1993; the Ablatherm™ (Edap-Technomed, Lyon, France) and the Sonablate500™ (Focus Surgery, Inc., Indianapolis, IN, USA). Basic features of these devices are identical; differences are mainly with respect to patient position, technical details, and safety systems. In both cases, the operation is performed as a day case, under general or regional anesthesia with a rectal probe containing the transducer. The focal length of the Sonablate500 transducer can be adjusted according to the operation needs.

This technology was first employed in urology by Madersbacher in 1995 to treat bladder outlet obstruction due to prostate enlargement [40]. Both the high rate of temporary urinary retention and the development of other less-invasive techniques to treat benign prostate hypertrophy decreased the use of this technology for this indication. The same group from Vienna employed HIFU before surgery to investigate the feasibility and the ablative effect of this procedure [41]. The main finding of this study was the thin and demarcated layer between the target zone and adjacent tissue. Thereby HIFU has been widely employed by different groups in the setting of localized prostate cancer. The debate is still open within Europe with some national societies considering HIFU as an option for the treatment of localized prostate cancer, that is, France, Italy, United Kingdom (as part of a registry or trials) and others such as Germany still considering HIFU as fully experimental.

## Whole-gland results

As in cryotherapy, HIFU has been mainly employed in a whole-gland approach both in primary and salvage cases. The largest series described until now comes from the multicenter HIFU registry, the @-registry where 356 patients with localized prostate cancer were treated in several centers [42]. Biochemical failure was reported according to Phoenix criteria. Negative biopsies were found in 80.5% patients and bDFS at 5 and 7 years was 85% and 79%, respectively. When other small series are considered, the 5-year bDFS after primary treatment is between 55% and 95% and negative biopsy rate varies between 35% and 95%, although some of these include for-cause biopsy cases as the denominator [43]. Regarding adverse events, most of the concerns since the early use of HIFU have been for large glands. Indeed in the first series, 65–100% underwent concomitant or pretreatment TURP to avoid urinary retention following treatment. Severe incontinence was found in 0–5%, impotence in 30–77%, and recto-urethral fistula in 0.5–5% of patients with higher rates reported in earlier case series using earlier prototypes [26]. In modern series fistula is rare.

## Focal therapy results

Given the ability of HIFU to focus the target zone and spare the adjacent tissue, this energy source has been considered an ideal way to target focal disease in the prostate (Figure 10.4, Plate 10.4). Muto *et al.* published a retrospective case series on extended hemi-ablation HIFU on 29 patients in 2008. Cancer control rates were encouraging, although the study was limited by its lack of detailed outcome reporting and mixture of cases with another 31 men which had whole-gland HIFU. Learning from shortcomings of previous case series, great efforts have been carried out by several groups to explore this approach in a systematic prospective manner [39]. Several small studies using focal HIFU in patients having localized, low-, intermediate-, and high-risk prostate cancer have been published to date [44–47]. The first was a proof-of-concept prospective development study of 20 men treated in a hemi-ablation manner following verification of unilateral disease on multiparametric MRI and TPM [45]. Trifecta rates (no incontinence, erections sufficient for penetration, absence of clinically significant disease on biopsy) was 89%. In a subsequent larger trial including 42 patients, there was 92% absence of significant prostate cancer and 84% overall achieved the trifecta status after 12 months [44]. Trifecta rates after surgery vary from 30% to 60%. This trial highlighted that erectile function and continence are affected in the first 3–6 months, but recovery of these functions is nearly complete after 12 months. Regarding concerns about longer-term cancer control, a small series of only 12 patients reported by El Fegoun *et al.* achieved a median follow-up after focal HIFU of 10 years [47]. Negative prostate biopsy rate was of 91%; bDFS at 5 and 10 years were 90% and 38%, respectively, with prostate-cancer-specific survival at 100%. Another multi-institutional trial (NCT01194648) is currently recruiting patients with the aim to treat only clinically significant prostate cancer through focal manner. For the first time, the primary endpoint will be ablative efficacy and not safety as in previous trials. With this purpose, TPM biopsy will be performed after 3 years of biochemical and MRI surveillance.

## Photodynamic therapy

Photodynamic therapy (PDT) is based on the activation of a photosensitizer by light of a given wavelength, specific for each photosensitizer. The

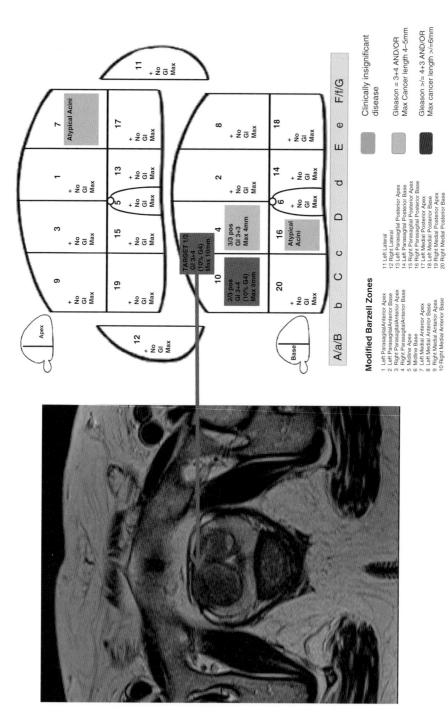

**Figure 10.4** Right anterior location of a tumor (*red arrow*) on multiparametric MRI and TPM biopsy in a man who subsequently underwent focal HIFU. (See also Plate 10.4.)

interaction between light transmitted by a laser fiber and the activated drug leads to the formation of reactive oxygen species. The cell death is due to vascular damage or induction of apoptosis and/or necrosis. This technique is routinely used in other fields such as dermatology. In urology, the amino laevulinic acid (ALA) is used as photosensitizer to detect bladder cancer during cystoscopy. The increasing use of PDT in malignancy is related to the property of some photosensitizers to accumulate preferentially in tumor cells. As for other techniques some innovations have been needed to develop their use in prostate cancer. To precisely position the laser fiber within the prostate, a transperineal approach using the brachytherapy template is now employed. The placement is carried out under TRUS control. Usually the photosensitizers have long light intervals meaning that the drug and the treatment need to be delivered in different sessions. In addition, several weeks are necessary to completely clear the body from the photosensitizer; initially patients had to be protected from the sun to avoid skin damage for a number of days. The development of vascular photosensitizers having short light intervals and a rapid clearance from the body has notably facilitated the use of PDT in clinical practice.

PDT was first used in prostate cancer in 1990 when Windahl *et al.* reported in a letter to *Lancet* the treatment of two patients after the finding of prostate cancer on TURP tissue [48]. The histological results were encouraging with negative biopsy after 3 months in one patient and absence of residual tumor in the other patient, who died of lung cancer 6 months later. After other studies in the salvage setting, the first phase I trial was carried out in 2006 by Moore *et al.* in six men affected by low-risk prostate cancer [49]. The design of this trial aimed to demonstrate the feasibility and the safety profile of this therapy. Focal treatment was delivered to areas of biopsy-proven prostate cancer. All patients undergoing biopsy had residual or recurrent prostate cancer. However, the procedure seemed safe with rectal toxicity being very low. The International Prostate Symptoms Score (IPSS) questionnaire remained stable 3 months after the procedure and one patient had urinary sepsis managed by intravenous antibiotics. Regarding erectile function, one patient reported decreased potency.

The latest two multi-institutional phase II trials using a new water-soluble photosensitizer (WST-11 Tookad® Soluble) have been completed and results have been presented at international meetings [50]. Intermediate results highlighted the low genitourinary side-effects rate with stable IPSS and International Index of Erectile Function-15 (IIEF-15) scores after the procedure. The overall results of these trials are awaited for full publication. In the meantime, a phase III randomized control trial is ongoing in Europe and will compare PDT using the same photosensitizer with patients on active surveillance (NCT01310894). The first endpoint is the ablative efficacy of PDT verified by prostate biopsy at 2 years.

## Irreversible electroporation

Irreversible electroporation (IRE) uses electrical current at frequencies that do not cause heat effect but lead to cell death by the formation of nano-sized pores within the cellular membrane. The energy is passed from the generator to electrode probes inserted within the target area in the prostate via a transperineal approach under TRUS guidance. Its first use in the prostate was reported by Onik *et al.* in 2007 in a canine model [51]. Histology showed no viable tissue within the treated area with a clear demarcation between the target tissue and the surrounding prostate parenchyma. A feasibility study using IRE in a focal manner was recently presented to the European Association of Urology Congress in 2011 from Brausi *et al.* [52]. Focal IRE was performed in 11 patients affected by unilateral low-risk prostate cancer on TPM. Control biopsy showed residual tumor in three patients. At 19.2 months follow-up, continence was preserved in 100% of patients and mean IIEF-15 score returned to baseline. Urinary retention was reported in one patient, transient urgent incontinence in three. No major complications were noticed in this study. The study has yet to be fully published in a peer-reviewed journal.

This technology is seen as a promising technique in focal therapy since it has unique characteristics. Indeed, the ablative effect appears to be confined to the exact limits of the target tissue and adjacent healthy tissue beyond 1 mm safety zone seems unaffected. Further studies needed are currently in set-up stage (NCT01726894).

## Laser photothermal therapy

Another emerging technology is laser therapy where thermal damage is achieved by the use of laser fibers within the prostate tissue through needles placed via a transperineal or transrectal approach. After two studies in a canine model, Lindner *et al.* performed focal laser therapy 1 week before radical prostatectomy in four patients [53]. Histology showed complete ablation with no viable tissue within the target area. In the same study, the authors found a good correlation between ablation tissue on MRI and histology. The same group performed a pilot study on 12 patients affected by low-risk prostate cancer using MRI to target the tumor area [54]. At follow-up, patients maintained continence and potency as measured by validated questionnaires. At 6 months, the biopsy negative rate in the treated area was 67%.

## Conclusions

The lack of well-designed comparative effectiveness research evaluating different techniques in the treatment of localized prostate cancer makes it difficult to draw recommendations based on level I evidence about the management of prostate cancer. However, there is enough evidence that the current care of prostate cancer leads to overtreatment which is harmful with little benefit in a significant proportion of men, given the knowledge acquired in recent years about the natural history of the disease and morbidity related to radical treatments. The use of alternative energy sources in a focal manner might provide the solution to address the shortcomings of the traditional approach, but there is a strong need for further validating studies evaluating medium- and long-term outcomes across a number of centers to assess its reproducibility.

## Acknowledgments

Mark Emberton and Hashim U. Ahmed received funding from USHIFU, GlaxoSmithKline, and Advanced Medical Diagnostics for clinical trials. Mark Emberton is a paid consultant to Steba Biotech and has received funding from USHIFU/Focused Surgery (manufacturers and distributors of the Sonablate500 HIFU device). Both of them have previously received medical consultancy payments from Oncura/GE Healthcare. All other authors declare no conflicts of interest.

## References

1  Thompson I, Thrasher JB, Aus G, *et al.* Guideline for the management of clinically localized prostate cancer: 2007 update. *J Urol* 2007;177(6):2106–2131.
2  Bill-Axelson A, Holmberg L, Ruutu M, *et al.* Radical prostatectomy versus watchful waiting in early prostate cancer. *N Engl J Med* 2011;364(18):1708–1717.

3 Wilt TJ, Brawer MK, Jones KM, *et al.* Radical prostatectomy versus observation for localized prostate cancer. *N Engl J Med* 2012;367(3):203–213.

4 Andriole GL, Crawford ED, Grubb RL, 3rd, *et al.* Mortality results from a randomized prostate-cancer screening trial. *N Engl J Med* 2009;360(13):1310–1319.

5 Schroder FH, Hugosson J, Roobol MJ, *et al.* Screening and prostate-cancer mortality in a randomized European study. *N Engl J Med* 2009;360(13):1320–1328.

6 Klotz L, Zhang L, Lam A, *et al.* Clinical results of long-term follow-up of a large, active surveillance cohort with localized prostate cancer. *J Clin Oncol* 2010;28(1):126–131.

7 Barzell WE, Melamed MR, Cathcart P, *et al.* Identifying candidates for active surveillance: an evaluation of the repeat biopsy strategy for men with favorable risk prostate cancer. *J Urol* 2012;188(3):762–767.

8 Ahmed HU, Pendse D, Illing R, *et al.* Will focal therapy become a standard of care for men with localized prostate cancer? *Nat Clin Pract Oncol* 2007;4(11):632–642.

9 Mouraviev V, Villers A, Bostwick DG, *et al.* Understanding the pathological features of focality, grade and tumour volume of early-stage prostate cancer as a foundation for parenchyma-sparing prostate cancer therapies: active surveillance and focal targeted therapy. *BJU Int* 2011;108(7):1074–1085.

10 Ahmed HU. The index lesion and the origin of prostate cancer. *N Engl J Med* 2009;361(17):1704–1706.

11 Liu W, Laitinen S, Khan S, *et al.* Copy number analysis indicates monoclonal origin of lethal metastatic prostate cancer. *Nat Med* 2009;15(5):559–565.

12 Ahmed HU, Arya M, Freeman A, Emberton M. Do low-grade and low-volume prostate cancers bear the hallmarks of malignancy? *Lancet Oncol* 2012;13(11):e509–e517.

13 Carter HB, Partin AW, Walsh PC, *et al.* Gleason score 6 adenocarcinoma: should it be labeled as cancer? *J Clin Oncol* 2012;30(35):4294–4296.

14 Dickinson L, Ahmed HU, Allen C, *et al.* Magnetic resonance imaging for the detection, localisation, and characterisation of prostate cancer: recommendations from a European consensus meeting. *Eur Urol* 2011;59(4):477–494.

15 Villers A, Lemaitre L, Haffner J, Puech P. Current status of MRI for the diagnosis, staging and prognosis of prostate cancer: implications for focal therapy and active surveillance. *Curr Opin Urol* 2009;19(3):274–282.

16 Yerram NK, Volkin D, Turkbey B, *et al.* Low suspicion lesions on multiparametric magnetic resonance imaging predict for the absence of high-risk prostate cancer. *BJU Int* 2012;110:E783–E788.

17 Turkbey B, Mani H, Aras O, *et al.* Correlation of magnetic resonance imaging tumor volume with histopathology. *J Urol* 2012;188(4):1157–1163.

18 Crawford ED, Wilson SS, Torkko KC, *et al.* Clinical staging of prostate cancer: a computer-simulated study of transperineal prostate biopsy. *BJU Int* 2005;96(7):999–1004.

19 Ahmed HU, Hu Y, Carter T, *et al.* Characterizing clinically significant prostate cancer using template prostate mapping biopsy. *J Urol* 2011;186(2):458–464.

20 Lecornet E, Ahmed HU, Hu Y, *et al.* The accuracy of different biopsy strategies for the detection of clinically important prostate cancer: a computer simulation. *J Urol* 2012;188(3):974–980.

21 Hu Y, Ahmed HU, Carter T, *et al.* A biopsy simulation study to assess the accuracy of several transrectal ultrasonography (TRUS)-biopsy strategies compared with

template prostate mapping biopsies in patients who have undergone radical prosta-tectomy. *BJU Int* 2012;110(6):812–820.

22  Crawford ED, Rove KO, Barqawi AB, *et al*. Clinical-pathologic correlation between transperineal mapping biopsies of the prostate and three-dimensional reconstruction of prostatectomy specimens. *Prostate* 2012;73(7):778–887.

23  Huo AS, Hossack T, Symons JL, *et al*. Accuracy of primary systematic template guided transperineal biopsy of the prostate for locating prostate cancer: a comparison with radical prostatectomy specimens. *J Urol* 2012;187(6):2044–2049.

24  Taira AV, Merrick GS, Galbreath RW, *et al*. Performance of transperineal template-guided mapping biopsy in detecting prostate cancer in the initial and repeat biopsy setting. *Prostate Cancer Prostatic Dis* 2010;13(1):71–77.

25  Babaian RJ, Donnelly B, Bahn D, *et al*. Best practice statement on cryosurgery for the treatment of localized prostate cancer. *J Urol* 2008;180(5):1993–2004.

26  Wein AJ, Kavoussi LR, Campbell MF. *Campbell-Walsh Urology*, 10th edn. Philadel-phia, PA: Elsevier Saunders; 2012.

27  Donnelly BJ, Saliken JC, Ernst DS, *et al*. Prospective trial of cryosurgical ablation of the prostate: five-year results. *Urology* 2002;60(4):645–649.

28  Jones JS, Rewcastle JC, Donnelly BJ, *et al*. Whole gland primary prostate cryoabla-tion: initial results from the cryo on-line data registry. *J Urol* 2008;180(2):554–558.

29  Long JP, Bahn D, Lee F, *et al*. Five-year retrospective, multi-institutional pooled anal-ysis of cancer-related outcomes after cryosurgical ablation of the prostate. *Urology* 2001;57(3):518–523.

30  Bahn DK, Lee F, Badalament R, *et al*. Targeted cryoablation of the prostate: 7-year outcomes in the primary treatment of prostate cancer. *Urology* 2002;60(2 Suppl. 1):3–11.

31  Donnelly BJ, Saliken JC, Brasher PM, *et al*. A randomized trial of external beam radiotherapy versus cryoablation in patients with localized prostate cancer. *Cancer* 2010;116(2):323–330.

32  Robinson JW, Donnelly BJ, Siever JE, *et al*. A randomized trial of external beam radiotherapy versus cryoablation in patients with localized prostate cancer: quality of life outcomes. *Cancer* 2009;115(20):4695–4704.

33  Ward JF, Jones JS. Focal cryotherapy for localized prostate cancer: a report from the national Cryo On-Line Database (COLD) Registry. *BJU Int* 2012;109(11):1648–1654.

34  Onik G, Vaughan D, Lotenfoe R, *et al*. "Male lumpectomy": focal therapy for prostate cancer using cryoablation. *Urology* 2007;70(Suppl. 6):16–21.

35  Lambert EH, Bolte K, Masson P, Katz AE. Focal cryosurgery: encouraging health outcomes for unifocal prostate cancer. *Urology* 2007;69(6):1117–1120.

36  Truesdale MD, Cheetham PJ, Hruby GW, *et al*. An evaluation of patient selection criteria on predicting progression-free survival after primary focal unilateral nerve-sparing cryoablation for prostate cancer: recommendations for follow up. *Cancer J* 2010;16(5):544–549.

37  Ellis DS, Manny TB, Jr., Rewcastle JC. Focal cryosurgery followed by penile reha-bilitation as primary treatment for localized prostate cancer: initial results. *Urology* 2007;70(Suppl. 6):9–15.

38  Bahn D, de Castro Abreu AL, Gill IS, *et al*. Focal cryotherapy for clinically unilat-eral, low-intermediate risk prostate cancer in 73 men with a median follow-up of 3.7 years. *Eur Urol* 2012;62(1):55–63.

39 McCulloch P, Altman DG, Campbell WB, *et al.* No surgical innovation without evaluation: the IDEAL recommendations. *Lancet* 2009;374(9695):1105–1112.

40 Madersbacher S, Kratzik C, Susani M, *et al.* [Minimally invasive therapy of benign prostatic hyperplasia with focussed ultrasound]. *Urologe A* 1995;34(2):98–104.

41 Madersbacher S, Pedevilla M, Vingers L, *et al.* Effect of high-intensity focused ultrasound on human prostate cancer in vivo. *Cancer Res* 1995;55(15):3346–3351.

42 Blana A, Robertson CN, Brown SC, *et al.* Complete high-intensity focused ultrasound in prostate cancer: outcome from the @-Registry. *Prostate Cancer Prostatic Dis* 2012;15(3):256–259.

43 Lukka H, Waldron T, Chin J, *et al.* High-intensity focused ultrasound for prostate cancer: a systematic review. *Clin Oncol (R Coll Radiol)* 2011;23(2):117–127.

44 Ahmed HU, Hindley RG, Dickinson L, *et al.* Focal therapy for localised unifocal and multifocal prostate cancer: a prospective development study. *Lancet Oncol* 2012;13(6):622–632.

45 Ahmed HU, Freeman A, Kirkham A, *et al.* Focal therapy for localized prostate cancer: a phase I/II trial. *J Urol* 2011;185(4):1246–1254.

46 Muto S, Yoshii T, Saito K, *et al.* Focal therapy with high-intensity-focused ultrasound in the treatment of localized prostate cancer. *Jpn J Clin Oncol* 2008;38(3):192–199.

47 El Fegoun AB, Barret E, Prapotnich D, *et al.* Focal therapy with high-intensity focused ultrasound for prostate cancer in the elderly. A feasibility study with 10 years follow-up. *Int Braz J Urol* 2011;37(2):213–219; discussion 20-2.

48 Windahl T, Andersson SO, Lofgren L. Photodynamic therapy of localised prostatic cancer. *Lancet* 1990;336(8723):1139.

49 Moore CM, Nathan TR, Lees WR, *et al.* Photodynamic therapy using meso tetra hydroxy phenyl chlorin (mTHPC) in early prostate cancer. *Lasers Surg Med* 2006;38(5):356–363.

50 Azzouzi A-R, Barret E, Villers A, *et al.* Results of TOOKAD® soluble vascular targeted photodynamic therapy (VTP) for low risk localized prostate cancer (PCM201/PCM203). *Eur Urol Suppl* 2011;10(2):54.

51 Onik G, Mikus P, Rubinsky B. Irreversible electroporation: implications for prostate ablation. *Technol Cancer Res Treat* 2007;6(4):295–300.

52 Brausi MA, Giliberto GL, Simonini GL, *et al.* Irreversible electroporation (IRE), a novel technique for focal ablation of prostate cancer (PCa): Results of a interim pilot safety study in low risk patients with PCa. *Eur Urol Suppl* 2011;10(2):300.

53 Lindner U, Lawrentschuk N, Weersink RA, *et al.* Focal laser ablation for prostate cancer followed by radical prostatectomy: validation of focal therapy and imaging accuracy. *Eur Urol* 2010;57(6):1111–1114.

54 Lindner U, Weersink RA, Haider MA, *et al.* Image guided photothermal focal therapy for localized prostate cancer: phase I trial. *J Urol* 2009;182(4):1371–1377.

## CHAPTER 11

# Posttherapy Follow-up and First Intervention

*Ernesto R. Cordeiro, Anastasios Anastasiadis, Matias Westendarp, Jean J.M.C.H. de la Rosette, and Theo M. de Reijke*

Academic Medical Center, Amsterdam, The Netherlands

## Introduction

Cancer of the prostate (PCa) is now recognized as one of the most important medical problems the male population is facing, being the most frequently diagnosed cancer in men [1, 2]. The benefit of prostate-specific antigen (PSA)-based screening on PCa mortality and overall mortality remains one of the hottest and most intensively debated topics in modern urology. To date, the main diagnostic tools to obtain evidence of PCa include digital rectal examination (DRE), serum concentration of PSA, and prostate biopsy through transrectal ultrasonography (TRUS). Following a diagnosis of PCa, the goal of staging is the accurate determination of disease extent for management decisions and prognosis.

The management of PCa remains controversial because of its variable natural history, the diversity of available treatments, and the lack of randomized controlled trials (RCTs) comparing the different treatment approaches, especially in localized PCa. The choice of an adequate therapy option for PCa depends on several factors, including tumour stage, PSA value, Gleason score, lower urinary tract symptoms (LUTS), patients' age, concomitant diseases, life expectancy, and ultimately, patients' preferences. Stage, Gleason score, and PSA have been collated into three risk strata: low-, intermediate-, and high risk, establishing the basis for different therapeutic approaches according to each risk group [3]. Abundant literature can be found on the established therapies for different stages of PCa: radical prostatectomy (RP), radiation therapy (RT), androgen

*Prostate Cancer: Diagnosis and Clinical Management*, First Edition.
Edited by Ashutosh K. Tewari, Peter Whelan and John D. Graham.
© 2014 John Wiley & Sons, Ltd. Published 2014 by John Wiley & Sons, Ltd.

deprivation therapy (ADT), and deferred treatment (active surveillance [AS] and watchful waiting [WW]). In addition, emerging minimally invasive technologies, still investigational or experimental, have been developed during the last years with the potential for focal therapy and include high-intensity focused ultrasound (HIFU), cryoablation (CA), photodynamic therapy, photothermal therapy, and radiofrequency interstitial tumour ablation [4].

Following treatment, routine follow-up is advised in order to: (1) identify local recurrent disease at a stage when further radical treatment might be effective; (2) identify and treat the complications of therapy; (3) give information and address concerns; and (4) assess the outcomes of treatment. Patients' follow-up will vary depending on the treatment given, patients' age, co-morbidity, and the patients' own wishes. In general, patients are followed at periodic intervals with measurement of serum PSA levels and DRE, despite low reliability of DRE in evaluating local recurrent disease [5]. Recurrences will occur in a substantial number of patients who received treatment with curative intent at various time points after the primary therapy. Although RP and RT are considered definitive therapies, 30–50% of patients will have biochemical PSA relapse by 5 years [6]. Therefore, follow-up is intended not only as responsible care of patients but also to have the possibility of initiating second line of treatment with curative intent, possibility of early hormonal therapy after failure, or as part of a study protocol in selected cases [7].

To date, great efforts have been made to reach international consensus on *best-practice guidelines* for PCa monitoring and posttreatment follow-up. However, it remains a topic of discussion [8]. The aim of this work is to present a review on the strategies for monitoring patients after different types of therapies for PCa, and to define when a decision for intervention has to be taken during follow-up.

## Evidence acquisition

A literature search was conducted up to August 2012, using MEDLINE and EMBASE via Ovid databases, to identify best-practice guidelines on *posttherapy follow-up of PCa and first intervention*, by combining and exploding the terms "prostate neoplasms" and "practice guidelines" and "follow-up." In addition, major international guidelines such as EAU Guidelines (www.uroweb.org/guidelines) [7], American Urological Association (www.auanet.org/guidelines) [9], National Guidelines

Clearinghouse (www.guideline.gov), National Comprehensive Cancer Network (www.nccn.org) [10], National Cancer Institute (www.cancer. gov), American Society of Clinical Oncologists (www.asco.org), European Society for Medical Oncology (ESMO) [11], National Institute for Health and Clinical Excellence (NICE) (http://www.nice.org.uk/guidance/) [12], and American Society for Therapeutic Radiology and Oncology (www.astro.org) were investigated in order to identify key elements of existing models of follow-up care to establish recommendations for evaluating future interventions. Only English-language and human-based full manuscripts concerning clinical evidence of the best practice for PCa diagnosis, treatment, and follow-up were included. References of recently published review articles were also checked in order to add any relevant paper missed by the bibliographic search.

## Evidence synthesis

### Monitoring tools
#### PSA
Prostate-specific antigen (PSA) is a glycoprotein produced almost exclusively by the epithelial cells of the prostate gland and is considered specific for prostatic tissue. A rise in PSA is detected in the serum when the prostate gland has been disrupted, as with PCa, benign prostatic hyperplasia, and acute prostatitis or after prostate biopsy. PSA is widely used as a tumor marker for PCa, both for detection and for monitoring response to therapy; thus, measurement of PSA level represents the cornerstone in the follow-up after treatment with curative intent.

An increasing PSA level after curative therapy is referred to as *biochemical recurrence* (BCR). Approximately one-third to half of patients treated with curative intent will experience BCR during the course of their follow-up, regardless of modality of treatment [13]. The significance of a BCR is in itself unclear, as not all men who have experienced BCRs will develop metastatic disease. However, BCR precedes clinical recurrence after radical treatment, in some cases by many years [14–16]. Although PSA alone does not differentiate local from distant disease recurrence, the patterns of PSA increase after local therapy have been incorporated into clinical nomograms to predict whether recurrence is more likely local or distant metastatic disease. Patients with late BCR following RP (>24 months after local treatment), low PSA velocity (change in PSA over time), and/or prolonged PSA doubling time (PSADT >6 months) most likely have recurrent local disease. Conversely, patients with an early PSA recurrence (<24 months after local treatment), high PSA velocity, or short PSADT (<6 months) are more likely to have distant disease recurrence [17]. For these reasons, PSA monitoring after treatment is useful for implementation of effective salvage therapeutic strategies or systemic treatment in those patients whose recurrences are deemed to be local and metastatic, respectively. The definition of BCR varies depending on the type of treatment that a patient has undergone and is continually being re-evaluated as more data become available. Definitions of BCR according to each treatment are explained later in this chapter.

## DRE

Digital rectal examination (DRE) is performed to assess whether or not there is any sign of local disease recurrence. It is very difficult to interpret the findings of DRE after curative therapy, especially after radiotherapy. The utility of DRE in follow-up after radiotherapy has been questioned, as scar tissue can be difficult to differentiate from neoplastic nodules, and any residual tumor might not be palpable [18]. On the other hand, detection of a newly onset nodule during DRE may suggest local disease recurrence, even without a concomitant rise in PSA level, especially in undifferentiated tumors [19]. However, in asymptomatic patients, a disease-specific history and a serum PSA measurement supplemented by DRE are the recommended tests for routine follow-up, as they act synergistically to increase the positive predictive value of findings [7].

On the other hand, routine DRE following RP with undetectable PSA is not considered to be useful, but in case of a BCR it might be helpful to detect a local recurrence [20].

## TRUS and biopsy

Routine transrectal ultrasonography (TRUS) imaging should not be performed; however, in cases of BCR, the use of imaging in evaluating local tumor recurrence is controversial. Biopsy of the prostatic bed should not be performed in men with PCa who have had a RP. Negative results of TRUS-guided biopsy may be inconclusive because of sampling error. The use of biopsy has been questioned in the face of a rising PSA level because the negative results are unreliable and elevated PSA levels usually precede clinical evidence of local recurrence by ≥1 year [21].

The main purpose of the investigation is to confirm a histological diagnosis of local disease recurrence, in which this finding may affect the treatment decision. This is the case that occurs after radiotherapy failure, in patients who are being considered for local salvage therapy (mostly in the context of clinical trials).

In conclusion, TRUS and biopsy have no place in the routine follow-up of asymptomatic patients. These tests are therefore not advised as standard protocol, leaving PSA testing as the primary tool for monitoring disease recurrence. Following radiotherapy, TRUS-guided biopsy is advised in patients with a BCR, where a salvage treatment is considered.

### Bone scintigraphy

Whole-body bone scans are frequently performed to detect skeletal metastases in patients with rising PSA after treatment. If the results of a bone scan are positive for metastatic disease, no other imaging is indicated. Because bone scan results are rarely positive without symptoms or without abnormal PSA levels, the routine use of this study after treatment is considered unproductive [22]. Therefore, it should be considered in symptomatic patients and if serum PSA levels are above 20 ng/mL. The results of a bone scan may be inconclusive, because it is a sensitive but not specific examination. However, it should be indicated in patients with symptoms arising from the skeleton, since metastatic disease may occur even if PSA is undetectable [23].

### Computed tomography, positron emission tomography, and magnetic resonance imaging

Computed tomography (CT) and magnetic resonance imaging (MRI) have no place in the routine follow-up of asymptomatic patients. A CT scan can recognize only local recurrences that are $\geq 2$ cm [24]. In the evaluation of nodal disease, using 1 cm as a cut-off, studies have reported sensitivities between 27% and 75% and specificities between 66% and 100% [24]. CT is useful in detecting bone and visceral metastases, (although bone scan and MRI are superior in the diagnosis and follow-up of bone metastases), preferably when other examinations are conflicting, and it can be used to determine response to hormonal treatment [25]. Positron emission tomography (PET) has proven to be useful for early identification of local or systemic recurrences in several human cancers. In PCa, there are a few promising studies on the clinical efficacy of PET in detecting local recurrences after RP [26–30].

PSA values can also be used as a guide when radiologic investigations are appropriate. Bone and lymph node metastases rarely occur before PSA levels rise above 20 ng/mL, and CT and MRI has been found to have a low yield when PSA is <25 ng/mL [31]. It is believed to be of little utility in ordering any imaging studies in an asymptomatic patient with PSA <30 ng/mL, but a patient with bone pain should have a bone scan done irrespective of PSA level [31].

## Oncological follow-up after different therapies for PCa
### After AS
Patients being monitored under active surveillance (AS) are those who are still candidates for curative therapy but opt not to have immediate treatment with curative intent owing to the indolent characteristics of their tumors, with the expectation of intervening if the cancer progresses (i.e., short PSADT and deteriorating histopathological factors on repeat biopsy). AS is intended to reduce the ratio of overtreatment in patients with clinically confined very low risk PCa. Active surveillance as initial therapy for PCa might be considered for patients with clinically localized disease at a lowest risk of progression: cT1-2a, PSA <10 ng/mL, biopsy Gleason score ≤6 (at least 10 cores), ≤2 positive biopsies, and minimal biopsy core involvement (<50% cancer per biopsy) [7].

It is noteworthy that follow-up schedules regarding AS differ in several research groups. Although some recommend regular performing DRE every 3–6 months for 2 years [32], others do not suggest it as long as the PSA remains at baseline levels [12]. Follow-up typically consists of serum PSA levels every 3–6 months, DRE every 6–12 months, and repeat prostate biopsy as often as annually to ensure that there is no up-staging of the disease [7, 32]. The trigger for patients being moved to active treatment is based mainly on grade progression on repeat biopsies or at the patients' request [7].

In those patients opting for AS, imaging is generally not a component of follow-up, but a few recent studies have suggested that MRI may help in better staging of the tumor and also in guiding patients who are considering AS and how the surveillance is conducted [33, 34].

### After RP for localized tumor
Surgical excision of the prostate should remove all the PSA-producing tissue within the body. It is therefore expected that after RP, PSA should decline to undetectable levels within 3–6 weeks. Any persistent elevation of PSA beyond this time is suggestive of residual local or distant disease [35], but can also reflect the presence of benign glandular tissue at the resection margin. This situation occurs more frequently in cases of nerve-sparing surgery.

According to available data, patients whose PSA levels fail to fall to undetectable levels or with detectable PSA increases on two subsequent measurements (two consecutive values of 0.2 ng/mL or greater appear to represent an international consensus defining recurrent cancer) should undergo a search for the presence of distant metastatic disease or local recurrent disease, each requiring different forms of systemic or local therapy [36,37]. As it was described above, a rapidly increasing PSA level (high PSA velocity, short PSADT) indicates distant metastases, while a later and slowly increasing concentration of PSA is most likely to indicate local disease recurrence. In addition, it has been stated that tumor differentiation and time to PSA recurrence may also play a role as predictive factors for local and systemic recurrence [17].

In asymptomatic patients, PSA levels for all men with PCa who are having radical treatment should be checked at the earliest 6 weeks following treatment, at least every 6 months for the first 2–3 years, and then at least once a year thereafter. Routine DRE is not recommended in men with PCa while the PSA remains at baseline levels. When metastasis is suspected, pelvic CT/MRI or bone scan should be considered; however, these examinations may be omitted if the serum PSA level is <20 ng/mL. If the patient has bone pain, a bone scan should be considered irrespective of the serum PSA level [7].

Regarding positive surgical margins (PSMs) status, to date there are no solid recommendations for follow-up in these patients. The prognostic impact of PSMs on outcome after RP is still controversial. In general terms, PSMs are an independent predictor of biochemical progression in patients with intermediate- and high-risk PCa. Patients with low-risk disease have a favorable long-term outcome regardless of margin status and may be candidates for expectant management even with PSMs [38], while high-risk patients may benefit from early adjuvant radiotherapy [39,40].

## After external beam radiotherapy

PSA levels are not expected to decline to undetectable levels after external beam radiotherapy (EBRT), as prostate tissue is left in place. It is expected, however, that there should be a substantial decline in PSA level to a *nadir* level, the lowest PSA value after treatment, which generally oscillates between 0.2 and 0.5 ng/mL [37]. This phenomenon occurs in the majority of patients during the first year but may not reach a nadir until 18–30 months after treatment [37]. Thus, each treated individual will have a nadir characterized by the lowest PSA measurement recorded after treatment completion. In addition, the nadir value may predict treatment efficacy, as values <0.5 ng/mL are consistent with a 5-year disease-free survival in 93% of patients, compared with only 26% of patients having disease-free status at 5 years when they have a nadir of ≥1.0 ng/mL [41].

In 10–30% of patients who have been treated with EBRT, a transitory PSA rise of at least 0.4 ng/mL or a 15% rise in the previous PSA value can occur that resolves spontaneously. This phenomenon is referred to as a *PSA bounce* and generally appears within 9 months of treatment, but can occur up to 60 months after completion of therapy [42]. The etiology of this phenomenon is not well understood. Therefore, at the 2005 Phoenix Consensus Conference, ASTRO and RTOG described a new definition of radiation failure in order to better correlate between the definition and clinical outcome. The new definition of biochemical failure after RT is a rise of ≥2 ng/mL above the nadir PSA level [43].

As it was stated above, follow-up in asymptomatic patients after treatment with curative intent, both serum PSA measurement and DRE are the recommended tests for routine follow-up. According to the EAU guidelines, these should be performed at 3, 6, 9, and 12 months after treatment, then every 6 months until 3 years, and then annually.

An increasing serum PSA level will prompt a radionuclide bone scan. If the results are positive, no further evaluation is necessary. If the results are negative or inconclusive, TRUS-directed biopsy of the prostate is indicated if this has implications for further salvage treatment. If the results of the bone scan are inconclusive, MRI may be helpful. MRI may also be indicated to depict local recurrence after radiotherapy.

### After brachytherapy

PSA response after brachytherapy is not extensively described in the literature. It appears that a PSA bounce might be more common among these patients [44]. In some studies, patients experiencing PSA bounces were less likely to have BCRs [45].

As for follow-up after brachytherapy, the same definitions of BCR and the same surveillance strategies are employed as in EBRT.

### After other therapies (HIFU and CA)

After HIFU or cryotherapy, a variety of definitions for PSA relapse have been used. Most of these are based on a cut-off of around 1 ng/mL, eventually combined with a negative posttreatment biopsy. To date, none of these endpoints have been validated against clinical progression or survival and therefore it is not possible to give firm recommendations on the definition of biochemical failure [46, 47].

## Functional follow-up after different therapies for PCa

Assessment of side effects in terms of functional areas (urinary, bowel, and sexual) after different therapies for PCa has become an important focus of investigation. These functional domains are encompassed by the term *quality of life* (QoL). Disease-specific domains focus on the impact of particular organic dysfunctions associated with the disease that may affect *health-related quality of life* (HRQOL). This term is typically used to refer to the impact that disease and treatment have on a persons' well-being and physical, emotional, and social functioning [48, 49]. PCa-specific domains include areas such as bony pain; anxiety regarding cancer recurrence; urinary, sexual, and bowel dysfunction; and distress from these dysfunctions. However, recommendations for follow-up on this topic cannot be found yet in the urological practice guidelines.

In most cases, physician ratings of PCa patients' symptoms do not correlate well with patients' assessment of those clinical domains [50]. Therefore, to evaluate HRQOL from the patients' perspective, several self-administered instruments or questionnaires have been developed [51–54]. In addition, posttreatment symptoms are strongly associated with patient age [55]. Thus, while mild symptoms can lead to important bother in younger men, severe symptoms can generate minimal bother in the elderly. Moreover, HRQOL is not a steady state but can progressively change owing to anatomical and clinical responses, as well as the natural history of ageing [56]. Therefore, both time since treatment and age at HRQOL assessment are important to evaluate these patients. Besides, pretreatment factors such as clinical stage, Gleason score, and total PSA levels and also posttreatment outcomes such as BCR and hormonal status are important variables that may influence the HRQOL assessment.

### After RP for localized tumor

To date, there is abundant evidence proving that RP may have a negative impact on two primary QoL domains: sexual and urinary functions. Erectile dysfunction (ED) and incontinence are the two prostate-specific domains that decline most after surgery and remain most affected after 1 year [57]. The recovery of sexual dysfunction and urinary incontinence occurs over 2–3 years [58]. During the recent years, certain advances have been achieved on surgical techniques in order to diminish these side effects, such as nerve-sparing RP, either by open, laparoscopic, or robotic-assisted radical prostatectomy (RALP); however, their impact on HRQOL remains controversial [59].

Recently, two new concepts emerged for reporting outcomes after RP: *trifecta* (continence, potency, and cancer control) and *pentafecta* (trifecta plus peri-operative complications and PSMs). The use of these two concepts could improve HRQOL assessment; nevertheless, further validation in future trials will determine its true value [60, 61].

As for the management of these side effects, if incontinence is present, pelvic floor exercises as well as biofeedback may be beneficial. Since improvement in urinary continence may occur between 1 and 3 years following surgery, it is suggested that invasive treatments for incontinence should be delayed for at least 1 year after prostatectomy [62]. Once incontinence is noted to persist, several modalities, including cystoscopy, uroflowmetry, and urodynamics, can be implemented to diagnose the cause and exclude potentially treatable etiologies. Final treatment decisions can then be based on findings from these investigations [63]. When the decision to proceed with surgical treatment is taken, several therapeutic options can be offered to patients: injection therapy, slings, and an artificial urinary sphincter (AUS). Injectable therapy for postprostatectomy incontinence has been notoriously associated with low success rates of 20–35%. Data regarding postprostatectomy sling procedures are preliminary and will require long-term confirmation. It seems that some patients will eventually benefit from the procedure, which is not free of complications. The AUS is considered by many to be the gold standard for treating postprostatectomy incontinence resulting in continence rates as high as 79–96% [58].

As for ED, patients who are immediately impotent after surgery may develop erections adequate for intercourse up to 24 months after surgery. Furthermore, with the use of phosphodiesterase inhibitors up to 80% of previously potent men who had no erections after RP will eventually recover [64].

### After EBRT and brachytherapy

Patients undergoing EBRT and brachytherapy may have urinary, sexual, and bowel dysfunction after treatment [65]. Both methods can result in irritative voiding symptoms, such as urgency, frequency, and urge incontinence, that negatively affect overall urinary function and HRQOL. The most predominant severe acute toxicity after brachytherapy is urinary retention requiring catheterization [66]. Nevertheless, it has been shown that these effects tend to disappear at 12 months after treatment [67].

Obstructive and irritative urinary symptoms during and after radiation are often effectively managed with alpha-blockers, such as tamsulosin or terazosin, or by anticholinergics [68, 69]. However, months or years after external radiation, late sequelae may develop. These are the result of changes in the small vessels of the irradiated tissues that lead to chronic hypoxia, mucosal thinning, and aberrant vessel development (telangiectasia). Patients may experience painless hematuria, or a cystitis-like syndrome referred to as radiation cystitis [68, 70].

Besides the urinary symptoms, bowel and rectal disorders appear to have an overall negative impact on HRQOL. The onset of symptoms usually occurs during or early after treatment, and sometimes persists longer into follow-up. These include rectal urgency, frequency, pain, fecal incontinence, and rectorrhagia [67]. Most of mild to moderate symptoms are treated effectively with simple dietary changes, especially fiber, or by the use of hydrocortisone suppositories or foam. Rarely, some patients with persistent bleeding, despite conservative medical management, should undergo endoscopic evaluation and eventually coagulation of abnormal vessels [67].

In the era of high-tech radiotherapy such as intensity-modulated radiotherapy, image-guided radiotherapy, and particle therapy, the incidence of radiation-induced cystitis and proctitis has been decreasing. However, serious radiation-induced injuries still persist in a number of patients. The safety and efficacy of hyperbaric oxygen (HBO) in the treatment of radiation-induced hemorrhagic lesions has been shown by several groups. Low level of oxygen concentration and hypovascularity of the irradiated tissue can be effectively reversed by HBO treatment. Future randomized clinical trials will confirm its long-term efficacy for both conditions: radiation cystitis and proctitis [71, 72].

A rare but serious complication of irradiating normal tissues is the induction of second (bladder and rectal) cancers. It has been described that PCa patients treated by RT have a 1% additional absolute risk of cancer 10 or more years later [73]. Although this has become certainly lower with contemporary techniques, it should be taken in consideration when treating younger men (Figure 11.1).

## First intervention against treatment failure
### After RP

As it was described before, there is an international consensus for recurrent cancer after RP, and it is defined by two consecutive values of PSA >0.2 ng/mL [74]. Once the BCR has been diagnosed, the type of relapse has to be determined in order to indicate the most suitable treatment. Several parameters help to differentiate between local or distant relapse and

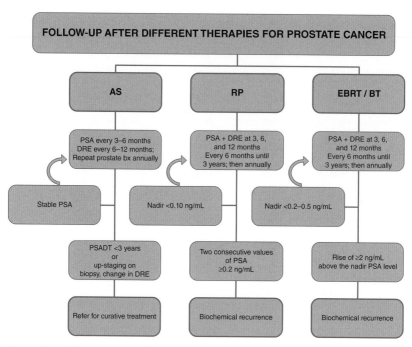

**Figure 11.1** Follow-up after different therapies for prostate cancer.

have been described previously; it include (1) interval between BCR and treatment; (2) PSA velocity; (3) PSADT; (4) pathological stage; and (5) Gleason score of the prostatectomy specimen.

In general, low pretreatment PSA levels, lower-grade tumors, low clinical or pathologic staging, late time from definitive local therapy to PSA relapse, and long PSADTs generally indicate a low likelihood of developing distant radiographically apparent metastases [74]. Thus, PSMs, Gleason score <7, stage <pT3a N0, PSADT >11 months, and time to recurrence >3 years are highly suggestive of local recurrence. Conversely, seminal vesicles invasion in the pathology specimen, Gleason score 8–10, stage pT3b, PSADT of 4–6 months, PSA relapse <1 year are highly suggestive of systemic failure.

Imaging studies have low sensitivity and specificity and can be safely omitted in the routine workup of relapsing cases, unless the PSA serum levels are >20 ng/mL. A few promising studies have been conducted on the capability of *endorectal MRI (eMRI)* and *PET* to identify local recurrences following RP. Nevertheless, to date they cannot be recommended as routine imaging modalities [75, 76].

Patients with local recurrences are candidates for local salvage treatment with RT at a PSA serum level of <0.5 ng/mL. Immediate postoperative radiotherapy after RP is not routinely recommended, even in men with positive-margin disease. For patients with presumed local recurrence who are too unfit or unwilling to undergo RT, expectant management can be offered.

Patients with systemic relapse are best treated by early ADT, as it resulted in decreased frequency of clinical metastases.

### After RT

According to the 2005 Phoenix Consensus Conference, ASTRO and RTOG definition, biochemical failure after RT is a rise of ≥2 ng/mL above the nadir PSA level. Once the BCR has been diagnosed, the type of relapse has to be determined in order to indicate the treatment accordingly. A suspicious DRE, Gleason <7, and high PSADT (>10 months) will be highly suggestive of local relapse. Instead, a Gleason score of 8–10 and a low PSADT (<10 months) will be suggestive of distant relapse. Therapeutic options in these patients are local procedures, such as salvage RP, cryotherapy, and interstitial RT or ADT for local and distant relapses, respectively.

Salvage RP for local recurrence should be indicated in carefully selected patients, who presumably demonstrate organ-confined disease. When patients are not suitable for surgery, CA of the prostate and interstitial brachytherapy may be therapeutic alternatives. In addition, HIFU may be an alternative option, as long as patients are well informed about the investigational nature of this treatment modality.

It is noteworthy that after HIFU or cryotherapy, a variety of definitions for PSA relapse have been used. Most of these are based on a cut-off of around 1 ng/mL, eventually combined with a negative posttreatment biopsy. As yet, none of these endpoints have been validated against clinical progression or survival and therefore it is not possible to give firm recommendations on the definition of biochemical failure [46] (Figure 11.2).

## Conclusion

Abundant literature can be found on the established therapies for different stages of PCa. Conversely, solid recommendations on follow-up for its wide range of oncological manifestations are still lacking. On the other hand, given the heterogeneity of the disease and its variable natural history, one

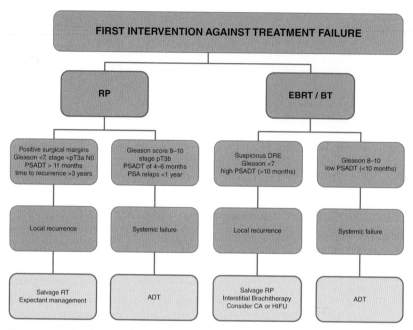

**Figure 11.2** First intervention against treatment failure.

should consider that at a certain point, follow-up needs to be individually tailored to patients with PCa.

Although monitoring PSA remains the cornerstone of follow-up for men with PCa, the diversity of guideline recommendations on the frequency and duration of PSA testing, and components of follow-up other than PSA testing, reflects the current lack of research evidence on which to base firm conclusions. Therefore, robust research models are needed to improve the evidence base for PCa follow-up in order to establish *best-practice* models of care.

## References

1 Jemal A, Bray F, Center MM, *et al.* Global cancer statistics. *CA Cancer J Clin* 2011; 61(2):69–90.
2 Siegel R, Naishadham D, Jemal A. Cancer statistics, 2012. *CA Cancer J Clin* 2012; 62(1):10–29.
3 D'Amico AV, Whittington R, Malkowicz SB, *et al.* Biochemical outcome after radical prostatectomy, external beam radiation therapy, or interstitial radiation therapy for clinically localized prostate cancer. *J Am Med Assoc* 1998;280(11):969–974.

4  Cordeiro ER, Cathelineau X, Thuroff S, *et al.* High-intensity focused ultrasound (HIFU) for definitive treatment of prostate cancer. *BJU Int* 2012;110(9):1228–1242.

5  Pound CR, Christens-Barry OW, Gurganus RT, *et al.* Digital rectal examination and imaging studies are unnecessary in men with undetectable prostate specific antigen following radical prostatectomy. *J Urol* 1999;162(4):1337–1340.

6  Pucar D, Sella T, Schoder H. The role of imaging in the detection of prostate cancer local recurrence after radiation therapy and surgery. *Curr Opin Urol* 2008;18(1):87–97.

7  Heidenreich A, Bellmunt J, Bolla M, *et al.* [EAU guidelines on prostate cancer. Part I: screening, diagnosis, and treatment of clinically localised disease]. *Actas Urol Esp* 2011;35(9):501–514.

8  McIntosh HM, Neal RD, Rose P, *et al.* Follow-up care for men with prostate cancer and the role of primary care: a systematic review of international guidelines. *Br J Cancer* 2009;100(12):1852–1860.

9  Thompson I, Thrasher JB, Aus G, *et al.* Guideline for the management of clinically localized prostate cancer: 2007 update. *J Urol* 2007;177(6):2106–2131.

10  Prostate cancer. NCCN Clinical Practice Guidelines in oncology. *J Natl Compr Canc Netw* 2004;2(3):224–248.

11  Horwich A, Parker C, Bangma C, Kataja V. Prostate cancer: ESMO Clinical Practice Guidelines for diagnosis, treatment and follow-up. *Ann Oncol* 2010;21 (Suppl. 5):v129–v133.

12  Graham J, Baker M, Macbeth F, Titshall V. Diagnosis and treatment of prostate cancer: summary of NICE guidance. *BMJ* 2008;336(7644):610–612.

13  Wilkinson AN, Brundage MD, Siemens R. Approach to primary care follow-up of patients with prostate cancer. *Can Fam Physician* 2008;54(2):204–210.

14  Han M, Partin AW, Pound CR, *et al.* Long-term biochemical disease-free and cancer-specific survival following anatomic radical retropubic prostatectomy. The 15-year Johns Hopkins experience. *Urol Clin North Am* 2001;28(3):555–565.

15  Horwitz EM, Thames HD, Kuban DA, *et al.* Definitions of biochemical failure that best predict clinical failure in patients with prostate cancer treated with external beam radiation alone: a multi-institutional pooled analysis. *J Urol* 2005;173(3):797–802.

16  Stephenson AJ, Kattan MW, Eastham JA, *et al.* Defining biochemical recurrence of prostate cancer after radical prostatectomy: a proposal for a standardized definition. *J Clin Oncol* 2006;24(24):3973–3978.

17  Partin AW, Pearson JD, Landis PK, *et al.* Evaluation of serum prostate-specific antigen velocity after radical prostatectomy to distinguish local recurrence from distant metastases. *Urology* 1994;43(5):649–659.

18  Johnstone PA, McFarland JT, Riffenburgh RH, Amling CL. Efficacy of digital rectal examination after radiotherapy for prostate cancer. *J Urol* 2001;166(5):1684–1687.

19  Oefelein MG, Smith N, Carter M, *et al.* The incidence of prostate cancer progression with undetectable serum prostate specific antigen in a series of 394 radical prostatectomies. *J Urol* 1995;154(6):2128–2131.

20  Chaplin BJ, Wildhagen MF, Schroder FH, *et al.* Digital rectal examination is no longer necessary in the routine follow-up of men with undetectable prostate specific antigen after radical prostatectomy: the implications for follow-up. *Eur Urol* 2005;48(6):906–910.

21 Foster LS, Jajodia P, Fournier G, Jr., *et al.* The value of prostate specific antigen and transrectal ultrasound guided biopsy in detecting prostatic fossa recurrences following radical prostatectomy. *J Urol* 1993;149(5):1024–1028.

22 Freitas JE, Gilvydas R, Ferry JD, Gonzalez JA. The clinical utility of prostate-specific antigen and bone scintigraphy in prostate cancer follow-up. *J Nucl Med* 1991;32(7):1387–1390.

23 Leibman BD, Dillioglugil O, Wheeler TM, Scardino PT. Distant metastasis after radical prostatectomy in patients without an elevated serum prostate specific antigen level. *Cancer* 1995;76(12):2530–2534.

24 Kramer S, Gorich J, Gottfried HW, *et al.* Sensitivity of computed tomography in detecting local recurrence of prostatic carcinoma following radical prostatectomy. *Br J Radiol* 1997;70(838):995–999.

25 Turner JW, Hawes DR, Williams RD. Magnetic resonance imaging for detection of prostate cancer metastatic to bone. *J Urol* 1993;149(6):1482–1484.

26 Alfarone A, Panebianco V, Schillaci O, *et al.* Comparative analysis of multiparametric magnetic resonance and PET-CT in the management of local recurrence after radical prostatectomy for prostate cancer. *Crit Rev Oncol Hematol* 2012;84(1):109–121.

27 Castellucci P, Fuccio C, Rubello D, *et al.* Is there a role for (1)(1)C-choline PET/CT in the early detection of metastatic disease in surgically treated prostate cancer patients with a mild PSA increase <1.5 ng/ml? *Eur J Nucl Med Mol Imaging* 2011;38(1): 55–63.

28 Tilki D, Reich O, Graser A, *et al.* 18F-fluoroethylcholine PET/CT identifies lymph node metastasis in patients with prostate-specific antigen failure after radical prostatectomy but underestimates its extent. *Eur Urol* 2013;63(5):792–796.

29 Rybalov M, Breeuwsma AJ, Leliveld AM, *et al.* Impact of total PSA, PSA doubling time and PSA velocity on detection rates of (11)C-Choline positron emission tomography in recurrent prostate cancer. *World J Urol* 2013;31(2):319–323.

30 Fuccio C, Castellucci P, Schiavina R, *et al.* Role of (11)C-choline PET/CT in the re-staging of prostate cancer patients with biochemical relapse and negative results at bone scintigraphy. *Eur J Radiol* 2012;81(8):e893-e896.

31 Carroll P, Coley C, McLeod D, *et al.* Prostate-specific antigen best practice policy–part II: prostate cancer staging and post-treatment follow-up. *Urology* 2001;57(2):225–229.

32 Active surveillance monitoring more stringent in updated NCCN Guidelines for prostate cancer. *J Natl Compr Canc Netw* 2011;9(5):xxxvii–xlii.

33 Fradet V, Kurhanewicz J, Cowan JE, *et al.* Prostate cancer managed with active surveillance: role of anatomic MR imaging and MR spectroscopic imaging. *Radiology* 2010;256(1):176–183.

34 van As NJ, de Souza NM, Riches SF, *et al.* A study of diffusion-weighted magnetic resonance imaging in men with untreated localised prostate cancer on active surveillance. *Eur Urol* 2009;56(6):981–987.

35 Moreira DM, Presti JC, Jr., Aronson WJ, *et al.* Postoperative prostate-specific antigen nadir improves accuracy for predicting biochemical recurrence after radical prostatectomy: results from the Shared Equal Access Regional Cancer Hospital (SEARCH) and Duke Prostate Center databases. *Int J Urol* 2010;17(11):914–922.

36 Moul JW. Biochemical recurrence of prostate cancer. *Curr Probl Cancer* 2003;27(5):243–272.

37 Boccon-Gibod L, Djavan WB, Hammerer P, *et al.* Management of prostate-specific antigen relapse in prostate cancer: a European consensus. *Int J Clin Pract* 2004;58(4):382–390.

38 Alkhateeb S, Alibhai S, Fleshner N, *et al.* Impact of positive surgical margins after radical prostatectomy differs by disease risk group. *J Urol* 2010;183(1):145–150.

39 Van der Kwast TH, Bolla M, van PH, *et al.* Identification of patients with prostate cancer who benefit from immediate postoperative radiotherapy: EORTC 22911. *J Clin Oncol* 2007;25(27):4178–4186.

40 Bolla M, van PH, Collette L. [Preliminary results for EORTC trial 22911: radical prostatectomy followed by postoperative radiotherapy in prostate cancers with a high risk of progression]. *Cancer Radiother* 2007;11(6–7):363–369.

41 Critz FA, Levinson AK, Williams WH, *et al.* The PSA nadir that indicates potential cure after radiotherapy for prostate cancer. *Urology* 1997;49(3):322–326.

42 Pickles T. Prostate-specific antigen (PSA) bounce and other fluctuations: which biochemical relapse definition is least prone to PSA false calls? An analysis of 2030 men treated for prostate cancer with external beam or brachytherapy with or without adjuvant androgen deprivation therapy. *Int J Radiat Oncol Biol Phys* 2006;64(5):1355–1359.

43 Roach M, III, Hanks G, Thames H, Jr., *et al.* Defining biochemical failure following radiotherapy with or without hormonal therapy in men with clinically localized prostate cancer: recommendations of the RTOG-ASTRO Phoenix Consensus Conference. *Int J Radiat Oncol Biol Phys* 2006;65(4):965–974.

44 Toledano A, Chauveinc L, Flam T, *et al.* [PSA bounce after permanent implant prostate brachytherapy may mimic a biochemical failure]. *Cancer Radiother* 2007; 11(3):105–110.

45 Toledano A, Chauveinc L, Flam T, *et al.* PSA bounce after permanent implant prostate brachytherapy may mimic a biochemical failure: a study of 295 patients with a minimum 3-year followup. *Brachytherapy* 2006;5(2):122–126.

46 Aus G. Current status of HIFU and cryotherapy in prostate cancer–a review. *Eur Urol* 2006;50(5):927–934.

47 Beerlage HP, Thuroff S, Madersbacher S, *et al.* Current status of minimally invasive treatment options for localized prostate carcinoma. *Eur Urol* 2000;37(1):2–13.

48 Schumacher M, Olschewski M, Schulgen G. Assessment of quality of life in clinical trials. *Stat Med* 1991;10(12):1915–1930.

49 Leplege A, Hunt S. The problem of quality of life in medicine. *J Am Med Assoc* 1997;278(1):47–50.

50 Litwin MS, Lubeck DP, Henning JM, Carroll PR. Differences in urologist and patient assessments of health related quality of life in men with prostate cancer: results of the CaPSURE database. *J Urol* 1998;159(6):1988–1992.

51 Penson DF, Litwin MS, Aaronson NK. Health related quality of life in men with prostate cancer. *J Urol* 2003;169(5):1653–1661.

52 Wei JT, Dunn RL, Litwin MS, *et al.* Development and validation of the expanded prostate cancer index composite (EPIC) for comprehensive assessment of health-related quality of life in men with prostate cancer. *Urology* 2000;56(6):899–905.

53 Giesler RB, Miles BJ, Cowen ME, Kattan MW. Assessing quality of life in men with clinically localized prostate cancer: development of a new instrument for use in multiple settings. *Qual Life Res* 2000;9(6):645–665.

54  van AG, Visser AP, Zwinderman AH, *et al.* A prospective longitudinal study comparing the impact of external radiation therapy with radical prostatectomy on health related quality of life (HRQOL) in prostate cancer patients. *Prostate* 2004;58(4):354–365.

55  Wang H, Huang E, Dale W, *et al.* Self-assessed health-related quality of life in men who have completed radiotherapy for prostate cancer: instrument validation and its relation to patient-assessed bother of symptoms. *Int J Cancer* 2000;90(3):163–172.

56  Lubeck DP, Litwin MS, Henning JM, *et al.* Changes in health-related quality of life in the first year after treatment for prostate cancer: results from CaPSURE. *Urology* 1999;53(1):180–186.

57  Ku J, Krahn M, Trachtenberg J, *et al.* Changes in health utilities and health-related quality of life over 12 months following radical prostatectomy. *Can Urol Assoc J* 2009;3(6):445–452.

58  Alivizatos G, Skolarikos A. Incontinence and erectile dysfunction following radical prostatectomy: a review. *ScientificWorldJournal* 2005;5:747–758.

59  Abel EJ, Masterson TA, Warner JN, *et al.* Nerve-sparing prostatectomy and urinary function: a prospective analysis using validated quality-of-life measures. *Urology* 2009;73(6):1336–1340.

60  Bianco FJ, Jr., Scardino PT, Eastham JA. Radical prostatectomy: long-term cancer control and recovery of sexual and urinary function ("trifecta"). *Urology* 2005;66(5 Suppl.):83–94.

61  Patel VR, Sivaraman A, Coelho RF, *et al.* Pentafecta: a new concept for reporting outcomes of robot-assisted laparoscopic radical prostatectomy. *Eur Urol* 2011;59(5):702–707.

62  Eastham JA, Scardino PT, Kattan MW. Predicting an optimal outcome after radical prostatectomy: the trifecta nomogram. *J Urol* 2008;179(6):2207–2210.

63  Michaelson MD, Cotter SE, Gargollo PC, *et al.* Management of complications of prostate cancer treatment. *CA Cancer J Clin* 2008;58(4):196–213.

64  Cooperberg MR, Koppie TM, Lubeck DP, *et al.* How potent is potent? Evaluation of sexual function and bother in men who report potency after treatment for prostate cancer: data from CaPSURE. *Urology* 2003;61(1):190–196.

65  Wei JT, Dunn RL, Sandler HM, *et al.* Comprehensive comparison of health-related quality of life after contemporary therapies for localized prostate cancer. *J Clin Oncol* 2002;20(2):557–566.

66  Roeloffzen EM, Hinnen KA, Battermann JJ, *et al.* The impact of acute urinary retention after iodine-125 prostate brachytherapy on health-related quality of life. *Int J Radiat Oncol Biol Phys* 2010;77(5):1322–1328.

67  Sanda MG, Dunn RL, Michalski J, *et al.* Quality of life and satisfaction with outcome among prostate-cancer survivors. *N Engl J Med* 2008;358(12):1250–1261.

68  Beard CJ, Propert KJ, Rieker PP, *et al.* Complications after treatment with external-beam irradiation in early-stage prostate cancer patients: a prospective multiinstitutional outcomes study. *J Clin Oncol* 1997;15(1):223–229.

69  Berkey FJ. Managing the adverse effects of radiation therapy. *Am Fam Physician* 2010;82(4):381–388, 394.

70  Smit SG, Heyns CF. Management of radiation cystitis. *Nat Rev Urol* 2010;7(4):206–214.

71 Nakada T, Nakada H, Yoshida Y, *et al.* Hyperbaric oxygen therapy for radiation cystitis in patients with prostate cancer: a long-term follow-up study. *Urol Int* 2012;89:208–214.

72 Oliai C, Fisher B, Jani A, *et al.* Hyperbaric oxygen therapy for radiation-induced cystitis and proctitis. *Int J Radiat Oncol Biol Phys* 2012;84(3):733–840.

73 Brenner DJ, Curtis RE, Hall EJ, Ron E. Second malignancies in prostate carcinoma patients after radiotherapy compared with surgery. *Cancer* 2000;88(2):398–406.

74 Pound CR, Partin AW, Eisenberger MA, *et al.* Natural history of progression after PSA elevation following radical prostatectomy. *J Am Med Assoc* 1999;281(17): 1591–1597

75 Cirillo S, Petracchini M, Scotti L, *et al.* Endorectal magnetic resonance imaging at 1.5 Tesla to assess local recurrence following radical prostatectomy using T2-weighted and contrast-enhanced imaging. *Eur Radiol* 2009;19(3):761–769.

76 Kotzerke J, Volkmer BG, Neumaier B, *et al.* Carbon-11 acetate positron emission tomography can detect local recurrence of prostate cancer. *Eur J Nucl Med Mol Imaging* 2002;29(10):1380–1384.

## CHAPTER 12

# Managing Rising PSA in Naive and Posttherapy Patients

*George Thalmann and Martin Spahn*

Department of Urology, University Hospital Bern, Inselspital Anna Seiler-Haus, Bern, Switzerland

## Introduction

Serum prostate-specific antigen (PSA) is an organ-specific tumor marker. The repeated measurement of PSA in men with prostate cancer (PCa) is an apparently successful example of a rule-based monitoring strategy. Although no prospective randomized trials are supporting such an approach, current guidelines recommend follow-up examinations every 6–12 months for 5 years and annually thereafter for men with localized PCa after conservative treatment, radical prostatectomy (RP), or radiation therapy (RT), including digital rectal examination and PSA-level measurement (Chapter 11). Although these follow-up examinations do not vary significantly for conservatively treated men and those treated with RP and RT, the definition of PSA recurrence varies among the treatment chosen and is still an issue of debate.

Currently, consensus exists that two consecutive values of 0.2 ng/mL or greater define recurrence after RP [1, 2]. Based on the 2–3 days of serum PSA half-life after removal of all prostatic tissue, serum PSA "normalization" can be calculated and serum PSA is expected to be undetectable within 6 weeks after successful RP [3, 4].

Following RT, the situation is more complex because the prostate is still in place. PSA level therefore falls slowly after RT when compared with RP. Because the serum PSA usually does not reach an undetectable state, the PSA nadir was chosen as a baseline parameter and recurrence was defined by a rising PSA above this nadir. However, the time to PSA nadir after RT is highly variable and the optimal cut-off value for a favorable PSA nadir is controversial. Some radiation therapists suggest a minimum 18 months

*Prostate Cancer: Diagnosis and Clinical Management*, First Edition.
Edited by Ashutosh K. Tewari, Peter Whelan and John D. Graham.
© 2014 John Wiley & Sons, Ltd. Published 2014 by John Wiley & Sons, Ltd.

period of observation for nadir and achieving a PSA nadir of <0.5 ng/mL seems to be associated to favorable outcome [5]. Several adaptations were made within the past to define PSA recurrence after RT. The initial ASTRO definition of three consecutive PSA raises was criticized for several reasons and the most widely used definition nowadays is the Phoenix definition (PSA value of 2 ng/mL above the nadir after RT) [6]. The date of PSA recurrence is at call, what means at the time of the first rise in PSA level above the PSA nadir. This definition can also be used for postbrachytherapy monitoring and in case of short-term neoadjuvant hormonal treatment. However, increasing use of the combination of RT with androgen deprivation therapy (ADT) makes it more difficult to use this approach to accurately measure the outcome of the patients. There might be lead time in some of these patients prolonging PSA recurrence-free interval, and others might even have castration-resistant PCa in case of PSA recurrence.

In treatment naive patients, PSA monitoring is even more complicated and no consensus exists on how to define PSA progression in these men. Although measuring PSA is somehow monitoring the disease and tumor progression can be detected by a rising PSA level, several other factors can be causative for increasing PSA levels (i.e., urinary tract infection, prostatitis). Rising PSA levels therefore should be carefully used to define tumor progression.

Although RP and RT are curative for most patients with low- and intermediate-risk PCa, up to 20–40% of these men will experience disease recurrence within 10 years after treatment [7–9]. This rate can be even higher for patients with locally advanced high-risk PCa (PSA >20 ng/ mL and/or Gleason score 8–10 and/or clinical stage T3/4) where up to 70% of the men treated by surgery or RT alone are reported to develop biochemical recurrence (BCR) [7–9].

The management of rising PSA in PCa under observation and after local therapy is one of the most challenging situations in urological oncology. Although it is generally accepted that treatment with ADT is the standard of care for metastatic disease, optimal management of patients with a rising PSA alone is unclear because the disease going forward is highly variable. PSA recurrence can be caused either by local recurrence or by metastatic disease. Unfortunately, currently no diagnostic test is available to accurately discriminate local from distant failure in case of low PSA levels and there are no prospective randomized studies defining when a local or systemic approach should be initiated and whether such an approach prolongs survival. However, several parameters can be helpful to differentiate local from distant metastatic relapse. Initial PSA level, tumor stage, Gleason score, time from RP/RT to PSA recurrence, PSA doubling time (PSADT), and PSA velocity are important factors to differentiate the presence of local or distant metastatic disease [10].

However, the natural course of the disease is highly variable. There might be some patients at highest risk of developing metastasis and dying of the disease. Such patients might benefit from early "salvage" treatment to prevent metastasis, to preserve quality of life (QOL) by delaying the complications of osseous lesions, and to prolong survival. On the other hand, in other patients the disease will have a rather benign behavior for which observation might be appropriate because the risk of cancer-related side effects might be low. This issue is becoming more and more important when considering the results of the SPCG-4 and PIVOT trial comparing the outcome of RP with watchful waiting/observation in the pre-PSA era and a more contemporary patients cohort diagnosed within the PSA era [11, 12]. Especially the results of the recently published PIVOT trial, which showed no survival benefit for patients with low-/intermediate-risk PCa undergoing surgery, when compared with observation—although limited by an underpowered study design—raise the question why BCR should matter in a patient cohort where the same excellent long-term cancer-specific survival rates of >97% at 10 years can be achieved even without any treatment. However, for a patient the situation of being diagnosed with recurrent PCa may provoke distress greater than the distress experienced after initial diagnosis of cancer [13]. Furthermore, although not very extensively studied, the psychological distress of tumor progression/recurrence in patients with PCa is most severe in men with urinary symptoms after initial treatment [14]. Both, cancer fear and fear of salvage-treatment-related side effects concern patients and might impact their QOL.

Therefore, the main question is not only how to discriminate local from distant cancer recurrence, but it is even more important to identify the high-risk and the low-risk patient and to determine the probabilities that a clinically significant event will occur. Treating only those patients at highest risk of metastasis and death would likely have the greatest impact on patient QOL and outcomes. Among these patients might be some men who would benefit from additional local treatment of the prostate/prostatic bed.

## Rising PSA in treatment naive patients

Active surveillance is currently recommended only for highly selected patients with low risk of tumor progression (Chapter 7). In healthy, younger patients with localized or locally advanced nonmetastatic PCa, usually curative treatment in terms of RP/RT is recommended. For elderly men and those with multiple co-morbidities, this might be different. The risk of dying of competing risks in this patient group exceeds the risk of dying of PCa several fold [15]. An observation strategy without any treatment in these men therefore is an appropriate alternative to RP or RT. Treatment-related side effects can be avoided and QOL is not diminished. However, the natural course of the disease even in these men is highly variable and the fact that some patients develop metastatic disease indicates the need to substratify this patient group. EORTC-30891 trial compared immediate versus delayed ADT at the time of symptomatic progression in men with localized T0-4 N0-2 M0 PCa who were not suitable for local treatment or refused curative treatment [16]. The median age of the study population was 73 years. Immediate ADT resulted in a modest, but significant, overall survival benefit, but no difference in PCa mortality or symptom-free survival was found. The median time for initiating ADT was 7 years and 25% of the patients died before becoming symptomatic. A subgroup analysis identified men with a baseline PSA of >50 ng/mL and/or a PSADT of <12 months to be at increased risk of death from PCa. These men might benefit from immediate ADT, whereas those men with a baseline PSA of <50 ng/mL and those with a PSADT of >12 months were likely to die of causes unrelated to PCa [17]. In these men, the burden of immediate ADT could be spared.

## Rising PSA in post-RP patients

Currently, no standard treatment exists for men with PSA recurrence after RP. Three randomized controlled trials analyzed the value of adjuvant RT in men with a high risk for progression after RP. Although some differences exist among the inclusion criteria, these studies demonstrated a benefit for immediate adjuvant RT in terms of BCR [18–20]. But only the SWOG study could show a significant improvement in metastasis-free and overall survival of 1.8 and 1.9 years, respectively [19]. Overtreatment is obvious. The number needed to treat was 12 to prevent metastasis in one patient at 12 years of follow-up and the number needed to treat was 9 to prevent one death at the same time. Therefore, Collette and van der Kwast tried to substratify the patients from EORTC trial 22911 and identified men with positive surgical margins to be at higher risk of biochemical progression (relative risk reduction of 62% for irradiated men, HR

0.38) [21,22]. Salvage RT (SRT) in men with PSA recurrence after RP was proposed to reduce overtreatment. However, the natural course of men with rising PSA after RP might be variable as well and should be considered before treatment initiation.

## Natural history

The natural history of the disease in patients with PSA recurrence whose course is not altered by additional therapies between the time of biochemical recurrence and the development of metastasis is highly variable. Therefore analysis like those performed at the Johns Hopkins Prostate Cancer Database has been used to estimate metastasis-free survival (MFS) in such patients [23]. Out of the 304 men with PSA recurrence after RP, 34% developed metastasis and out of these 43% of the men died due to disease-related effects after a median follow-up time of 5.3 years (0.5–15 years). The median time from PSA recurrence to metastasis was 8 years, and from metastasis to death was 5 years. In a follow-up study by Freedland *et al.* that included a slightly larger cohort, the median survival from PSA recurrence to PCa death was not reached after 16 years [24]. A recent report based on the data from the Center for Prostate Disease Research National Database confirmed these results reporting on an estimated 10-year MFS of almost 40% from the time at which PSA recurrence was diagnosed and overall survival reached 60% at 15 years [25]. The results obtained in these studies are important because they confirm that, even in the absence of additional therapy before metastasis, men with PSA-recurrent PCa generally have prolonged MFS and overall survival. The outcome of men with PSA recurrence is greatly influenced by some tumor-specific parameters. A time interval from RP to PSA recurrence of >3 years, PSADT >9 months after RP, specimen Gleason score ≤7, pathological stage pT2, and negative margin status are associated with favorable outcome even without additional therapy after PSA recurrence following RP (Table 12.1). These men might be selected for an observation strategy.

**Table 12.1** Factors associated with favorable outcome in men with PSA-recurrent disease after radical prostatectomy (RP) who did not receive any additional therapy until the development of metastases

- Interval to PSA recurrence >3 years
- PSA doubling time (PSADT) after primary therapy >9 months
- Gleason score <8
- No extraprostatic extension, seminal vesicle or lymph node involvement
- R0 resection

**Table 12.2** Metastasis-free survival (MFS) probability for patients with biochemical progression after RP

| Good prognosis | Poor prognosis |
| --- | --- |
| Gleason score ≤7<br>and/or<br>Interval to PSA recurrence >2 years<br>and/or<br>PSADT >9 months | Gleason score 8–10<br>and/or<br>Interval to PSA recurrence ≤2 years<br>and/or<br>± PSADT <10 months |
| | Gleason score ≤7<br>and<br>Interval to PSA recurrence <2 years<br>and<br>± PSADT <10 months |

MFS probability at 7 years from PSA recurrence: good prognosis group >75%; poor prognosis group <30%. (Modified from [23, 24]).

However, there is a significant overlap of these parameters to those reported to be associated with local recurrence: a specimen Gleason score ≤7, PSA elevations developing after 2 years following RP, PSADT >12 months, or a PSA velocity <0.75 ng/mL/year are more often associated with local recurrence [10, 26–28]. These men might be good candidates for SRT, although until now no prospective randomized trial has proven an overall survival benefit of SRT versus observation. At highest risk for metastatic disease are those men with a short time interval between RP and PSA recurrence (<2 years), short PSADT (<10 months), and specimen Gleason score ≥8. In addition to the aforementioned parameters to identify patients with very low risk of metastatic disease, a substratification into a good and poor prognosis group can be proposed which might be helpful to further stratify men with PSA recurrence after RP for SRT or systemic therapy (Table 12.2). However, such a substratification should be used carefully because mainly low- and intermediate-risk PCa patients were analyzed in the past. Comparable data for high-risk patients are lacking based on the high rate of early and delayed adjuvant and salvage treatments often used in these patients [23, 24, 29].

In summary, the natural course of PSA recurrence after RP is heterogeneous. Men with longer PSA free time interval after RP, a PSADT >9 months, specimen Gleason score ≤7, and favorable tumor stage are more likely to have local recurrence. These patients might be candidates for either observation or SRT. Men with high-grade tumor, or early PSA

**Table 12.3** Disease-free survival rates of salvage radiation therapy (SRT) for biochemical recurrence after RP

| Pre-RT PSA level (ng/mL) | Disease-free survival rate (%) | Literature |
|---|---|---|
| <0.5 | 48 | [30] |
| <1 | 58 | [31] |
| >1 | 21 | |
| <2 | 83 | [32] |
| >2 | 33 | |
| <2.5 | 76 | [33] |
| >2.5 | 26 | |

recurrence and a short PSADT, are at high risk for metastatic disease and therefore might be candidates for systemic salvage therapy.

## SRT for biochemical recurrent PCa

Salvage RT (SRT) is often used in curative intent for PSA progression after RP. The recommendation for percutaneous SRT in current guidelines is based on a controlled but nonrandomized study and case series [34, 35]. Various studies confirmed the relevance of the pre-RT PSA level for optimal treatment results (Table 12.3). Based on these data, ASTRO has published a consensus paper recommending a dose of at least 64 Gy when the PSA level is <1.5 ng/mL after RP [36]. In another study, Stephenson *et al.* evaluated prognostic models to predict the outcome of SRT on a cohort of 1603 men with PSA progression after RP and operated on in 17 North American tertiary referral centers [30]. The authors identified a significant relationship between serum PSA concentration at the time of RT and therapeutic outcome: the 6-year biochemical-free survival was 48% in men with PSA <0.5 ng/mL, but only 40%, 28%, and 18% in men with PSA levels of 0.51–1, 1.01–1.5, and > 1.5 ng/mL, respectively.

Whether SRT therapy improves overall survival has not yet been proven in prospective randomized trials. One retrospective comparative analysis showed improved cancer-specific survival rates after SRT when compared with a "wait-and-see" strategy. Notably, the three study groups analyzed (no salvage treatment, SRT, SRT+HT) differed significantly for all prognostic factors except surgical margin status and men with no salvage therapy had a much higher prevalence of positive lymph nodes (30% vs. 3–4%; $p$ < .001), thus limiting the value of this analysis [34]. A positive association

**Table 12.4** Parameters with positive association with treatment response to SRT for biochemical recurrence after RP

---

- PSA level before SRT <1 ng/mL
- PSA velocity before SRT <2 ng/mL/year
- Interval to PSA recurrence >2–3 years
- PSADT after primary therapy >12 months
- Gleason score <8
- No seminal vesicle or lymph node involvement
- R1 resection

---

with SRT treatment response was found for longer time intervals from RP to PSA recurrence (>2–3 years), lower PSA levels before SRT (Table 12.3), PSA velocity <2 ng/mL/year, PSADT after RP <12 months, Gleason score <7, pT2/3a tumors, positive surgical margins, and no lymph node invasion (Table 12.4).

These factors were used to determine whether the PSA recurrence is most likely caused by a local recurrence. In addition to the above listed parameters, it is recommended to initiate SRT at PSA level of <0.5 ng/mL [20, 30]. The reported dose used for percutaneous SRT varies between 64 and 70 Gy. A dose of >66 Gy is recommended as a standard nowadays [37]. Even if the rate of severe late complications is relatively low, SRT is an invasive approach and has several potential side effects (Table 12.5). The decision for local therapy should therefore be taken after careful consideration of the benefits against the adverse effects. Because the benefits cannot be fully evaluated, no general recommendation for SRT can be given.

In summary, men with longer time interval from RP to PSA recurrence, favorable PSA kinetics, and histopathological parameters and those with positive surgical margins are potential candidates for SRT. However, a

**Table 12.5** Acute and late toxicities in 173 patients who underwent percutaneous salvage 3D-conformal RT with 70 Gy [35]

|  | Grade 1+2 toxicity (%) | Grade 3 toxicity (%) |
| --- | --- | --- |
| Acute gastrointestinal | 42.2 | 1.2 |
| Acute genitourinary | 37.6 | 0.0 |
| Late gastrointestinal | 15.0 | 0.6 |
| Late genitourinary | 19.3 | 0.6 |

*Source:* Reproduced from Reference 35 with permission from Elsevier.

significant overlap exists to those parameters which can be used to identify men who have excellent outcome with observation alone. Careful patient selection is mandatory to avoid overtreatment.

## Rising PSA in post-RT patients

Currently no standard treatment for PSA recurrent PCa after RT exists. Treatment decisions are mainly based on the estimation whether local recurrence or distant metastases are present. Irrespective to whether local or distant recurrence is present, the natural history of the disease in RT recurrent PCa is important to be addressed.

### Natural history and risk stratification

The natural history of the disease in patients with PSA recurrence after RT is highly variable. Two retrospective series reported on this issue [38, 39]. Local recurrence-free and distant metastasis-free 5-year survival rates were reported to be 74% and 53%, respectively. Early recurrence (<12 months after the end of RT) and a PSADT <12 months significantly predicted the presence of distant metastasis. Overall and cancer-specific survival at 5 years ranged from 58% to 65% and from 73% to 76%, respectively. No parameters could be identified in these analyses to predict favorable outcome in men with rising PSA after RT. However, a pre-RT low-risk tumor, a time interval from RT to PSA recurrence >3 years, a PSADT >12 months, a PSA velocity <2 ng/mL/year, and <50% of positive prostate biopsies were defined to be associated with favorable outcome after salvage treatment (Table 12.6).

According to an ASTRO consensus recommendation, routine prostate biopsy should no longer be performed for the evaluation of PSA-only recurrences following RT [34]. However, prostate biopsy documenting local recurrence represents the main cornerstone in the decision-making

**Table 12.6** Parameters associated with a positive outcome after salvage local treatment for biochemical recurrence after RT [40, 41]

---

- Pre-RT "low-risk" tumor (T1c or T2a, Gleason score <6, PSA level <10 ng/mL)
- Interval to PSA recurrence >3 years
- PSADT after primary therapy >12 months
- PSA rise <2.0 ng/mL/J
- Percentage of positive biopsies <50%

---

process for salvage RP (SRP) in patients with rising PSA levels following a nadir after RT [42]. It is a general recommendation to wait for about 18 months following RT. Patients with rising PSA, viable cancer on biopsy 2 years after RT, and parameters listed in Table 12.6 have true locally recurrent disease and might be candidates for SRP.

## SRP

Salvage RP (SRP) is a curative treatment option for localized recurrence after initial RT. Irrespective of this, a recent review of the data of the Cancer of the Prostate Strategic Urologic Research Endeavor (CaPSURE) comprising 2336 patients with PCa demonstrated that 92% of patients initially irradiated received ADT for secondary treatment of PSA progression [43]. One of the reasons for the reluctant use of SRP is the high complication rates reported in several case series: incontinence 17–67%, rectal injury 0–10%, anastomotic strictures 0–41% [40, 44]. Recently, Chade *et al.* reported on the outcome of 404 men after SRP treated in multiple institutions [45]. The BCR reported after SRP was 48%, metastasis developed in 16% of the men, and 10% died due to PCa. Preoperative predictors for BCR and metastases after SRP were only the pre-SRP PSA and the biopsy Gleason score, whereas in the postoperative models lymph node invasion also predicted distant metastases. Pre-SRP PSA, clinical stage, biopsy and specimen Gleason score, and the presence of seminal vesicle invasion were associated with PCa-related death. A good prognosis group was identified by pre-SRP biopsy Gleason score ≤7 and PSA ≤4 ng/mL. In this group, 52 out of 93 patients had BCR recurrence but only 3 developed metastases and none died of PCa. The estimated 5- and 10-year BCR-free probability in this subgroup was 64% (95% CI = 52–74) and 51% (95% CI = 35–64), respectively.

In summary, SRP can be considered in patients with low co-morbidities and a life expectancy of more than 10 years who have an organ-confined tumor, Gleason score <7, pre-RT PSA level <10 ng/mL, and favorable PSA kinetics after RT. The benefits need to be balanced to the potential harms.

## Salvage cryosurgical ablation of the prostate for radiation failures

Salvage cryosurgery was proposed at the end of the 1990s as an alternative to SRP based on the potential to have less morbidity and equal efficacy. However, only few studies have been reported with mainly disappointing results. Pisters reported on BCR rates of 58% after a mean follow-up of

13.5 months [46]. Furthermore, the complications associated with cryoablation were significant (28–73% urinary incontinence, 67% obstructive symptoms, 72–90% impotence, 8–40% perineal/rectal pain) [46–48]. In addition, 4% of the patients had undergone surgical procedures for the management of treatment-related complications. The oncological outcome after salvage cryoablation is variable, the 5-year BCR-free survival rate was 54% (Phoenix definition), and one-third of the patients who underwent prostate biopsy after cryotherapy had positive biopsies [46].

Salvage cryosurgical ablation of the prostate for radiation failure should be further evaluated in prospective clinical trials and cannot be recommended at the current moment.

## Salvage high-intensity focused ultrasound

Only a few small retrospective studies with short follow-up reported on the outcome of salvage high-intensity focused ultrasound (HIFU) after RT. Thus, the oncological outcome cannot be fully assessed. Urinary tract infections (35%), dysuria (26%), and urinary incontinence (6%) were among the most frequently reported side effects. However, 7% of the men developed recto-urethral fistula as a mayor limitation that is difficult to handle after RT and HIFU therapy. Progression-free survival rate after 2 years was 43% [49]. Salvage HIFU must be considered experimental at the moment.

## Hormonal treatment for PSA recurrence after RP/RT

Although patients with PSA recurrence after RP and RT frequently undergo hormonal therapy, the benefit of this approach is uncertain. The only randomized controlled trial analyzing ADT for PSA-recurrent PCa after RP measured only surrogate endpoints and was underpowered [50]. Moul *et al.* demonstrated in a retrospective analysis that early ADT could delay the time to clinical metastasis only in men with Gleason score $>7$ and/or PSADT $>12$ months [51]. Tenenholz analyzed the effect of early ADT (PSA level $<15$ ng/mL and/or PSADT $>7$ months) versus delayed ADT after RT and found significantly better cancer-specific and overall survival in the early ADT group [52].

Men with high-grade tumor, high initial PSA ($>50$ ng/mL), early PSA recurrence, and a short PSADT are at increased risk for metastatic disease after RP and RT and therefore might be candidates for systemic salvage therapy.

## Summary

In PCa, the selection of further treatment for PSA recurrence depends on many factors, including previous treatment, site of recurrence, individual tumor-specific parameters, PSA kinetics, coexistent illnesses, and individual patient considerations. Observation can be chosen in men with favorable risk profiles, elderly patients, or those with severe co-morbidities. SRT and salvage prostatectomy are the preferred curative treatment options for men with local recurrence. However, these salvage treatments can be related to severe side effects. Patients therefore should be carefully selected for salvage treatment for rising PSA.

## References

1 Boccon-Gibod L, Djavan WB, Hammerer P, *et al.* Management of prostate-specific antigen relapse in prostate cancer: a European Consensus. *Int J Clin Pract* 2004;58(4):382–390.

2 Moul JW. Prostate specific antigen only progression of prostate cancer. *J Urol* 2000;163(6):1632–1642.

3 Stamey TA, Kabalin JN, McNeal JE, *et al.* Prostate specific antigen in the diagnosis and treatment of adenocarcinoma of the prostate. II. Radical prostatectomy treated patients. *J Urol* 1989;141(5):1076–1083.

4 Oesterling JE, Chan DW, Epstein JI, *et al.* Prostate specific antigen in the preoperative and postoperative evaluation of localized prostatic cancer treated with radical prostatectomy. *J Urol* 1988;139(4):766–772.

5 Ray ME, Thames HD, Levy LB, *et al.* PSA nadir predicts biochemical and distant failures after external beam radiotherapy for prostate cancer: a multi-institutional analysis. *Int J Radiat Oncol Biol Phys* 2006;64(4):1140–1150.

6 Horwitz EM, Thames HD, Kuban DA, *et al.* Definitions of biochemical failure that best predict clinical failure in patients with prostate cancer treated with external beam radiation alone: a multi-institutional pooled analysis. *J Urol* 2005;173(3):797–802.

7 Yossepowitch O, Eggener SE, Bianco FJ, Jr., *et al.* Radical prostatectomy for clinically localized, high risk prostate cancer: critical analysis of risk assessment methods. *J Urol* 2007;178(2):493–499; discussion 9.

8 Grimm P, Billiet I, Bostwick D, *et al.* Comparative analysis of prostate-specific antigen free survival outcomes for patients with low, intermediate and high risk prostate cancer treatment by radical therapy. Results from the Prostate Cancer Results Study Group. *BJU Int* 2012;109 (Suppl. 1):22–29.

9 Spahn M, Joniau S, Gontero P, *et al.* Outcome predictors of radical prostatectomy in patients with prostate-specific antigen greater than 20 ng/ml: a European multi-institutional study of 712 patients. *Eur Urol* 2010;58(1):1–7; discussion 10-1.

10 Consensus statement: guidelines for PSA following radiation therapy. American Society for Therapeutic Radiology and Oncology Consensus Panel. *Int J Radiat Oncol Biol Phys* 1997;37(5):1035–1041.

11 Bill-Axelson A, Holmberg L, Ruutu M, *et al.* Radical prostatectomy versus watchful waiting in early prostate cancer. *N Engl J Med* 2011;364(18):1708–1717.

12 Wilt TJ, Brawer MK, Jones KM, *et al.* Radical prostatectomy versus observation for localized prostate cancer. *N Engl J Med* 2012;367(3):203–213.

13 Cella DF, Mahon SM, Donovan MI. Cancer recurrence as a traumatic event. *Behav Med* 1990;16(1):15–22.

14 Ullrich PM, Carson MR, Lutgendorf SK, Williams RD. Cancer fear and mood disturbance after radical prostatectomy: consequences of biochemical evidence of recurrence. *J Urol* 2003;169(4):1449–1452.

15 Lu-Yao GL, Albertsen PC, Moore DF, *et al.* Outcomes of localized prostate cancer following conservative management. *J Am Med Assoc* 2009;302(11):1202–1209.

16 Studer UE, Whelan P, Albrecht W, *et al.* Immediate or deferred androgen deprivation for patients with prostate cancer not suitable for local treatment with curative intent: European Organisation for Research and Treatment of Cancer (EORTC) Trial 30891. *J Clin Oncol* 2006;24(12):1868–1876.

17 Studer UE, Collette L, Whelan P, *et al.* Using PSA to guide timing of androgen deprivation in patients with T0-4 N0-2 M0 prostate cancer not suitable for local curative treatment (EORTC 30891). *Eur Urol* 2008;53(5):941–949.

18 Bolla M, van Poppel H, Collette L, *et al.* Postoperative radiotherapy after radical prostatectomy: a randomised controlled trial (EORTC trial 22911). *Lancet* 2005;366(9485):572–578.

19 Thompson IM, Tangen CM, Paradelo J, *et al.* Adjuvant radiotherapy for pathological T3N0M0 prostate cancer significantly reduces risk of metastases and improves survival: long-term followup of a randomized clinical trial. *J Urol* 2009;181(3):956–962.

20 Wiegel T, Lohm G, Bottke D, *et al.* Achieving an undetectable PSA after radiotherapy for biochemical progression after radical prostatectomy is an independent predictor of biochemical outcome–results of a retrospective study. *Int J Radiat Oncol Biol Phys* 2009;73(4):1009–1016.

21 Collette L, van Poppel H, Bolla M, *et al.* Patients at high risk of progression after radical prostatectomy: do they all benefit from immediate post-operative irradiation? (EORTC trial 22911). *Eur J Cancer* 2005;41(17):2662–2672.

22 van der Kwast TH, Bolla M, Van Poppel H, *et al.* Identification of patients with prostate cancer who benefit from immediate postoperative radiotherapy: EORTC 22911. *J Clin Oncol* 2007;25(27):4178–4186.

23 Pound CR, Partin AW, Eisenberger MA, *et al.* Natural history of progression after PSA elevation following radical prostatectomy. *J Am Med Assoc* 1999;281(17):1591–1597.

24 Freedland SJ, Humphreys EB, Mangold LA, *et al.* Risk of prostate cancer-specific mortality following biochemical recurrence after radical prostatectomy. *J Am Med Assoc* 2005;294(4):433–439.

25 Antonarakis ES, Chen Y, Elsamanoudi SI, *et al.* Long-term overall survival and metastasis-free survival for men with prostate-specific antigen-recurrent prostate cancer after prostatectomy: analysis of the Center for Prostate Disease Research National Database. *BJU Int* 2011;108(3):378–385.

26 Roach M, Hanks G, Thames H, Jr, *et al.* Defining biochemical failure following radiotherapy with or without hormonal therapy in men with clinically localized prostate cancer: recommendations of the RTOG-ASTRO Phoenix Consensus Conference. *Int J Radiat Oncol Biol Phys* 2006;65(4):965–974.

27  Trapasso JG, deKernion JB, Smith RB, Dorey F. The incidence and significance of detectable levels of serum prostate specific antigen after radical prostatectomy. *J Urol* 1994;152(5 Pt 2):1821–1825.

28  Lange PH, Ercole CJ, Lightner DJ, *et al.* The value of serum prostate specific antigen determinations before and after radical prostatectomy. *J Urol* 1989;141(4):873–879.

29  Freedland SJ, Humphreys EB, Mangold LA, *et al.* Death in patients with recurrent prostate cancer after radical prostatectomy: prostate-specific antigen doubling time subgroups and their associated contributions to all-cause mortality. *J Clin Oncol* 2007;25(13):1765–1771.

30  Stephenson AJ, Scardino PT, Kattan MW, *et al.* Predicting the outcome of salvage radiation therapy for recurrent prostate cancer after radical prostatectomy. *J Clin Oncol* 2007;25(15):2035–2041.

31  Nudell DM, Grossfeld GD, Weinberg VK, *et al.* Radiotherapy after radical prostatectomy: treatment outcomes and failure patterns. *Urology* 1999;54(6):1049–1057.

32  Forman JD, Meetze K, Pontes E, *et al.* Therapeutic irradiation for patients with an elevated post-prostatectomy prostate specific antigen level. *J Urol* 1997;158(4):1436–1439; discussion 9-40.

33  Schild SE, Buskirk SJ, Wong WW, *et al.* The use of radiotherapy for patients with isolated elevation of serum prostate specific antigen following radical prostatectomy. *J Urol* 1996;156(5):1725–1729.

34  Trock BJ, Han M, Freedland SJ, *et al.* Prostate cancer-specific survival following salvage radiotherapy vs observation in men with biochemical recurrence after radical prostatectomy. *J Am Med Assoc* 2008;299(23):2760–2769.

35  Jereczek-Fossa BA, Zerini D, Vavassori A, *et al.* Sooner or later? Outcome analysis of 431 prostate cancer patients treated with postoperative or salvage radiotherapy. *Int J Radiat Oncol Biol Phys* 2009;74(1):115–125.

36  Cox JD, Gallagher MJ, Hammond EH, *et al.* Consensus statements on radiation therapy of prostate cancer: guidelines for prostate re-biopsy after radiation and for radiation therapy with rising prostate-specific antigen levels after radical prostatectomy. American Society for Therapeutic Radiology and Oncology Consensus Panel. *J Clin Oncol* 1999;17(4):1155.

37  Mottet N, Bellmunt J, Bolla M, *et al.* EAU guidelines on prostate cancer. Part II: Treatment of advanced, relapsing, and castration-resistant prostate cancer. *Eur Urol* 2011;59(4):572–583.

38  Lee WR, Hanks GE, Hanlon A. Increasing prostate-specific antigen profile following definitive radiation therapy for localized prostate cancer: clinical observations. *J Clin Oncol* 1997;15(1):230–238.

39  Sandler HM, Dunn RL, McLaughlin PW, *et al.* Overall survival after prostate-specific-antigen-detected recurrence following conformal radiation therapy. *Int J Radiat Oncol Biol Phys* 2000;48(3):629–633.

40  Nguyen PL, D'Amico AV, Lee AK, Suh WW. Patient selection, cancer control, and complications after salvage local therapy for postradiation prostate-specific antigen failure: a systematic review of the literature. *Cancer* 2007;110(7):1417–14128.

41  Heidenreich A, Richter S, Thuer D, Pfister D. Prognostic parameters, complications, and oncologic and functional outcome of salvage radical prostatectomy for locally recurrent prostate cancer after 21st-century radiotherapy. *Eur Urol* 2010;57(3):437–443.

42 Heidenreich A, Semrau R, Thuer D, Pfister D. [Radical salvage prostatectomy: treatment of local recurrence of prostate cancer after radiotherapy]. *Urologe A* 2008;47(11):1441–1446.

43 Grossfeld GD, Li YP, Lubeck DP, *et al.* Predictors of secondary cancer treatment in patients receiving local therapy for prostate cancer: data from cancer of the prostate strategic urologic research endeavor. *J Urol* 2002;168(2):530–535.

44 Leonardo C, Simone G, Papalia R, *et al.* Salvage radical prostatectomy for recurrent prostate cancer after radiation therapy. *Int J Urol* 2009;16(6):584–586.

45 Chade DC, Shariat SF, Cronin AM, *et al.* Salvage radical prostatectomy for radiation-recurrent prostate cancer: a multi-institutional collaboration. *Eur Urol* 2011; 60(2):205–510.

46 Pisters LL, Rewcastle JC, Donnelly BJ, *et al.* Salvage prostate cryoablation: initial results from the cryo on-line data registry. *J Urol* 2008;180(2):559–563; discussion 63-4.

47 Pisters LL, Leibovici D, Blute M, *et al.* Locally recurrent prostate cancer after initial radiation therapy: a comparison of salvage radical prostatectomy versus cryotherapy. *J Urol* 2009;182(2):517–525; discussion 25-7.

48 Cespedes RD, Pisters LL, von Eschenbach AC, McGuire EJ. Long-term followup of incontinence and obstruction after salvage cryosurgical ablation of the prostate: results in 143 patients. *J Urol* 1997;157(1):237–240.

49 Ahmed HU, Cathcart P, McCartan N, *et al.* Focal salvage therapy for localized prostate cancer recurrence after external beam radiotherapy: a pilot study. *Cancer* 2012;118(17):4148–4155.

50 Goluboff ET, Prager D, Rukstalis D, *et al.* Safety and efficacy of exisulind for treatment of recurrent prostate cancer after radical prostatectomy. *J Urol* 2001;166(3):882–886.

51 Moul JW, Wu H, Sun L, *et al.* Early versus delayed hormonal therapy for prostate specific antigen only recurrence of prostate cancer after radical prostatectomy. *J Urol* 2004;171(3):1141–1147.

52 Tenenholz TC, Shields C, Ramesh VR, *et al.* Survival benefit for early hormone ablation in biochemically recurrent prostate cancer. *Urol Oncol* 2007;25(2):101–109.

# CHAPTER 13

# Diagnosis and Management of Metastatic Prostate Cancer

*Bertrand Tombal[1] and Frederic Lecouvet[2]*

[1]Division of Urology, Cliniques universitaires Saint Luc, Institut de Recherche clinique, Université catholique de Louvain, Brussels, Belgium
[2]Division of Radiology, Cliniques universitaires Saint Luc, Institut de Recherche clinique, Université catholique de Louvain, Brussels, Belgium

## Introduction

In men over the age of 50 years, prostate cancer (PCa) is the most commonly diagnosed cancer and the second leading cause of death by cancer [1]. Because of intense use of prostate-specific antigen (PSA) testing, most PCa are diagnosed at an early stage. Recent updated results of the European Randomized Study of Screening for Prostate Cancer (ERSPC) have indicated that screening reduces the cumulative incidence of metastatic PCa from 0.86% to 0.67% after a median follow-up of 12 years [2]. In a sub-analysis of the Goteborg section of ERSPC, Aus *et al.* have reported an incidence of lymph node metastases of 3.2% and 9.3% and an incidence of bone metastases of 8.5% and 22%, in the screened and nonscreened cohort, respectively [3]. Therefore, it can be assumed that the incidence of metastases in a given practice will vary within these boundaries according to the intensity of opportunistic PSA testing. Nonlymphatic visceral metastases (VM) are detected in around 10% of castration-resistant prostate cancer (CRPC) patients, but rarely at initial diagnosis.

Consequently, most patients are treated with radical prostatectomy, external beam radiation therapy, or seeds implant. Despite major advances, a proportion of these patients will recur. Because PSA is used to monitor these patients, most will receive androgen deprivation therapy (ADT) at an earlier stage when metastases are not yet detectable. Many of

---

*Prostate Cancer: Diagnosis and Clinical Management*, First Edition.
Edited by Ashutosh K. Tewari, Peter Whelan and John D. Graham.
© 2014 John Wiley & Sons, Ltd. Published 2014 by John Wiley & Sons, Ltd.

these patients will have already entered CRPC stage when the first metastasis is detected.

Although the epidemiologists view metastatic PCa as a rare event, it still bears most of the lethality and most of the morbidity of the disease. PCa cells spreading out of the prostate show an exquisite tropism for pelvic and retroperitoneal lymph nodes and the skeleton. Bone metastases represent the initial and main metastatic site in about 80% of PCa patients, therefore being one of the most important prognostic factors [4]. Skeletal complications of bone metastases, most commonly designed as "skeletal-related events" (SRE), account for most of the PCa morbidity and mortality [5]. Replacement of hematopoietic tissues in the bone marrow by metastatic cells leads to anemia, whereas abnormal tissue growing in the bone marrow can lead to pain, fractures, and spinal cord compression. As for today, bone metastases are still considered incurable [6].

In this chapter, we will focus on timing and modality of diagnostic procedures for metastases and treatment of hormone-naïve metastases. We will not address the treatment of bone metastasis in the CRPC setting, as well as palliative treatment of SRE.

## Proper diagnosis of metastases: when and how?

Practice guidelines recommend $^{99m}$Tc bone scintigraphy (BS) and contrast-enhanced computed tomography (CT) or magnetic resonance imaging (MRI) of the pelvis and abdomen to define metastatic status [7, 8].

### When is bone imaging required?

Because PSA testing has shifted the diagnosis of PCa toward early stage of the disease, there is no need to perform an initial CT or a $^{99m}$Tc BS in every new patient. In a study conducted on 60 patients with newly diagnosed PCa, a PSA >100 ng/mL, a PSA, cT$_{3-4}$ stage, and a Gleason score >7 were the strongest predictors of bone metastases [9]. Based on this trial and others, the EAU guidelines recommend that [ ... ] *Patients with stage T2 or less, PSA <10 ng/ml, a Gleason score ≤6, and <50% positive biopsy cores have <10% likelihood of having node metastases and can be spared nodal evaluation* [ ... ] and a $^{99m}$Tc BS is indicated [ ... ] *if the serum PSA level is <20 ng/ml in the presence of well-differentiated or moderately differentiated tumours* [ ... ] [7]. Briganti *et al.* have developed a risk stratification tool to select patients requiring initial imaging [10]. Low-risk (biopsy Gleason ≤7, cT$_{1-2}$, and PSA <10 ng/mL) patients have a risk of bone metastases of 1.8% and do not need any evaluation. Intermediate-risk (biopsy Gleason $\leq$7, cT$_{2-3}$, and PSA >10 ng/mL) and high-risk (biopsy Gleason >7) patients have a risk of metastases of 8.5% and 16.4%, respectively, and should be imaged.

Later in the course of the disease, imaging will be discussed in case of PSA recurrence after radical treatment. However, physicians should keep in mind that the rate of metastatic progression is very low and occurs over several years; therefore, many imaging modalities can be spared [11]. Patients at risk of bone metastases are those with a short time to biochemical progression ($\leq$2 years), a Gleason score $\geq$8, and PSA doubling time (PSADT) $\leq$10 months.

## Present and future imaging technologies
### Lymph nodes and visceral metastases

Guidelines traditionally recommend contrast-enhanced abdomino-pelvic CT and/or MRI [7, 8]. Based on limited comparative studies, it appears that CT and MRI perform similarly in the detection of pelvic lymph nodes, with limited value and questioned diagnostic performance of size criteria used for screening [12]. In the future, MRI will certainly outperform CT as a diagnostic technique, because MRI has become a central tool in the evaluation of the primary tumor [13] and that specific contrast agents, such as lymphotropic paramagnetic iron particles will become available [14].

Positron emission tomography combined with computed tomography (PET-CT), especially with [11]C-choline, has emerged as a potential candidate to replace CT and/or MRI. However, results for lymph node detections are still contradictory, reporting sensitivities, specificities, and negative predictive (NPV) and positive predictive values (PPV) ranging from 9.4% to 60.0%, 97.6% to 99.7%, and 87.0% to 87.2%, and 91%, respectively [15, 16].

### Detection of bone metastases
### Is [99m]Tc bone scanning still the gold standard?

[99m]Tc methylene diphosphonate (MDP) BS has been used for decades as the first-line modality for the screening of PCa bone metastases [17]. [99m]Tc-MDP is a nonspecific marker of osteoblastic activity, which accumulates in response to tumor, but also to degenerative joint disease, benign fractures, and inflammation [18]. Sensitivities are acceptable and range between 62% and 89% [19]. In contrast, [99m]Tc BS has a low specificity [20]. In many cases, regions of increased uptake cannot be definitively characterized as negative or positive for malignancy. Routinely, it will end up in reading characterized bone as "equivocal," "possible," "suspicious,"

"likely," "highly suspicious," and "almost certain," a series of definitions encompassing all cases in which imaging findings could not be categorized confidently as metastatic or benign, regardless of the level of incertitude. Usually, equivocal BS uptakes will be characterized by targeted X-rays to distinguish benign (fracture, Paget, degenerative joint disease, etc.) from malignant (metastatic) origin [21].

Whole-body single-photon emission computerized tomography (SPECT) enhances both sensitivity and specificity of $^{99m}$Tc BS [22]. Even-Sapir *et al.* have reported sensitivity, specificity, PPV, and NPV for planar $^{99m}$Tc BS of 70%, 57%, 64%, and 55%, respectively, and for SPECT of 92%, 82%, 86%, and 90%, respectively. However, because whole-body SPECT is time-consuming and not widely available, it is not yet recognized as the "optimal state-of-the-art" screening technique, although it is available on most standard BS machines and be performed at minimal cost increased.

### Position emission tomography

Positron emission tomography combined with computed tomography (PET-CT) has demonstrated higher sensitivity for the early detection of bone metastases in various malignancies [23]. Unfortunately, the most widely used metabolic marker, $^{18}$F-FDG PET, has little or even no interest in PCa patients [24]. Other metabolic markers seem more appropriate for detecting bone metastases from PCa, including $^{18}$F-fluoride, $^{11}$C-acetate, and $^{18}$F-fluorocholine. In the aforementioned study, Even-Sapir *et al.* has reported sensitivity, specificity, PPV, and NPV of 100% for $^{18}$F-fluoride PET/CT. Beheshti *et al.* have reported sensitivity, specificity, and accuracy of 81%, 93%, and 86% for $^{18}$F-fluoride PET/CT and 74%, 99%, and 85% for $^{18}$F-fluorocholine PET/CT, respectively [25].

### Magnetic resonance imaging of the skeleton

Magnetic resonance imaging (MRI) is highly sensitive for detecting bone metastases in cancer patients and its superiority over $^{99m}$Tc BS has been repeatedly demonstrated [26]. It has been used as a *"gold standard"* to evaluate PET for detecting bone metastases, and more recently to quantify PCa metastases and measure tumor response to therapy [27, 28]. The superiority of MRI lies in its ability to detect early tumor cells seeding into the hematopoietic compartment, thus identifying bone metastases at an early stage, before host reaction of the osteoblasts becomes visible on $^{99m}$Tc BS and X-rays [19]. Our group has evaluated the diagnostic performance and impact on therapy of one-step MRI of the axial skeleton (MRIas) for detecting bone metastases in high-risk PCa [29]. MRIas has been compared to a routine workup based on $^{99m}$Tc BS completed with targeted X-rays in cases of equivocal BS findings, and with MRI "on request" (MRIor) in case of inconclusive $^{99m}$Tc BS/X-rays findings. Sensitivities were 46% for $^{99m}$Tc BS alone, 63% for $^{99m}$Tc BS/X-rays, 83% for $^{99m}$Tc BS/X-rays/MRI, and 100% for MRIas. Corresponding specificities were 32%, 64%, 100%, and 88%, respectively. MRIas correctly identified metastases in 7/23 (30%) patients considered negative and 8/17 (47%) considered equivocal by other strategies, which resulted in altering the initially planned therapy. These results were confirmed by other studies [30–32].

## The future of diagnosis and treatment of bone metastases

The imaging technique of the future should enable accurate detection and monitoring of lymph node, visceral and bone metastases. This should be done in a single visit, without contrast injection and minimal exposure to radiations.

Whole-body MRI (WB-MRI) and PET-CT compete for whole-body single-step assessment of metastatic burden in solid cancers. The performance of PET largely depends on the affinity of the tumor cells for the PET tracer. Axial skeleton and WB-MRI have better sensitivity and specificity than $^{99m}$Tc BS, and allow monitoring of tumor response [28, 29, 31]. Eschmann *et al.* have compared the diagnostic accuracy of $^{11}$C-choline PET-CT to WB-MRI for the staging workup of PCa and reported sensitivity, specificity, and accuracy of 96.6%, 76.5%, and 93.3%, respectively, for $^{11}$C-choline PET-CT and 78.4%, 94.1%, and 81.0%, respectively, for MRI [33].

Addition of diffusion-weighted imaging (DWI) to WB-MRI also enables the study of extraskeletal involvement, including lymph nodes and other soft tissue metastases, without requiring intravenous contrast agents [34]. Our group has compared the performance of DWI/WB-MRI to the standard CT + $^{99m}$TC BS approach in 100 high-risk PCa patients, including 68 patients with metastases [30]. In that study, WB-MRI outperformed $^{99m}$Tc BS in detecting more bone metastases and performed equally to CT for the detection of lymph node and VM.

# Initial treatment of bone metastases

## Androgen deprivation therapy: 60 years of existence and still so much to learn

Since the seminal work of Charles Huggins in the early 1940s, androgen deprivation therapy (ADT) has been the cornerstone treatment of advanced and metastatic PCa [35]. Huggins indeed showed that depriving

PCa cells of androgens by surgical castration or estrogens induces apoptotic death, resulting in major shrinkage of the prostate tumor and its metastases. After 60 years of intense pharmacological research, hormone therapy is still used basically as Huggins described it. Although gonadotropin-releasing hormone (GnRH) agonists and peripheral antiandrogens have been developed and different timing and modalities have been investigated, physicians still remain today with more questions than answers.

## Timing of ADT

Symptomatic PCa patients need rapid and effective treatment [36]. With the modern migration toward earlier disease stages, the question of when to start ADT is frequently asked for minimally symptomatic and/or oligometastatic patients. The duration of ADT, if started at time of diagnosis, will be much longer, and its burden (side effects and cost) much heavier. It is therefore imperative to prove that the potential benefits positively balance the expected inconveniences; that is, improved survival compensates the side effects of ADT.

Until now, no study has unequivocally demonstrated a significant survival advantage when ADT is given early. Three studies have been conducted by the Veterans Administration Cooperative Urological Research Group (VACURG) between 1960 and 1975, evaluating diethylstilbestrol (DES) 5 mg and 1 mg, orchiectomy + placebo, and orchiectomy + DES versus placebo. When the results of the first VACURG study were published, it was concluded that early ADT delayed progression but does not prolong survival, the cardiovascular mortality of 5 mg DES negating the benefit of treatment [37]. The second VACURG study with 1 mg of DES showed an improvement in survival with immediate treatment [38]. However, a re-analysis of the data revealed the importance of selection factors since only high-grade tumors are benefited from early ADT, providing the first evidence that the decision to treat should be tailored to the patient's characteristics [39]. The Medical Research Council (MRC) has conducted a randomized study to compare immediate (started at diagnosis) with deferred (started at clinical progression) ADT [40]. Clinical progression was delayed by immediate group treatment, so that severe complications from disease progression were less frequent. The mortality rate was not statistically significantly different between immediate and deferred ADT.

Unfortunately, the relevance of these studies in the modern era is limited because many patients in the deferred group never received ADT, Gleason scores were not used to stratify risk groups, $^{99m}$Tc BS was not available to detect metastasis, and PSA was not available to ascertain disease progression. In 2006, a Cochrane Review on early versus delayed treatment concluded that *"the evidence from randomized controlled trials is limited by the variability in study design, stage of cancer and subjects enrolled, interventions utilized, definitions and reporting of outcomes and the lack of PSA testing for diagnostic and monitoring purposes. However, the available information suggests that early androgen suppression for treatment of advanced prostate cancer reduces disease progression and complications due to progression. Early androgen suppression may provide a small but statistically significant improvement in overall survival at 10 years. There was no statistically significant difference in prostate cancer specific survival but a clinically important difference could not be excluded"* [41].

Inconclusive recommendations and intense commercial support have resulted in the "conventional wisdom" that every metastatic patient needs ADT. But as pointed by Galbraith, these are [ … ] *ideas which are esteemed at any time for their acceptability* [ … ] and there may be important differences between what is acceptable and what is true.

There are several arguments in favor of early ADT:

1  Early experimental animal models indicate that ADT is more effective when started early in the development of a tumor [42].

2  The need for ancillary procedures (i.e., transurethral resection of the prostate (TURP), JJ stent) and the emergence of life-threatening complications (i.e. pathological fractures, spinal cord compression, and paraplegia) are less likely to occur when the patient is treated early [40].

3  Progression of PCa is painful; most patients will suffer from malaise, fatigue, and a sense of unhealthiness. In addition, some patients will die without having the opportunity to receive treatment [38].

But here are also several arguments in favor of delaying ADT:

1  As ADT has showed minimal benefit on survival, it should be considered palliative. Asymptomatic patients have no symptoms to palliate; delaying treatment avoids side effects. When symptomatic progression occurs—and it inevitably will—effective treatment still exists.

2  Observation means "active surveillance" and not neglect: rapid progression and complications can be detected early by PSA-based follow-up and modern imaging technology; treatment can therefore be started early enough to anticipate catastrophic complications.

3  Sequential observation allows the determination of PSA velocity and PSADT, which have been demonstrated to be one of the most important parameters in the evaluation of the patient with nonmetastatic PCa [43].

In conclusion, although clear guidelines regarding timing of ADT are premature, practical recommendations can be made based on evaluable risk factors. Symptomatic patients and those at high risk of progression clearly should receive treatment, whereas compliant patients with a very low risk of progression can safely opt for watchful waiting.

## Modality of ADT
### GnRH agonists

Following the discovery by Schally *et al.*, in 1971, of the sequence of GnRH, GnRH analogs have become the standard approach to induce ADT [44]. GnRH first causes an increase in luteinizing hormone (LH) and testosterone before desensitizing the receptor so that the onset of ADT is delayed by about 3–6 weeks. The Leuprolide Study Group has compared leuprolide to DES in metastatic PCa. As expected from its agonist activity, leuprolide induced an initial increase in serum testosterone and required a longer time to achieve castration levels compared with DES [45]. The time to progression and survival plots were not significantly different between the two treatment groups, but the study was inadequately powered to detect a difference in survival or cardiovascular toxicity. Goserelin has been compared to orchiectomy in two trials on metastatic patients [46,47]. In the study conducted by Kaisary *et al.*, median survival time was 115 and 104 weeks ($p = .33$) in the goserelin and orchiectomy groups, respectively [47]. In the study conducted by Vogelzang *et al.*, median survival time was 119 and 136 weeks ($p = .42$) in the goserelin and orchiectomy groups, respectively [46]. These two studies have been used abundantly by the pharmaceutical industry to claim the equivalence of GnRH agonists to orchiectomy. The truth may be slightly different. The Vogelzang trial was stopped early, before recruitment was fully completed, leaving them 67% chances to detect a 30% difference. In the Kaisary trial, the dropout rate was so high that the number of patients analyzed was similar to the Vogelzang trial. Therefore, we are left with the question whether LH-releasing hormone (LHRH) agonists are equivalent to castration.

Because GnRH agonists induce an initial surge in serum testosterone, patients with advanced symptomatic PCa may experience transient worsening, or flare, of symptoms, leading in dramatic but rare cases of potential life-threatening complications [48]. Thus, physicians routinely use an antiandrogen during the first weeks of treatment to protect the patients against the consequence of the testosterone surge. However, nonsteroidal antiandrogens may not compensate effectively for the testosterone surge. In the study conducted by Kuhn *et al.*, bone pain appeared or worsened in

29% of metastatic patients receiving flutamide and GnRH agonist busere-lin [49]. In a trial comparing leuprolide alone or combined with flutamide, there was no change or worsening of pain in 73–77%, performance status in 88–90%, alkaline phosphatase in 65% of patients receiving flutamide [50].

### GnRH antagonists

In contrast with agonists, GnRH antagonists immediately suppress LH and follicle-stimulating hormone (FSH) without initial stimulation. Two GnRH antagonists are commercially available, abarelix and degarelix, and several others are in development. The efficacy and safety of degarelix has been tested against leuprolide [51]. Three days after starting treatment, testosterone levels were ≤0.5 ng/mL in 96.1% and 95.5% of patients in the degarelix 240/80 mg and 240/160 mg groups, respectively, and in none in the leuprolide group. No transient testosterone surge was seen in the degarelix arm. Preplanned sub-analysis showed degarelix to be significantly superior to leuprolide in decreasing the rate of PSA and alkaline phosphatase failure, especially in patients with bone metastases or a PSA ≥20 ng/mL [52,53]. Patients receiving degarelix showed a significantly lower risk of PSA progression or death compared with leuprolide ($p = .05$) [52]. Patients with metastatic disease had greater and more prolonged reduction in alkaline phosphatase levels with degarelix than with leuprolide [53]. Taken together, these data suggest that GnRH antagonists have become the agent of choice to induce ADT in metastatic patients.

### Monotherapy with antiandrogens

Thorpe *et al.* have compared goserelin to cyproterone acetate, and to a combination of the two [54]. Goserelin was clearly superior in delaying the time to progression ($p = .016$).

Bicalutamide 150 mg has been compared with ADT in patients with locally advanced nonmetastatic disease or metastatic disease [55]. The first analysis showed that the median survival of metastatic patients was 6 weeks shorter with bicalutamide [55]. By contrast, bicalutamide 150 mg has a more favorable side-effect profile, especially with respect to sexual interest and physical capacity ($p = .046$), with breast pain and gynecomastia being the most frequent side effects. Because of that more favorable toxicity profile, the EAU guidelines acknowledge that *"High-dose bicalutamide has emerged as an alternative to castration for patients with locally advanced (M0) if PFS is the target, and in highly selected, well-informed cases of M1 PCa with a low PSA"* [56].

## Complete androgen blockade

Complete androgen blockade (CAB) occurs in permanent association of a GnRH agonist or orchiectomy with an antiandrogen. Most patients studied had distant metastases; eight studies having included only patients with distant metastases. Two meta-analyses have showed that CAB improves significant but modest survival (2–3%) [57, 58]. However, nonsteroidal antiandrogens increased the rate of side effects versus castration alone, including diarrhea (10% vs. 2%), gastrointestinal pain (7% vs. 2%), and nonspecific ophthalmologic events (29% vs. 5%).

In the Cochrane meta-analysis, when only studies with more than 90% metastatic disease were included, the odds ratio for overall survival was significant only at 5 years, suggesting that CAB would benefit only patients with low-burden metastatic disease. This has been confirmed by a combined analysis of the two CAB phase III trials conducted by EORTC [59]. Sylvester *et al.* have stratified patients into risk groups based on their alkaline phosphatase, hemoglobin, performance status, pain score, T category, and G grade at entry on study [59]. Study 30853 showed that CAB with goserelin plus flutamide increased overall survival compared with orchiectomy, but the benefit was limited to 54% of patients with a good prognosis. In the second trial, 30843, that compared orchiectomy or buserelin to CAB with buserelin + cyproterone acetate, there was no observed difference in overall survival, but only 28% had a good prognosis. Hence, it appears that only patients with a good prognosis, that is, limited metastatic disease, could potentially benefit from CAB.

## Intermittent androgen deprivation therapy

The rationale for using intermittent androgen deprivation (IAD) therapy comes from studies conducted in an animal model of Shianogi mammary carcinoma in the early 1990s, suggesting that IAD prolonged the duration of androgen dependence [60]. This generated the hypothesis that IAD would delay the onset of CRPC and its associated debilitating and deathly complications. This seminal observation and the hope of clinicians to reduce side effects of ADT has motivated a series of phase II clinical trials that demonstrated IAD feasibility [61]. Unfortunately, phase III trials would prove otherwise.

The South European Uroncological Group (SEUG) trial has enrolled 766 patients with locally advanced or metastatic PCa [62]. After 3 months of induction ADT, 626 patients with a PSA <4 ng/mL or <80% of initial value were randomized between intermittent (IAD) or continuous treatment (CAD). There was no difference in overall survival, resulting however from a greater number of cancer deaths in the intermittent treatment arm (106 vs. 84) that was balanced by a greater number of cardiovascular deaths in the continuous arm (52 vs. 41). Salonen *et al.* have reported the results of FinnProstate VII study that has enrolled 852 locally advanced or metastatic patients. After induction, 554 patients with a PSA <10 ng/mL or <50% of initial value were randomized [63]. The study showed no difference in median times from randomization to progression, median times to death (all cause), to PCa death to treatment failure. The study demonstrates significant differences in quality of life in terms of activity limitation, physical capacity, and sexual functioning favoring IAD [64]. But interestingly, the study detected no significant differences in terms of cardiovascular adverse events, death from cardiovascular adverse events, and bone fractures.

More controversy on the role of IAD has risen after the release of the results of the Southwest Oncology Group (SWOG) trial S9346, an international phase III trial, designed to specifically investigate the benefit of IAD in metastatic patients [65]. The study was designed to show that IAD was not inferior to CAD in terms of overall survival postrandomization. In total, 3040 metastatic PCa patients were recruited, but after 7 months of CAB only 1535 patients had achieved a PSA of ≤4.0 ng/mL and were randomized to CAB or IAD. The median and 10-year overall survivals from randomization were 5.8 years and 29% for CAD and 5.1 years and 23% for IAD, therefore failing to prove that IAD was non-inferior to CAD (hazard ratio (HR): 1.09; 95% CI = 0.95–1.24). Patients were stratified by disease extent using an arbitrary definition of minimal disease (spine, pelvis bone metastases, and/or lymph nodes) versus Extensive disease (ribs, long bones metastases, and/or visceral organs). The median overall survival of patients with extensive disease patients was 4.9 years for IAD and 4.4 years for CAD; in patients with minimal disease, median overall survival was 5.4 years for IAD and 6.9 years for CAD. In 2006, Hussain *et al.* had already demonstrated that the absolute PSA value after 7 months of induction ADT was a strong predictor of survival. Median overall survival was 13 months for patients with a PSA >4 ng/mL, 44 months for patients with PSA >0.2– 4 ng/mL, and 75 months for patients with PSA ≤0.2 ng/mL or less.

This helps the clinician making recommendations about the role of IAD in metastatic patients: it should not be presented to the patient as an alternative to CAD in terms of survival, but should be discussed only with patients with a major PSA response, preferably those reaching near undetectable PSA; the benefit of IAD on side effects is limited to the off-treatment phase, and it seems that it does not help reducing cardio-vascular and skeletal morbidity.

## Side effects of ADT

Because testosterone is the principal male hormone, its withdrawal is asso-ciated with a series of side effects [66]. Until recently, most studies on ADT have focused on the "symptomatic" toxicity of testosterone withdrawal, such as hot flushes, loss of libido, emotional instability, or fatigue [66]. The morbidity of ADT, however, mainly results from devious toxicities such as the induction of metabolic syndrome leading to increased cardiovascular risk and osteoporosis [67–69]. It is interesting that sex hormones are play-ing an important role in promoting metabolic changes and determining cardiovascular risk since cardiovascular disease is the major cause of death among men worldwide [70]. In an observational population-based cohort study including 73,196 men, Keating *et al.* showed that ADT increased the risk of diabetes by 44%, coronary heart disease by 16%, myocardial infarc-tion by 11%, and sudden cardiac death by 16% [67].

Loss of bone mineral density is another complication that is induced by ADT. Using medical claims data from Medicare beneficiaries, Smith *et al.* calculated that the rate of any clinical fracture was 7.88 per 100 person-years at risk in men receiving a LHRH agonist compared with 6.51 per 100 person-years in matched controls (relative risk: 1.21; 95% CI = 1.14–1.29; $p < .001$) [71].

The physician prescribing ADT should spend sufficient time explaining the side effects of ADT to the patient and encourage him to adopt a lifestyle that is adapted to ADT (see Table 13.1) [66]. Physical activity should be tailored to the preexisting physical activity of the patient, including regular resistance exercise, and be associated with correct diet supplementation of calcium and vitamin D [66].

## The role of bone-targeted agents in first-line treatment of metastatic PCa

Because the skeleton is the most frequent metastatic site and bone metas-tases the main cause of morbidity and quality-of-life deterioration in patients with metastatic PCa, bone-targeted therapies represent a major therapeutic class. PCa cells seeding in the bone marrow disrupt the normal bone remodeling process, which may lead to abnormal bone destruction or deposit, leading respectively to osteolytic or osteoblastic metastases.

**Table 13.1** Proposed checklist for monitoring patients receiving ADT (adapted from [66])

Before initiating treatment:

**1** Inform the patient about the occurrence of hot flushes and provide lifestyle recommendations to avoid excessive triggering.

**2** Inform the patient and his partner about libido, mood and cognitive changes. Encourage maintaining and even increasing social activities and networking, possibly referring to patient support groups.

**3** Inform in due time the patient's general practitioner, cardiologist, and endocrinologist about initiation of ADT. Advise the patient to schedule a follow-up visit with these specialists within 6 months.

**4** Provide dietetic counseling and recommend resistance exercise. This will be done optimally by referring the patient to a dietician, physical therapist or by administrating a specifically designed coaching program.

**5** Search for risk factors of bone loss, and perform an immediate DEXA, if present.

During treatment:

**6** In addition to PSA and testosterone measurements and imaging studies that are required for oncological follow-up, it is recommended to assess weight and abdominal perimeter (or preferably body fatty tissue content by impedance technique), blood pressure, and fasting cholesterol (total and HDL), triglyceride and glucose levels. In case of abnormalities, refer the patient to a specialist.

**7** Advise a Dual-energy X-ray absorptiometry (DEXA) scan after 1–2 years of ADT. Low-dose denosumab can be initiated in osteopenic patients to lower the risk of fracture.

Bisphosphonates and RANK ligand inhibitor, denosumab, have been used to block bone remodeling induced by bone metastases. Bisphosphonates are pyrophosphate analogs that inhibit osteoclast function. They are taken up by osteoblasts and deposited within the skeleton in areas of active bone remodeling. Once incorporated within new bone, they likely exert long-lasting effects on osteoclasts that encounter them as they attempt to resorb bone. The receptor activator of nuclear factor (NF)-κB ligand (RANKL) is an essential mediator of osteoclast formation, function, and survival. Denosumab is a fully human monoclonal antibody against RANKL and a potent inhibitor of bone remodeling.

Zoledronic acid and denosumab have been tested and approved for the prevention of SRE in CRPC patients. In contrast, use of bone-targeted agents in combination with first-line ADT is not an established strategy. Clodronate failed to produce a benefit in the MRC "PR05" trial producing a nonsignificant reduction in symptomatic bone progression-free survival [72, 73]. Interestingly, long-term follow-up revealed a significant improvement in overall survival with clodronate treatment [73]. Interestingly enough, EMA and FDA have granted regulatory approvals for zoledronic acid and denosumab independently of the hormone-naïve or -resistant status, creating a registration gap that has been used intensively by the industry to promote these drugs in the hormone-naïve setting. In absence of specific evidence, these drugs should be restricted to CRPC patients, in the absence of a clearly demonstrated benefit in earlier setting. Metastatic PCa is unique in that it is so frequently responsive to first-line disease-modifying therapy. It is likely that effective cancer treatment in the absence of osteoclast inhibition prevents or delays SREs. Further, the natural history of PCa is longer than that of many other solid tumors and would lead to prolonged exposure to monthly osteoclast inhibition if given in conjunction with first-line ADT.

## Future therapeutic strategies

As mentioned already, ADT is mainly palliative and there is therefore an intense clinical activity to improve its efficacy by combining it with local treatment of the metastases and novel systemic strategies.

Berkovic *et al.* have investigated in patients with up to three synchronous metastases (bone and/or lymph nodes) diagnosed on PET whether repeated stereotactic body radiotherapy (SBRT) was able to defer ADT. The study has included 24 patients with a median follow-up of 24 months. Ten patients started with ADT resulting in a median ADT-free survival of 38 months. The 2-year local control and clinical progression-free survival was 100% and 42%, respectively. This promising approach should lead to larger phase III trial.

The integration of systemic treatment with ADT is under intense scrutiny. Systemic Therapy for Advanced or Metastatic Prostate cancer: Evaluation of Drug Efficacy (STAMPEDE) is a randomized controlled trial that follows a novel multiarm, multistage (MAMS) design [74]. The study is running mostly in the United Kingdom and enrolls locally advanced and metastatic patients. The original arms comprised ADT alone or combined with docetaxel, zoledronic acid, celecoxib, docetaxel + zoledronic acid, or zoledonic acid + celecoxib. A recent analysis of the study has concluded in the absence of efficacy of celecoxib. Consequently, the two celecoxib-containing arms were closed. More recently two new arms have been added. The first one is ADT combined with androgen biosynthesis inhibitor abiraterone acetate and the second will investigated adding prostate bed radiotherapy in metastatic patients.

## Summary overview

Patient diagnosed with low-risk PCa (PSA <10 ng/mL, Gleason ≤6, and stage ≤T2) do not need a metastatic workup.

Recommended metastatic workup is still based on $^{99m}$Tc bone scanning for the detection of bone metastases, and CT or MRI for the detection of lymph nodes and VM. However, both techniques lack specificity and underestimate the true incidence of metastases. Whenever a higher level of specificity is required, PET-CT or WB-MRI with diffusion should be recommended.

The standard treatment of metastatic PCa is ADT.

ADT can be delayed in patients with low-burden slowly progressing disease. PSA kinetic may help selecting the patients.

Preliminary studies indicate that GnRH antagonist degarelix delay PSA and alkaline phosphatase progression in metastatic patients. CAB confers limited if any additional benefit.

Intermittent ADT should be used with caution and only in patients with a major PSA response.

There is no role for bone-targeted therapies such as zoledronic acid or denosumab in the hormone-naïve stage.

Proper monitoring of cardiovascular and skeletal complications is compulsory, including appropriate life-style recommendations.

## References

1 Ferlay J, Shin HR, Bray F, *et al.* Estimates of worldwide burden of cancer in 2008: GLOBOCAN 2008. *Int J Cancer* 2010;127(12):2893–2917.

2 Schroder FH, Hugosson J, Carlsson S, *et al.* Screening for prostate cancer decreases the risk of developing metastatic disease: findings from the European Randomized Study of Screening for Prostate Cancer (ERSPC). *Eur Urol* 2012;62(5):745–752.

3 Aus G, Bergdahl S, Lodding P, *et al.* Prostate cancer screening decreases the absolute risk of being diagnosed with advanced prostate cancer–results from a prospective, population-based randomized controlled trial. *Eur Urol* 2007;51(3):659–664.

4 Soloway MS, Hardeman SW, Hickey D, *et al.* Stratification of patients with metastatic prostate cancer based on extent of disease on initial bone scan. *Cancer* 1988;61(1):195–202.

5 Norgaard M, Jensen AO, Jacobsen JB, *et al.* Skeletal related events, bone metastasis and survival of prostate cancer: a population based cohort study in Denmark (1999 to 2007). *J Urol* 2010;184(1):162–167.

6 Loberg RD, Logothetis CJ, Keller ET, Pienta KJ. Pathogenesis and treatment of prostate cancer bone metastases: targeting the lethal phenotype. *J Clin Oncol* 2005;23(32):8232–8241.

7  Heidenreich A, Bellmunt J, Bolla M, *et al.* EAU guidelines on prostate cancer. Part 1: screening, diagnosis, and treatment of clinically localised disease. *Eur Urol* 2011;59(1):61–71.

8  Clinical practice guidelines in oncology. Prostate cancer. V.1. 2013. Available at http://www.nccn.org/professionals/physician˙gls/PDF/prostate.pdf. Last accessed December 1, 2012.

9  Rana A, Karamanis K, Lucas MG, Chisholm GD. Identification of metastatic disease by T category, gleason score and serum PSA level in patients with carcinoma of the prostate. *Br J Urol* 1992;69(3):277–281.

10  Briganti A, Passoni N, Ferrari M, *et al.* When to perform bone scan in patients with newly diagnosed prostate cancer: external validation of the currently available guidelines and proposal of a novel risk stratification tool. *Eur Urol* 2009;57(4):551–558.

11  Pound CR, Partin AW, Eisenberger MA, *et al.* Natural history of progression after PSA elevation following radical prostatectomy. *J Am Med Assoc* 1999;281(17):1591–1597.

12  Hovels AM, Heesakkers RA, Adang EM, *et al.* The diagnostic accuracy of CT and MRI in the staging of pelvic lymph nodes in patients with prostate cancer: a meta-analysis. *Clin Radiol* 2008;63(4):387–395.

13  Barentsz JO, Richenberg J, Clements R, *et al.* ESUR prostate MR guidelines 2012. *Eur Radiol* 2012;22(4):746–757.

14  Heesakkers RA, Hovels AM, Jager GJ, *et al.* MRI with a lymph-node-specific contrast agent as an alternative to CT scan and lymph-node dissection in patients with prostate cancer: a prospective multicohort study. *Lancet Oncol* 2008;9(9):850–856.

15  Schiavina R, Scattoni V, Castellucci P, *et al.* 11C-choline positron emission tomography/computerized tomography for preoperative lymph-node staging in intermediate-risk and high-risk prostate cancer: comparison with clinical staging nomograms. *Eur Urol* 2008;54(2):392–401.

16  Budiharto T, Joniau S, Lerut E, *et al.* Prospective evaluation of 11C-choline positron emission tomography/computed tomography and diffusion-weighted magnetic resonance imaging for the nodal staging of prostate cancer with a high risk of lymph node metastases. *Eur Urol* 2011;60(1):125–130.

17  Condon BR, Buchanan R, Garvie NW, *et al.* Assessment of progression of secondary bone lesions following cancer of the breast or prostate using serial radionuclide imaging. *Br J Radiol* 1981;54(637):18–23.

18  Eustace S, Tello R, DeCarvalho V, *et al.* A comparison of whole-body turbo-STIR MR imaging and planar 99mTc-methylene diphosphonate scintigraphy in the examination of patients with suspected skeletal metastases. *AJR Am J Roentgenol* 1997;169(6):1655–1661.

19  Daldrup-Link HE, Franzius C, Link TM, *et al.* Whole-body MR imaging for detection of bone metastases in children and young adults: comparison with skeletal scintigraphy and FDG PET. *AJR Am J Roentgenol* 2001;177(1):229–236.

20  Jacobson AF, Fogelman I. Bone scanning in clinical oncology: does it have a future? *Eur J Nucl Med* 1998;25(9):1219–1223.

21  Gosfield E, 3rd, Alavi A, Kneeland B. Comparison of radionuclide bone scans and magnetic resonance imaging in detecting spinal metastases. *J Nucl Med* 1993;34(12):2191–2198.

22  Venkitaraman R, Sohaib A, Cook G. MRI or bone scan or both for staging of prostate cancer? *J Clin Oncol* 2007;25(36):5837–5838; author reply 8–9.

23  Schirrmeister H, Kuhn T, Guhlmann A, *et al.* Fluorine-18 2-deoxy-2-fluoro-D-glucose PET in the preoperative staging of breast cancer: comparison with the standard staging procedures. *Eur J Nucl Med* 2001;28(3):351–358.

24  Ghanem N, Uhl M, Brink I, *et al.* Diagnostic value of MRI in comparison to scintigraphy, PET, MS-CT and PET/CT for the detection of metastases of bone. *Eur J Radiol* 2005;55(1):41–55.

25  Beheshti M, Vali R, Waldenberger P, *et al.* Detection of bone metastases in patients with prostate cancer by 18F fluorocholine and 18F fluoride PET-CT: a comparative study. *Eur J Nucl Med Mol Imaging* 2008;35(10):1766–1774.

26  Haubold-Reuter BG, Duewell S, Schilcher BR, *et al.* The value of bone scintigraphy, bone marrow scintigraphy and fast spin-echo magnetic resonance imaging in staging of patients with malignant solid tumours: a prospective study. *Eur J Nucl Med* 1993;20(11):1063–1069.

27  Schirrmeister H, Guhlmann A, Elsner K, *et al.* Sensitivity in detecting osseous lesions depends on anatomic localization: planar bone scintigraphy versus 18F PET. *J Nucl Med* 1999;40(10):1623–1629.

28  Tombal B, Rezazadeh A, Therasse P, *et al.* Magnetic resonance imaging of the axial skeleton enables objective measurement of tumor response on prostate cancer bone metastases. *Prostate* 2005;65(2):178–187.

29  Lecouvet FE, Geukens D, Stainier A, *et al.* Magnetic resonance imaging of the axial skeleton for detecting bone metastases in patients with high-risk prostate cancer: diagnostic and cost-effectiveness and comparison with current detection strategies. *J Clin Oncol* 2007;25(22):3281–3287.

30  Lecouvet FE, El Mouedden J, Collette L, *et al.* Can whole-body magnetic resonance imaging with diffusion-weighted imaging replace Tc 99m bone scanning and computed tomography for single-step detection of metastases in patients with high-risk prostate cancer? *Eur Urol* 2012;62(1):68–75.

31  Lecouvet FE, Simon M, Tombal B, *et al.* Whole-body MRI (WB-MRI) versus axial skeleton MRI (AS-MRI) to detect and measure bone metastases in prostate cancer (PCa). *Eur Radiol* 2010;20(12):2973–2982.

32  Venkitaraman R, Cook GJ, Dearnaley DP, *et al.* Whole-body magnetic resonance imaging in the detection of skeletal metastases in patients with prostate cancer. *J Med Imaging Radiat Oncol* 2009;53(3):241–247.

33  Eschmann SM, Pfannenberg AC, Rieger A, *et al.* Comparison of 11C-choline-PET/CT and whole body-MRI for staging of prostate cancer. *Nuklearmedizin* 2007;46(5):161–168; quiz N47–N48.

34  Khoo MM, Tyler PA, Saifuddin A, Padhani AR. Diffusion-weighted imaging (DWI) in musculoskeletal MRI: a critical review. *Skeletal Radiol* 2011;40(6):665–681.

35  Huggins C. Endocrine-induced regression of cancers. *Cancer Res* 1967;27(11):1925–1930.

36  Heidenreich A. Consensus criteria for the use of magnetic resonance imaging in the diagnosis and staging of prostate cancer: not ready for routine use. *Eur Urol* 2011;59(4):495–497.

37  The Veterans Administration Co-operative Urological Research Group. Treatment and survival of patients with cancer of the prostate. *Surg Gynecol Obstet* 1967;124(5):1011–1017.

38 Byar DP. Proceedings of the Veterans Administration Cooperative Urological Research Group's studies of cancer of the prostate. *Cancer* 1973;32:1126–1130.

39 Byar DP, Green SB. The choice of treatment for cancer patients based on covariate information: application to prostate cancer. *Bull Cancer (Paris)* 1980;67: 477–490.

40 The Medical Research Council Prostate Cancer Working Party Investigators Group. Immediate versus deferred treatment for advanced prostatic cancer: initial results of the Medical Research Council Trial. *Br J Urol* 1997;79(2):235–246.

41 Nair B, Wilt T, MacDonald R, Rutks I. Early versus deferred androgen suppression in the treatment of advanced prostatic cancer. *Cochrane Database Syst Rev* 2002(1):CD003506.

42 Isaacs JT. The timing of androgen ablation therapy and/or chemotherapy in the treatment of prostatic cancer. *Prostate* 1984;5(1):1–17.

43 Studer UE, Collette L, Whelan P, *et al.* Using PSA to guide timing of androgen deprivation in patients with T0-4 N0-2 M0 prostate cancer not suitable for local curative treatment (EORTC 30891). *Eur Urol* 2008;53(5):941–949.

44 Schally AV, Arimura A, Baba Y, *et al.* Isolation and properties of the FSH and LH-releasing hormone. *Biochem Biophys Res Commun* 1971;43(2):393–399.

45 The Leuprolide Study Group. Leuprolide versus diethylstilbestrol for metastatic prostate cancer. *N Engl J Med* 1984;311(20):1281–1286.

46 Vogelzang NJ, Chodak GW, Soloway MS, *et al.* Goserelin versus orchiectomy in the treatment of advanced prostate cancer: final results of a randomized trial. Zoladex Prostate Study Group. *Urology* 1995;46(2):220–226.

47 Kaisary AV, Tyrrell CJ, Peeling WB, Griffiths K. Comparison of LHRH analogue (Zoladex) with orchiectomy in patients with metastatic prostatic carcinoma. [Published erratum appears in *Br J Urol* 1993 May;71(5):632] [see comments]. *Br J Urol* 1991;67(5):502–508.

48 Thompson IM. Flare associated with LHRH-agonist therapy. *Rev Urol* 2001;3(Suppl. 3):S10–S14.

49 Kuhn JM, Billebaud T, Navratil H, *et al.* Prevention of the transient adverse effects of a gonadotropin-releasing hormone analogue (buserelin) in metastatic prostatic carcinoma by administration of an antiandrogen (nilutamide). *N Engl J Med* 1989;321(7):413–418.

50 Crawford ED, Eisenberger MA, McLeod DG, *et al.* A controlled trial of leuprolide with and without flutamide in prostatic carcinoma. *N Engl J Med* 1989;321(7):419–424.

51 Klotz L, Boccon-Gibod L, Shore ND, *et al.* The efficacy and safety of degarelix: a 12-month, comparative, randomized, open-label, parallel-group phase III study in patients with prostate cancer. *BJU Int* 2008;102(11):1531–1538.

52 Tombal B, Miller K, Boccon-Gibod L, *et al.* Additional analysis of the secondary end point of biochemical recurrence rate in a phase 3 trial (CS21) comparing degarelix 80 mg versus leuprolide in prostate cancer patients segmented by baseline characteristics. *Eur Urol* 2010;57(5):836–842.

53 Schroder FH, Tombal B, Miller K, *et al.* Changes in alkaline phosphatase levels in patients with prostate cancer receiving degarelix or leuprolide: results from a 12-month, comparative, phase III study. *BJU Int* 2010;106(2):182–187.

54 Thorpe SC, Azmatullah S, Fellows GJ, *et al.* A prospective, randomised study to compare goserelin acetate (Zoladex) versus cyproterone acetate (Cyprostat) versus a combination of the two in the treatment of metastatic prostatic carcinoma. *Eur Urol* 1996;29(1):47–54.

55 Tyrrell CJ, Kaisary AV, Iversen P, *et al.* A randomised comparison of 'Casodex' (bicalutamide) 150 mg monotherapy versus castration in the treatment of metastatic and locally advanced prostate cancer. *Eur Urol* 1998;33(5):447–456.

56 Mottet N, Bellmunt J, Bolla M, *et al.* EAU guidelines on prostate cancer. Part II: Treatment of advanced, relapsing, and castration-resistant prostate cancer. *Eur Urol* 2011;59(4):572–583.

57 Schmitt B, Bennett C, Seidenfeld J, *et al.* Maximal androgen blockade for advanced prostate cancer. *Cochrane Database Syst Rev* 2000(2):CD001526.

58 Prostate Cancer Trialists' Collaborative Group. Maximum androgen blockade in advanced prostate cancer: an overview of the randomised trials. *Lancet* 2000;355(9214):1491–1498.

59 Sylvester RJ, Denis L, de Voogt H. The importance of prognostic factors in the interpretation of two EORTC metastatic prostate cancer trials. European Organization for Research and Treatment of Cancer (EORTC) Genito-Urinary Tract Cancer Cooperative Group. *Eur Urol* 1998;33(2):134–143.

60 Akakura K, Bruchovsky N, Goldenberg SL, *et al.* Effects of intermittent androgen suppression on androgen-dependent tumors. Apoptosis and serum prostate-specific antigen. *Cancer* 1993;71(9):2782–2790.

61 Bhandari MS, Crook J, Hussain M. Should intermittent androgen deprivation be used in routine clinical practice? *J Clin Oncol* 2005;23(32):8212–8218.

62 Calais da Silva FE, Bono AV, Whelan P, *et al.* Intermittent androgen deprivation for locally advanced and metastatic prostate cancer: results from a randomised phase 3 study of the South European Uroncological Group. *Eur Urol* 2009;55(6):1269–1277.

63 Salonen AJ, Taari K, Ala-Opas M, *et al.* The FinnProstate Study VII: intermittent versus continuous androgen deprivation in patients with advanced prostate cancer. *J Urol* 2012;187(6):2074–2081.

64 Salonen AJ, Taari K, Ala-Opas M, *et al.* Advanced prostate cancer treated with intermittent or continuous androgen deprivation in the randomised FinnProstate Study VII: quality of life and adverse effects. *Eur Urol* 2013;63(1):111–120.

65 Hussain M, Tangen CM, Higano CS, *et al.* Intermittent (IAD) versus continuous androgen deprivation (CAD) in hormone sensitive metastatic prostate cancer (HSM1PC) patients (pts): results of S9346 (INT-0162), an international phase III trial. *J Clin Oncol* 2012;30(Suppl.; abstract 4).

66 Tombal B. A holistic approach to androgen deprivation therapy: treating the cancer without hurting the patient. *Urol Int* 2009;83(4):373–378.

67 Keating NL, O'Malley AJ, Freedland SJ, Smith MR. Diabetes and cardiovascular disease during androgen deprivation therapy: observational study of veterans with prostate cancer. *J Natl Cancer Inst* 2010;102(1):39–46.

68 Smith MR, Egerdie B, Hernandez Toriz N, *et al.* Denosumab in men receiving androgen-deprivation therapy for prostate cancer. *N Engl J Med* 2009;361(8):745–755.

69 Smith MR, O'Malley AJ, Keating NL. Gonadotrophin-releasing hormone agonists, diabetes and cardiovascular disease in men with prostate cancer: which metabolic syndrome? *BJU Int* 2008;101(11):1335–1336.

70 Smith MR, Lee H, Nathan DM. Insulin sensitivity during combined androgen blockade for prostate cancer. *J Clin Endocrinol Metab* 2006;91(4):1305–1308.

71 Smith MR, Lee WC, Brandman J, *et al.* Gonadotropin-releasing hormone agonists and fracture risk: a claims-based cohort study of men with nonmetastatic prostate cancer. *J Clin Oncol* 2005;23(31):7897–7903.

72 Dearnaley DP, Sydes MR, Mason MD, *et al.* A double-blind, placebo-controlled, randomized trial of oral sodium clodronate for metastatic prostate cancer (MRC PR05 Trial). *J Natl Cancer Inst* 2003;95(17):1300–1311.

73 Dearnaley DP, Mason MD, Parmar MK, *et al.* Adjuvant therapy with oral sodium clodronate in locally advanced and metastatic prostate cancer: long-term overall survival results from the MRC PR04 and PR05 randomised controlled trials. *Lancet Oncol* 2009;10(9):872–876.

74 Sydes MR, Parmar MK, Mason MD, *et al.* Flexible trial design in practice - stopping arms for lack-of-benefit and adding research arms mid-trial in STAMPEDE: a multi-arm multi-stage randomized controlled trial. *Trials* 2012;13:168.

## CHAPTER 14

# New Therapies in Hormone Relapsed Disease*

*Carmel Pezaro, Aurelius Omlin, Diletta Bianchini, and Johann de Bono*

Prostate Cancer Targeted Therapy Group and Drug Development Unit, The Royal Marsden NHS Foundation Trust and The Institute of Cancer Research, Surrey, UK

## Introduction

Since the pioneering work of Charles Huggins, recognized in a Nobel Prize for Medicine in 1966, prostate cancer has been known to be hormone dependent. Men with relapsed or metastatic prostate cancer are treated with androgen deprivation therapy (ADT) to achieve surgical or medical castration. However, while metastatic prostate cancer is incurable, progression on ADT therapy no longer signals the end of therapeutic options. Five novel treatments proven to prolong survival in castration-resistant prostate cancer (CRPC) have been reported in the past 2 years. These novel therapies comprise abiraterone acetate and enzalutamide, which act to inhibit androgen receptor (AR) signaling, sipuleucel-T immunotherapy, the bone targeting radionuclide radium[223], and second-line cabazitaxel chemotherapy, as summarized in Table 14.1 and Figures 14.1, Plate 14.1 and 14.2. These new CRPC treatments and other promising agents will be reviewed, including practical management issues. The therapeutic landscape of CRPC is changing rapidly, and this chapter will outline the current options and discuss emerging strategies.

---

*All authors are employees of the Institute of Cancer Research (ICR). The ICR has a commercial interest in abiraterone and PI3K and AKT inhibitors. Johann de Bono has served as a paid consultant for J&J, Sanofi-Aventis, Medivation, Astellas, AstraZeneca, Dendreon, Genetech, Pfizer, and GSK.

---

*Prostate Cancer: Diagnosis and Clinical Management*, First Edition.
Edited by Ashutosh K. Tewari, Peter Whelan and John D. Graham.
© 2014 John Wiley & Sons, Ltd. Published 2014 by John Wiley & Sons, Ltd.

**Table 14.1** Phase III CRPC trials with positive overall survival endpoints

| Mechanism of action | Drug | Trial name | Patient population, intervention | Median overall survival | Reference |
|---|---|---|---|---|---|
| CYP17 inhibitor | Abiraterone acetate | COU-AA-301 | 1195 CRPC patients, post-docetaxel Abiraterone + prednisone vs. placebo + prednisone | Final analysis: 15.8 vs. 11.2 months HR 0.74, 95% CI = 0.64–0.86 | [1] |
| CYP17 inhibitor | Abiraterone acetate | COU-AA-302 | 1088 CRPC patients, asymptomatic or minimally symptomatic, pre-chemotherapy Abiraterone + prednisone vs. placebo + prednisone | Preliminary analysis: NR vs. 27.2 months HR 0.75, 95% CI = 0.61–0.93 | [2] |
| Taxane chemotherapy | Cabazitaxel | TROPIC | 755 CRPC patients, post-docetaxel Cabazitaxel + prednisone vs. mitoxantrone + prednisone | 15.1 vs. 12.7 months HR 0.70; 95% CI = 0.59–0.83 | [3] |
| Taxane chemotherapy | Docetaxel | TAX-327 | 1006 CRPC patients Docetaxel + prednisone vs. mitoxantrone + prednisone | 18.9 vs. 16.5 months HR 0.76; 95% CI = 0.62–0.94 | [4] |
| Antiandrogen | Enzalutamide (MDV3100) | AFFIRM | 1199 CRPC patients, post-docetaxel Enzalutamide vs. placebo | 18.4 vs. 13.6 months HR 0.63, 95% CI = 0.53–0.75 | [5] |
| Alpha-emitting radionuclide | Radium[223] | ALSYMPCA | 922 CRPC patients, post-docetaxel or unfit for docetaxel Radium[223] vs. placebo | 14.9 vs. 11.3 months HR 0.70, 95% CI = 0.55–0.86 | [6] |
| Immunotherapy | Sipuleucel-T | IMPACT | 512 CRPC patients, minimally symptomatic, pre-chemotherapy Sipuleucel-T vs. placebo | 25.8 vs. 21.7 months HR 0.78, 95% CI = 0.61–0.98 | [7] |

CRPC, castration-resistant prostate cancer; HR, hazard ratio; CI, confidence interval; NR, not reached.

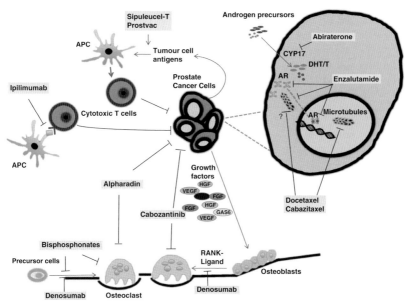

**Figure 14.1** Targets of current/emerging treatments for advanced prostate cancer. Abiraterone, CYP17 inhibitor; enzalutamide, antiandrogen, blocks AR shuttling into the nucleus, blocks interaction of activated AR with DNA; docetaxel and cabazitaxel, microtubule inhibitors, potentially also block AR shuttling into the nucleus; denosumab, RANK-ligand inhibitor; bisphosphonates, antiresorptive activity by osteoclast inhibition; alpharadin, α-radiation emitting radioisotope; cabozantinib, c-MET and VEGFR2 inhibitor; sipuleucel-T and PROSTVAC, vaccine therapies; ipilimumab, anti-CTLA-4 antibody. APC, antigen-presenting cell; DHT, dihydrotestosterone; T, testosterone; HGF, hepatocyte growth factor; FGF, fibroblast growth factor; IGF-1, insulin-like growth factor; VEGF, vascular endothelial growth factor; GAS6, growth arrest-specific 6. (See also Plate 14.1.)

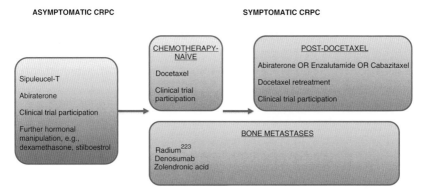

**Figure 14.2** Treatment paradigm for men with CRPC.

# Targeting androgen receptor signaling

Medical or surgical castration causes interruption of AR signaling. Unfortunately, the response to ADT is not durable and is followed by disease progression, with rising prostate-specific antigen (PSA) despite castrate levels of testosterone, indicating a "castration-resistant" state. Laboratory and clinical research undertaken over the past two decades has changed our understanding of prostate cancer biology and it is now recognized that advanced prostate cancer remains dependent on AR signaling [8, 9]. Several mechanisms are involved, including intratumoral androgen synthesis from peripheral adrenal androgens [10, 11] and *de novo* synthesis directly from cholesterol [12, 13]. Additionally, androstenediol (a progesterone derivative) can be converted to dehydrotestosterone (DHT) via the "backdoor pathway" [14].

Novel therapies have been designed recognizing AR activation as a key target in advanced prostate cancer. Successful strategies to overcome AR activation include novel androgen biosynthesis inhibitors and potent AR inhibitors.

## CYP17 inhibition

The enzyme CYP17, which has dual functions as a 17α-hydroxylase and 17,20 lyase, has an essential role in androgen biosynthesis. Clinical research demonstrated that ketoconazole and aminoglutethimide, which are nonspecific inhibitors of CYP17, had modest antitumor activity in advanced prostate cancer [15, 16]. Both agents were limited by significant drug interactions and toxicities.

## Abiraterone acetate

Abiraterone acetate (abiraterone; Zytiga®, Janssen Pharmaceuticals, Titusville, New Jersey, USA) was rationally designed at the Institute of Cancer Research, in a partnership with Cancer Research, UK. The molecular structure of pregnenolone was modified to identify a potent, irreversible, and selective inhibitor of CYP17A1 [17]. Early-phase testing of abiraterone was encouraging, with a favorable toxicity profile at doses up to 2000 mg daily and evidence of PSA and radiological activity (reviewed in [18]). Two Phase III trials have now been completed. COU-AA-301 was performed in men with progressive CRPC following docetaxel chemotherapy. In total, 797 men received abiraterone 1000 mg plus prednisone or prednisolone 10 mg daily, and 398 received placebo with prednisone or prednisolone. The trial was unblinded when a planned interim analysis showed unequivocal survival benefit with abiraterone and at final analysis there was a 4.6-month improvement in median overall survival (OS), giving a hazard ratio (HR) of 0.74 ($p<$.0001) [1, 19]. Secondary endpoints favored abiraterone, including time to PSA progression (10.2 vs. 6.6 months; $p<$.001), progression-free survival (PFS; 5.6 vs. 3.6 months; $p<$.001), PSA response rate (defined as $\geq$50% PSA decline; 29% vs. 6%; $p<$.001), and quality of life as judged by brief pain and fatigue scores [20]. COU-AA-301 also included translational studies, including enumeration of circulating tumor cells (CTCs). Conversion from unfavorable (defined as $\geq$5 CTC/7.5 mL) to favorable ($<$5 CTC/7.5 mL) counts was strongly associated with improved OS [19]. On the basis of the COU-AA-301 results, abiraterone has been approved by the United States Food and Drug Administration (US FDA) for use after docetaxel.

Androgen biosynthesis inhibition with abiraterone results in accumulation of androgen precursor molecules and a positive feedback loop, causing high ACTH levels and increased mineralocorticoid activity. Although concomitant prednisone can cover most of the mineralocorticoid excess, the most common side effects in patients receiving abiraterone on COU-AA-301 were fluid retention and edema (seen in 31% of patients receiving abiraterone, compared with 22% placebo patients), hypokalemia (seen in 17% and 8% patients, respectively), and hypertension (10% and 8%, respectively). These toxicities were generally easily managed with increased glucocorticoid doses or by adding the specific mineralocorticoid antagonist eplerenone.

Preliminary results of the Phase III COU-AA-302 trial were presented at ASCO 2012. This study was performed in asymptomatic or minimally symptomatic chemotherapy-naïve CRPC patients with rising PSA. Participants were randomized 1:1 between abiraterone and placebo in combination with prednisone or prednisolone. This was the first Phase III trial in prostate cancer to apply a co-primary endpoint of OS and radiographic PFS. The study was unblinded when a planned interim analysis showed significant improvement in radiographic PFS (not reached in abiraterone arm vs. 8.3 months in placebo arm, HR 0.43, 95% confidence interval (CI) = 0.35–0.52), accompanied by a strong trend to improved survival (median not reached in abiraterone arm vs. 27.2 months in placebo arm, HR 0.75, $p$ = .0097) [2]. More mature results are awaited, but there is need for a well-tolerated and highly active oral alternative to first-line chemotherapy.

## Practical considerations

Abiraterone is a well-tolerated oral therapy that is very suitable for outpatient administration, although regular review for toxicities associated with mineralocorticoid excess and transaminase elevation is recommended. The health implications of the concomitant corticosteroid must be considered when undertaking routine monitoring on treatment. Potential drug interactions must be considered, as abiraterone is a CYP3A4 substrate and therefore pharmacokinetics may be altered with administration of concurrent CYP3A4 inducers or inhibitors. Abiraterone exposure is also significantly increased if taken with food. Premature assessment of activity should be avoided, particularly in view of the described incidence of radiographic bone flares [21]. It is worth noting that both Phase III studies recommended that, in the absence of clinical progression, patients with rising PSA continued on treatment until radiographic evidence of progression was documented. Finally, it is important to point out that abiraterone has impressive antitumor activity in patients with visceral metastases, who benefited just as much from CYP17 inhibition in the COU-AA-301 subanalysis [1, 19].

*Orteronel* (TAK-700, Takeda Pharmaceuticals, Osaka, Japan) is more selective for 17,20 lyase compared with abiraterone. Phase I testing showed activity for doses of $\geq$300 mg twice daily [22]. A Phase II expansion enrolled 97 patients to one of four doses with or without concomitant prednisone and showed $\geq$50% PSA declines of 60–63% without prednisone and 41–50% with prednisone, accompanied by radiographic partial responses in 10 of 51 evaluable patients [23]. Large Phase III studies are underway in pre- and post-chemotherapy patients (NCT01193244 and NCT01193257, respectively) and also in combination with radiotherapy for high-risk localized disease (NCT01546987).

*Galeterone* (TOK-001, Tokai Pharmaceuticals, Cambridge, MA, USA) combines CYP17 inhibition with AR downregulation and AR antagonism and is currently in Phase I–II testing (NCT00959959). Preliminary results in 49 men with chemotherapy-naïve CRPC suggested evidence of PSA activity, but also reported mild liver transaminase elevations [24].

*VT-464* (Viamet Pharmaceuticals, Durham, North Carolina, USA) is an oral CYP inhibitor that is 10-fold more selective for 17,20 lyase compared with hydroxylase inhibition. Preclinical testing suggested abrogation of the effect on upstream steroids and cortisol [25], which may allow therapeutic dosing without concurrent corticosteroids. Early-phase clinical testing is underway.

## Next-generation antiandrogens

Antiandrogens are agents that compete with endogenous androgen ligand for the ligand-binding pocket of the AR. Mutations in the AR can cause older "first-generation" antiandrogens to become agonistic, which can contribute to cancer progression. Second-generation oral antiandrogens have been rationally designed as potent AR antagonists with currently no evidence of agonistic activity.

## Enzalutamide

Enzalutamide (MDV3100, Medivation, San Francisco, CA, USA) binds the AR with approximately fivefold greater avidity compared with bicalutamide. In preclinical studies, enzalutamide showed activity in bicalutamide-resistant models, preventing AR nuclear translocation, DNA binding, and AR co-activator recruitment [26]. A Phase I/II trial in 140 men with metastatic CRPC suggested antitumor activity at doses between 30 and 600 mg/day, with ≥50% PSA decline in 78 (56%) participants [27]. Common terminology criteria for adverse events (CTCAE) grade 3 fatigue and concern regarding a possible link between enzalutamide and seizures limited dose escalation beyond 240 mg/day.

Subsequently, a large Phase III study was conducted in men with metastatic CRPC and disease progression following docetaxel chemotherapy. The AFFIRM study enrolled 800 men to enzalutamide 160 mg/day and 399 to matched placebo. A preplanned analysis after 520 events showed significant benefit from enzalutamide, with a median 4.8-month improvement in OS and an estimated HR of 0.631 ($p$<.0001) [5]. Secondary endpoints significantly favored enzalutamide, including PSA and radiological response, clinical response as judged by time to first skeletal-related event (SRE), and quality of life, measured using the functional assessment of cancer therapy—prostate (FACT-P). Treatment was well tolerated, with generally mild side effects including fatigue, diarrhea, and hot flushes. Grade 3–4 adverse events were rare, without excessive occurrence of fatigue compared with placebo. Seizure rate did appear higher, occurring in five men (0.6%) in the enzalutamide arm, compared with none in the placebo arm.

Ongoing single-agent studies are examining the efficacy of enzalutamide in earlier-stage disease, including a Phase III study in chemotherapy-naïve patients (PREVAIL; NCT01212991) and a Phase II study in men with hormone-naïve disease (NCT01302041). A combination study with docetaxel is underway (NCT01565928) and further combination studies are likely.

It is not yet clear how enzalutamide therapy should best be sequenced with older antiandrogens, with other AR-targeted treatments such as abiraterone, or with chemotherapy. Much remains to be understood about the best use of this agent.

### Practical considerations

Although corticosteroids may be used concurrently with enzalutamide, they are not mandated. Toxicity is mild and dose reduction is rarely required, allowing for outpatient administration with regular clinic reviews. Concern about seizure risk was raised in early-phase clinical testing, and in the AFFIRM trial, despite excluding men with a seizure history or known CNS metastases, 5 men (0.6%) receiving enzalutamide had seizures. Several of the cases were associated with diagnosis of CNS metastases or with concomitant medications known to increase the risk of seizures. Nonetheless, outside of clinical trials, it is recommended to avoid enzalutamide in men with a history of seizures and to consider the risk of lowered seizure threshold in the context of their disease and medications.

The survival benefit in AFFIRM was achieved in a study designed to evaluate benefit rather than response, and so participants continued treatment until combined PSA, radiological and clinical progression. If possible, patients who remain well despite PSA progression should therefore be continued on enzalutamide.

*ARN-509* (Janssen Pharmaceuticals, Titusville, New Jersey, USA) is another rationally designed oral antiandrogen, with structural similarity to enzalutamide. Testing in preclinical models suggested superior characteristics and lesser penetration of the blood–brain barrier compared with related agents [28]. ARN-509 is currently in early-phase clinical studies, including in CRPC patients who have progressed on abiraterone (NCT01171898).

### Mechanisms of resistance to targeting the androgen receptor

Some patients treated with abiraterone or enzalutamide in the postchemotherapy setting are primarily refractory (progress immediately) and eventually almost all patients develop secondary resistance. Increasing preclinical evidence suggests that resistance occurs due to continued AR activation. A number of mechanisms have been elucidated.

## AR mutations

Mutations in the ligand-binding domain of the AR can confer resistance to AR-antagonists [29]. Additionally, mutations that increase sensitivity of the AR can turn AR-antagonists into stimulating agents and promote prostate cancer cell growth, observed clinically in the "androgen withdrawal" response on discontinuing first-generation AR-antagonists [30, 31]. These "gain of function" AR mutations may be present but not easily detectable in treatment-naïve patients but are more commonly observed in later-stage castration-resistant disease [32]. Several steroidal compounds such as prednisolone or prednisone, eplerenone and spironolactone have been shown to bind and activate mutant AR [33, 34]. Based on these findings, spironolactone should not be used to treat fluid retention or edema in CRPC patients and eplerenone be used with caution.

## AR amplification

In preclinical models, antiandrogen treatment resulted in AR overexpression and increased sensitivity to low levels of androgens [35]. Furthermore, AR overexpression was shown to enhance binding to chromatin, facilitating transcription of AR-regulated genes [36].

## AR splice variants

In the AR protein, several key domains can be defined such as the NH2 terminal transactivation domain, a hinge region, a central DNA-binding domain, and a COOH-terminal ligand-binding domain [37]. AR splice variants (AR-V) are AR proteins that generally lack the ligand-binding domain but have been associated with prostate cancer progression through ligand-independent constitutive activation [38]. In preclinical models, resistance to treatment with abiraterone has been associated with increased expression of AR-Vs [39]. Novel AR targeting drugs such as enzalutamide have been shown to overcome AR-V mediated growth in preclinical models [40].

## Other mechanisms of AR activation

Continued AR signaling can also be a result of up- or downregulation in cofactors. Heat-shock protein 90 (Hsp90) is a chaperone protein that folds and stabilizes client proteins such as AR. Hsp90 is commonly overexpressed in prostate cancer cells [41]. Other key proteins that regulate the binding of ligands to the AR are the co-chaperones FKBP51 and FKBP52 [42]. Preclinical experiments also proved reciprocal feedback mechanisms between the AR and the important PTEN-PI3K-AKT-mTOR signaling pathway, suggesting that AR blockade can result in AKT activation and conversely, that blockade of the PI3K-AKT-mTOR pathway can result in AR activation through activation of HER2/3 [43].

# Immune targeting in advanced prostate cancer

Harnessing the immune system against cancer cells has proven difficult, but immunotherapies have met with some success in metastatic CRPC. Promising strategies include specific vaccines and more general immune system modulation to decrease cancer immune tolerance by blocking immune checkpoints such as CTLA4 and PD1.

## Sipuleucel-T

Sipuleucel-T (APC8015, Provenge®, Dendreon, Seattle, WA, USA) is a vaccine therapy developed for the treatment of CRPC. It is prepared using a sample of a patients' own dendritic cells, which are pulsed *ex vivo* with a recombinant fusion protein of granulocyte macrophage colony stimulating factor (GM-CSF) and prostatic acid phosphatase (PAP). Collection of dendritic cells by apheresis usually requires insertion of a "long line" central venous catheter. A series of three treatments is administered over 1 month.

Two small Phase III studies suggested that sipuleucel-T improved survival [44, 45]. This finding was confirmed by the larger Phase III IMPACT study [7], leading to FDA approval. IMPACT enrolled 512 men with progressive but mainly low-volume and asymptomatic CRPC. Participants were randomized 2:1 between sipuleucel-T and placebo, which consisted the same process of dendritic cell harvest and reinfusion, without GM-CSF and PAP culture. Although there was no observed difference in radiographic or PSA response, sipuleucel-T was associated with improved median OS (25.8 vs. 21.7 months, HR 0.78, $p = .03$). Antibody response, judged by high levels of antibodies to PA2024 (immunizing antigen) or PAP, appeared associated with improved survival. Sipuleucel-T was well tolerated, with most adverse events due to temporary grade 1/2 post-infusion toxicities. There is ongoing debate regarding the effectiveness of sipuleucel-T, including concern that the isolated difference in OS related to chance imbalance or, more seriously, to flawed trial design [46].

Utility of sipuleucel-T in earlier hormone-sensitive disease was tested in a randomized trial of 117 men with rising PSA 3 or more months after radical prostatectomy. The study failed to meet the primary endpoint of improved time to biochemical failure [47]. Longer follow-up is required to acquire mature survival data.

The manufacture and administration of sipuleucel-T is only available in the United States at present and manufacturing capacity continues to limit supply. The cost, at US$ 93,000 for the course of three infusions, is also a limitation for many patients without private health insurance. Sipuleucel-T is not yet licensed in Europe.

## Ipilimumab

Cytotoxic T-lymphocyte antigen-4 (CTLA-4) is a protein expressed by cytotoxic T cells. T cell activation requires binding of CD28, but CTLA-4 competes for binding with a higher efficiency, and thus acts as an immune inhibitor. Ipilimumab (Ipi; Yervoy$^{TM}$, Bristol-Myers Squibb, New York, USA) is a humanized monoclonal antibody to CTLA-4 that has been trialed as a nonspecific immunotherapy and is approved for use in advanced melanoma.

*In vitro* testing of CTLA-4 blockade in a transgenic mouse prostate cancer model showed that CTLA-4-specific antibody treatment resulted in slowed tumor growth or rejection, whereas placebo treatment caused uniform tumor growth [48]. When administered after resection of an established tumor, CTLA-4 antibody treatment decreased the development of metastases [49].

A Phase I trial tested a single intravenous dose of Ipi 3 mg/kg in 14 men with metastatic CRPC. Two patients had $\geq$50% PSA decline and a further 8 patients had lesser PSA declines [50]. Additional Phase I and II studies have examined the safety of Ipi combined with immunotherapy, radiotherapy, antiandrogens, and chemotherapy [51]. Adverse effects related to immune activation were observed, with severe inflammatory events reported in 10–24% of patients in metastatic CRPC trials, particularly at doses $\geq$3 mg/kg. Affected systems included the colon, skin, liver, eye, and endocrine organs. In addition, arthralgias and bone pain, malaise and fatigue were commonly reported. Of interest, Ipi therapy has been associated with hypophysitis and hypogonadism, which may contribute to an antitumor effect in men with CRPC through reduction in androgen levels [52].

Two Phase III trials are examining the impact of Ipi on survival in CRPC. In 600 chemotherapy-naïve men, Ipi will be tested against placebo (NCT 01057810), whereas in more advanced disease, 800 men who have previously received docetaxel will receive palliative radiotherapy followed by Ipi or placebo (NCT00861614).

*PROSTVAC-VF®* (PROSTVAC®-VF/TRICOM™, Bavarian Nordic, Kvistgaard, Denmark) is a recombinant viral PSA-targeted vaccine regimen. Treatment comprises an initial recombinant vaccinia virus vaccine, followed by six boosters using a fowlpox vector. The vaccines contain transgenes for PSA and T-cell co-stimulatory molecules and are accompanied by adjuvant GM-CSF. Early studies showed preliminary evidence of activity when PROSTVAC was given without co-stimulatory molecules and/or GM-CSF [53–55]. A randomized Phase II study of 125 men with minimally symptomatic metastatic CRPC showed no difference in the primary endpoint of PSA progression, but suggested a survival advantage to PROSTVAC-VF therapy compared with placebo, with median OS 25.1 months and 16.6 months, respectively, giving an estimated HR 0.56 ($p = .0061$) [56]. Survival will be further examined in a large Phase III trial with three-way blinded randomization between PROSTVAC-VF with GM-CSF, PROSTVAC-VF alone, or placebo (NCT01322490).

*Anti-PD1 therapy* aims to block the inhibitory PD1 (programmed cell death 1) receptor expressed on activated T-cells. The most advanced inhibitor in clinical development for solid cancers is the monoclonal antibody BMS-936558 (MDX-1106), which was reported as showing preliminary antitumor activity against a number of advanced malignancies [57]. Although no objective responses were reported in patients with advanced prostate cancer, there is strong rationale, both preclinically and in view of the intriguing Ipi data, to further explore PD1 inhibition in CRPC.

## Bone-targeting agents in advanced prostate cancer

Bone metastases are the most common metastatic site in prostate cancer, occurring in up to 90% of patients with advanced disease [1, 4]. SREs are also common, with a cumulative incidence of 30–50%, and impact morbidity and quality of life [58, 59]. The main cancer-related SREs are fractures, spinal cord compressions, and painful bone metastases requiring radiotherapy or surgery.

*Bisphosphonates* are bone-seeking agents that bind to hydroxyapatite crystals in the bone and inhibit osteoclast activity. The bisphosphonate zoledronic acid is approved for the prevention of SREs in patients with prostate cancer and bone metastases. The pivotal Phase III trial randomized 643 patients to 3-weekly infusions of zoledronic acid or placebo for 15 months. The primary endpoint was the proportion of patients who developed SREs. Overall zoledronic acid significantly reduced the risk of

SREs compared with placebo (HR 0.64, 95% CI = 0.485–0.845; $p$ = .002) and time to first SRE was significantly longer in patients on zoledronic acid (488 days vs. 321 days with placebo, $p$ = .009); however, survival was not different between the two arms [60]. Due to renal elimination, bisphosphonate dosing needs to be adjusted to renal function. Osteonecrosis of the jaw is a characteristic side effect of bisphosphonate treatment, occurring in 2–4% of patients, particularly those with poor dentition or undergoing invasive dental procedures.

The receptor activator of nuclear factor kappa-B ligand (RANKL) has been identified as key molecule in the regulation of bone turnover. RANKL activates osteoclasts to undergo differentiation and maturation and suppresses apoptosis [61, 62].

*Denosumab* (Xgeva®, Amgen, Thousand Oaks, CA, USA) is a monoclonal antibody against RANKL that was tested in a randomized double-blind Phase III trial in 1904 men with CRPC and bone metastases. Denosumab 120 mg subcutaneously every 4 weeks was compared with zoledronic acid 4 mg intravenously every 4 weeks [63]. In the primary endpoint of time to first SRE, denosumab was superior to zoledronic acid (20.7 vs. 17.1 months, HR 0.82, 95% CI = 0.71—0.95; $p$ = .0002 for non-inferiority; $p$ = .008 for superiority). Nevertheless, OS and PFS were not statistically different in the two treatment arms. Despite active treatment in both study arms, however, 41% of patients on zoledronic acid and 36% on denosumab experienced SREs (radiation to bone 21% vs. 19%, pathological fracture 15% vs. 14%, spinal cord compression 4% vs. 3%, and surgery to bone <1%). Adverse events were evenly distributed between the two treatments apart from hypocalcaemia, which occurred in 13% of patients on denosumab versus 6% on zoledronic acid ($p$<.0001) and osteonecrosis of the jaw (2.3% vs. 1.3%; $p$ = .09). Dose adjustments of zoledronic acid were necessary in 22% of patients due to impaired renal function. The main advantages of denosumab are the subcutaneous administration and lack of dose adjustments based on renal function.

The optimal timing of agents to prevent SREs or delay bone metastases needs to be investigated. In a randomized placebo-controlled Phase III trial, reported at ASCO 2012, 1432 patients with non-metastatic CRPC and a PSA doubling time of ≤10 months were randomized 1:1 to denosumab or placebo. The median bone metastasis-free survival was 29.5 months on denosumab versus 25.2 months on placebo (HR 0.85, 95% CI = 0.73–0.98, $p$ = .028) [64]. Subgroup analysis suggested that the treatment effect was greater in men with PSA doubling time of ≤6 months (25.2 vs. 18.7 months). With the advent of novel agents that both improve OS and decrease SRE rate, it is not clear what the role of bone targets such as denosumab will be in clinical practice.

## Alpharadin

Several beta-emitting radionuclides are bone-seeking agents that have been investigated in men with prostate cancer and bone metastases. Two drugs have been approved by the FDA: $^{89}$Sr (Strontium-89) and $^{153}$Sm (Samarium-153), based on trial results showing improved pain control when compared with placebo. Samarium and Strontium have no proven survival benefit; however, the trials were not powered to detect improvements in survival [65, 66].

Radium$^{223}$ chloride (Alpharadin, Bayer, Leverkusen, Germany) is a novel agent that acts as a calcium mimetic and is preferentially integrated into areas of new bone formation such as bone growth around metastases [67]. Radium$^{223}$ emits alpha particles, which have a high linear energy transfer in a very short range of $<100$ μm, causing irreparable amounts of DNA double-strand breaks in cells within that range [68]. Following promising results from a randomized Phase II clinical trial, the double-blind Phase III ALSYMPCA trial randomized 921 patients in a 2:1 ratio to radium$^{223}$ (50 kBq/kg IV) q4wks or matching placebo [6, 69]. Eligible patients had progressive symptomatic CRPC with $\geq$2 bone metastases, no visceral metastases, and had either previously received docetaxel, were docetaxel ineligible or refused chemotherapy (total 40% chemotherapy naïve). Radium$^{223}$ significantly improved median OS by 3.6 months when compared with placebo (HR $= 0.695$; $p = .00007$). The favorable safety profile of radium$^{223}$ with low frequencies of myelosuppression (grade 3/4 neutropenia 2.2% on radium$^{223}$ vs. 0.7% on placebo, grade 3/4 thrombocytopenia 6.3% vs. 2%, respectively) support the use of radium$^{223}$ in patients with bone metastases in the absence of visceral disease. The integration of radium$^{223}$ into treatment sequences for CRPC patients and potential combination strategies needs to be investigated.

## Cabozantinib

Cabozantinib (XL184, Exelixis, South San Francisco, CA, USA) is a novel oral small molecule targeting multiple-key receptor tyrosine kinases, including the receptor of the hepatocyte growth factor (c-MET) and the vascular endothelial growth factor receptor 2 (VEGFR2), but also inhibits KIT, FLT3, and AXL [70]. Preclinical data indicated that MET was expressed on prostate cancer cells and also on both osteoblasts and osteoclasts [71]. Hepatocyte growth factor secretion by osteoblasts was associated with migration of cancer cells from the blood stream into the bone marrow space underlining a key role of MET [72].

Preliminary data reporting on a large Phase I/II trial of cabozantinib were presented at ASCO 2011. Of 100 patients with advanced CRPC who received cabozantinib 100 mg once daily, 56 of 65 evaluable patients (86%) had complete or partial resolution of lesions on bone scan and 18 of 28 patients (64%) on narcotics at baseline had improved pain. These effects correlated with >50% declines in bone markers including alkaline phosphatase (ALP) and c-telopeptide in 56% and 55% of patients, respectively [73]. Further results of 93 patients with CRPC and progressive disease on or within 6 months of docetaxel showed bone scan responses in 51 (60%) associated with improvement in pain scores in 46% of patients. In 59 patients with unfavorable CTC counts ($\geq$5), 92% had declines of $\geq$30% with conversions to favorable counts in 39% [74].

The common side effects were comparable to other tyrosine kinase inhibitors and included fatigue (all grades/grade3-4: 83%/28%), anorexia (73%/6%), diarrhea (70%/11%), hand–foot syndrome (25%/5%), hypertension (24%/9%), and venous thrombosis (13%/6%). A further dose expansion cohort evaluating cabozantinib 40 mg daily is currently ongoing. Based on these encouraging Phase II results, two large randomized Phase III trials have been initiated in patients with CPRC following docetaxel and either abiraterone or enzalutamide (NCT01605227 and NCT01522443).

## Second-line chemotherapy

A number of agents have been tested in men following first-line docetaxel chemotherapy. There is Phase II trial evidence to support docetaxel retreatment as a second-line strategy in selected men who responded well to initial docetaxel, with $\geq$50% PSA declines in 25–48% patients [75, 76], but to date there is no Phase III trial level I evidence for docetaxel retreatment. Other agents have been tested second line, but have met with limited success. Satraplatin was tested against placebo in a Phase III trial and although it was positive for the co-primary endpoint of PFS, it failed to show any improvement in OS [77].

### Cabazitaxel

Cabazitaxel (Jevtana, Sanofi, Paris, France) is a partially synthesized taxane compound. Preclinical studies suggested activity in docetaxel-resistant cell lines. In Phase I studies in patients with solid tumors, neutropenia was the primary dose-limiting toxicity at 25–30 mg/m$^2$ [78, 79]. Antitumor activity was observed in three men with CRPC, including two radiologic partial responses accompanied by >50% PSA declines.

Encouraging activity in Phase I trials led to the open-label Phase III TROPIC trial, which randomized 755 men 1:1 to prednisone with either cabazitaxel or mitoxantrone [3]. More than 70% of participants had progressed on or within 3 months of completing docetaxel. A median of six cycles of cabazitaxel and four cycles of mitoxantrone were administered. Cabazitaxel showed superiority in the primary survival endpoint, with a median OS improvement of 2.4 months (HR 0.70, $p$<.0001). The benefit of cabazitaxel was maintained across all subgroups, including patients who were docetaxel-refractory. Secondary endpoints including PFS, PSA and radiographic responses, and time to progression were all significantly improved by cabazitaxel. Pain palliation was also evaluated, but in this respect cabazitaxel was not superior to the active comparator of mitoxantrone. Quality of life was not examined in TROPIC, but data from an early access program within the United Kingdom suggested improvement in pain control and preservation of quality of life during treatment [80].

The toxicity profile of cabazitaxel in TROPIC included neutropenia (grade 3/4 in 303 patients; 82%) with febrile neutropenia in 28 patients (8%). Grade 3/4 diarrhea occurred in 23 patients (6%). These events were key contributors to treatment-related mortality of almost 5%, along with older age, prior radiotherapy, and geographical variation, likely reflecting differences in supportive care. Although the FDA has approved cabazitaxel for second-line treatment for men with metastatic CRPC, a further Phase III non-inferiority trial is being performed to compare 20 mg/m$^2$ to 25 mg/m$^2$ (NCT01308580) in an effort to preserve efficacy but improve the safety profile. Additionally, cabazitaxel is being tested in the first-line setting against docetaxel (NCT01308567) and combination treatments are also being investigated.

## Conclusion

Unlocking the biology of CRPC and discovering the ongoing importance of AR signaling has led to increasing therapeutic options for men with CRPC. In addition to docetaxel chemotherapy, five novel therapies have resulted in survival improvements in Phase III trials, including abiraterone, enzalutamide, sipuleucel-T, radium$^{223}$ and cabazitaxel. Additionally, multiple promising therapies are in clinical development. Men who are well should be encouraged to participate in clinical trials in addition to receiving standard therapies. Further advances in CRPC management are likely to result from deeper genomic testing of individual prostate cancers. Future trials will also define the role of sequencing of the novel treatment options in order to achieve maximal benefit for patients.

## References

1 de Bono JS, Logothetis CJ, Molina A, *et al.* Abiraterone and increased survival in metastatic prostate cancer. *N Engl J Med* 2011;364(21):1995–2005.

2 Ryan CJ, Smith MR, de Bono JS, *et al.* Abiraterone in metastatic prostate cancer without previous chemotherapy. *N Engl J Med* 2013;368(2):138–148.

3 de Bono JS, Oudard S, Ozguroglu M, *et al.* Prednisone plus cabazitaxel or mitoxantrone for metastatic castration-resistant prostate cancer progressing after docetaxel treatment: a randomised open-label trial. *Lancet* 2010;376(9747):1147–1154.

4 Tannock IF, de Wit R, Berry WR, *et al.* Docetaxel plus prednisone or mitoxantrone plus prednisone for advanced prostate cancer. *N Engl J Med* 2004;351(15):1502–1512.

5 Scher HI, Fizazi K, Saad F, *et al.* Increased survival with enzalutamide in prostate cancer after chemotherapy. *N Engl J Med* 2012;367(13):1187–1197.

6 Parker C, Nilsson S, Heinrich D, *et al.* Alpha emitter radium-223 and survival in metastatic prostate cancer. *N Engl J Med* 2013;369(3):213–223.

7 Kantoff PW, Higano CS, Shore ND, *et al.* Sipuleucel-T immunotherapy for castration-resistant prostate cancer. *N Engl J Med* 2010;363(5):411–422.

8 Mohler JL. Castration-recurrent prostate cancer is not androgen-independent. *Adv Exp Med Biol* 2008;617:223–234.

9 Attard G, Swennenhuis JF, Olmos D, *et al.* Characterization of ERG, AR and PTEN gene status in circulating tumor cells from patients with castration-resistant prostate cancer. *Cancer Res* 2009;69(7):2912–2918.

10 Stanbrough M, Bubley GJ, Ross K, *et al.* Increased expression of genes converting adrenal androgens to testosterone in androgen-independent prostate cancer. *Cancer Res* 2006;66(5):2815–2825.

11 Montgomery RB, Mostaghel EA, Vessella R, *et al.* Maintenance of intratumoral androgens in metastatic prostate cancer: a mechanism for castration-resistant tumor growth. *Cancer Res* 2008;68(11):4447–4454.

12 Locke JA, Guns ES, Lubik AA, *et al.* Androgen levels increase by intratumoral de novo steroidogenesis during progression of castration-resistant prostate cancer. *Cancer Res* 2008;68(15):6407–6415.

13 Cai C, Chen S, Ng P, *et al.* Intratumoral de novo steroid synthesis activates androgen receptor in castration-resistant prostate cancer and is upregulated by treatment with CYP17A1 inhibitors. *Cancer Res* 2011;71(20):6503–6513.

14 Mohler JL, Titus MA, Wilson EM. Potential prostate cancer drug target: bioactivation of androstanediol by conversion to dihydrotestosterone. *Clin Cancer Res* 2011;17(18):5844–5849.

15 Figg WD, Dawson N, Middleman MN, *et al.* Flutamide withdrawal and concomitant initiation of aminoglutethimide in patients with hormone refractory prostate cancer. *Acta Oncol* 1996;35(6):763–765.

16 Small EJ, Baron AD, Fippin L, Apodaca D. Ketoconazole retains activity in advanced prostate cancer patients with progression despite flutamide withdrawal. *J Urol* 1997;157(4):1204–1207.

17 Potter GA, Barrie SE, Jarman M, Rowlands MG. Novel steroidal inhibitors of human cytochrome P45017 alpha (17 alpha-hydroxylase-C17,20-lyase): potential agents for the treatment of prostatic cancer. *J Med Chem* 1995;38(13):2463–2471.

18 Pezaro CJ, Mukherji D, De Bono JS. Abiraterone acetate: redefining hormone treatment for advanced prostate cancer. *Drug Discov Today* 2012;17(5–6):221–226.

19 Scher HI, Heller G, Molina A, *et al.* Evaluation of circulating tumor cell (CTC) enumeration as an efficacy response biomarker of overall survival (OS) in metastatic castration-resistant prostate cancer (mCRPC): planned final analysis (FA) of COU-AA-301, a randomized double-blind, placebo-controlled phase III study of abiraterone acetate (AA) plus prednisone (P) post docetaxel. *J Clin Oncol* 2011;29:(Suppl;abstr LBA4517).

20 Sternberg CN, Molina A, North S, *et al.* Fatigue improvement/reduction with abiraterone acetate in patients with metastatic castration-resistant prostate cancer (mCRPC) post-docetaxel – results from the COU-AA-301 phase 3 study. *Eur J Cancer* 2011;47(Suppl. 1):S488–S489.

21 Ryan CJ, Shah S, Efstathiou E, *et al.* Phase II study of abiraterone acetate in chemotherapy-naive metastatic castration-resistant prostate cancer displaying bone flare discordant with serologic response. *Clin Cancer Res* 2011;17(14):4854–4861.

22 Dreicer R, Agus DB, MacVicar GR, *et al.* Safety, pharmacokinetics, and efficacy of TAK-700 in castration-resistant, metastatic prostate cancer: a phase I/II, open-label study. 2010 Genitourinary Cancers Symposium 2010. Abstract: p. 103.

23 Agus DB, Stadler WM, Shevrin DH, *et al.* Safety, efficacy, and pharmacodynamics of the investigational agent orteronel (TAK-700) in metastatic castration-resistant prostate cancer (mCRPC): updated data from a phase I/II study. *J Clin Oncol* 2012;30:(Suppl 5;abstr 98).

24 Montgomery RB, Eisenberger MA, Rettig M, *et al.* Phase I clinical trial of galeterone (TOK-001), a multifunctional antiandrogen and CYP17 inhibitor in castration resistant prostate cancer (CRPC). *J Clin Oncol* 2012;30:(Suppl;abstr 4665).

25 Eisner JR, Abbott DH, Bird IM, *et al.* VT-464: a novel, selective inhibitor of P450c17(CYP17)-17,20 lyase for castration-refractory prostate cancer (CRPC). *J Clin Oncol* 2012;30:(Suppl 5;abstr 198).

26 Tran C, Ouk S, Clegg NJ, *et al.* Development of a second-generation antiandrogen for treatment of advanced prostate cancer. *Science* 2009;324(5928):787–790.

27 Scher HI, Beer TM, Higano CS, *et al.* Antitumour activity of MDV3100 in castration-resistant prostate cancer: a phase 1-2 study. *Lancet* 2010;375(9724):1437–1446.

28 Clegg NJ, Wongvipat J, Joseph JD, *et al.* ARN-509: a novel antiandrogen for prostate cancer treatment. *Cancer Res* 2012;72(6):1494–1503.

29 Taplin ME, Bubley GJ, Ko YJ, *et al.* Selection for androgen receptor mutations in prostate cancers treated with androgen antagonist. *Cancer Res* 1999;59(11):2511–2515.

30 Taplin ME, Bubley GJ, Shuster TD, *et al.* Mutation of the androgen-receptor gene in metastatic androgen-independent prostate cancer. *N Engl J Med* 1995;332(21):1393–1398.

31 Sartor AO, Tangen CM, Hussain MH, *et al.* Antiandrogen withdrawal in castrate-refractory prostate cancer: a Southwest Oncology Group trial (SWOG 9426). *Cancer* 2008;112(11):2393–2400.

32 Steinkamp MP, O'Mahony OA, Brogley M, *et al.* Treatment-dependent androgen receptor mutations in prostate cancer exploit multiple mechanisms to evade therapy. *Cancer Res* 2009;69(10):4434–4442.

33 Richards J, Lim AC, Hay CW, *et al.* Interactions of abiraterone, eplerenone, and prednisolone with wild-type and mutant androgen receptor: a rationale for increasing abiraterone exposure or combining with MDV3100. *Cancer Res* 2012;72(9):2176–2182.

34 Sundar S, Dickinson PD. Spironolactone, a possible selective androgen receptor modulator, should be used with caution in patients with metastatic carcinoma of the prostate. *BMJ Case Rep* 2012;2012.

35 Kawata H, Ishikura N, Watanabe M, *et al.* Prolonged treatment with bicalutamide induces androgen receptor overexpression and androgen hypersensitivity. *Prostate* 2010;70(7):745–754.

36 Urbanucci A, Sahu B, Seppala J, *et al.* Overexpression of androgen receptor enhances the binding of the receptor to the chromatin in prostate cancer. *Oncogene* 2012;31(17):2153–2163.

37 Guo Z, Yang X, Sun F, *et al.* A novel androgen receptor splice variant is upregulated during prostate cancer progression and promotes androgen depletion-resistant growth. *Cancer Res* 2009;69(6):2305–2313.

38 Hornberg E, Ylitalo EB, Crnalic S, *et al.* Expression of androgen receptor splice variants in prostate cancer bone metastases is associated with castration-resistance and short survival. *PLoS One* 2011;6(4):e19059.

39 Mostaghel EA, Marck BT, Plymate SR, *et al.* Resistance to CYP17A1 inhibition with abiraterone in castration-resistant prostate cancer: induction of steroidogenesis and androgen receptor splice variants. *Clin Cancer Res* 2011;17(18):5913–5925.

40 Watson PA, Chen YF, Balbas MD, *et al.* Constitutively active androgen receptor splice variants expressed in castration-resistant prostate cancer require full-length androgen receptor. *Proc Natl Acad Sci U S A* 2010;107(39):16759–16765.

41 Cardillo MR, Ippoliti F. IL-6, IL-10 and HSP-90 expression in tissue microarrays from human prostate cancer assessed by computer-assisted image analysis. *Anticancer Res* 2006;26(5A):3409–3416.

42 Ni L, Yang CS, Gioeli D, *et al.* FKBP51 promotes assembly of the Hsp90 chaperone complex and regulates androgen receptor signaling in prostate cancer cells. *Mol Cell Biol* 2010;30(5):1243–1253.

43 Carver BS, Chapinski C, Wongvipat J, *et al.* Reciprocal feedback regulation of PI3K and androgen receptor signaling in PTEN-deficient prostate cancer. *Cancer Cell* 2011;19(5):575–586.

44 Small EJ, Schellhammer PF, Higano CS, *et al.* Placebo-controlled phase III trial of immunologic therapy with sipuleucel-T (APC8015) in patients with metastatic, asymptomatic hormone refractory prostate cancer. *J Clin Oncol* 2006;24(19):3089–3094.

45 Higano CS, Schellhammer PF, Small EJ, *et al.* Integrated data from 2 randomized, double-blind, placebo-controlled, phase 3 trials of active cellular immunotherapy with sipuleucel-T in advanced prostate cancer. *Cancer* 2009;115(16):3670–3679.

46 Huber ML, Haynes L, Parker C, Iversen P. Interdisciplinary critique of sipuleucel-T as immunotherapy in castration-resistant prostate cancer. *J Natl Cancer Inst* 2012;104(4):273–279.

47 Beer TM, Bernstein GT, Corman JM, *et al.* Randomized trial of autologous cellular immunotherapy with sipuleucel-T in androgen-dependent prostate cancer. *Clin Cancer Res* 2011;17(13):4558–4567.

48 Kwon ED, Hurwitz AA, Foster BA, *et al.* Manipulation of T cell costimulatory and inhibitory signals for immunotherapy of prostate cancer. *Proc Natl Acad Sci U S A* 1997;94(15):8099–8103.

49 Kwon ED, Foster BA, Hurwitz AA, *et al.* Elimination of residual metastatic prostate cancer after surgery and adjunctive cytotoxic T lymphocyte-associated antigen 4 (CTLA-4) blockade immunotherapy. *Proc Natl Acad Sci U S A* 1999;96(26):15074–15079.

50 Small EJ, Tchekmedyian NS, Rini BI, *et al.* A pilot trial of CTLA-4 blockade with human anti-CTLA-4 in patients with hormone-refractory prostate cancer. *Clin Cancer Res* 2007;13(6):1810–1815.

51 Kwek SS, Cha E, Fong L. Unmasking the immune recognition of prostate cancer with CTLA4 blockade. *Nat Rev Cancer* 2012;12(4):289–297.

52 Juszczak A, Gupta A, Karavitaki N, *et al.* Ipilimumab: a novel immunomodulating therapy causing autoimmune hypophysitis: a case report and review. *Eur J Endocrinol* 2012;167(1):1–5.

53 Kaufman HL, Wang W, Manola J, *et al.* Phase II randomized study of vaccine treatment of advanced prostate cancer (E7897): a trial of the Eastern Cooperative Oncology Group. *J Clin Oncol* 2004;22(11):2122–2132.

54 DiPaola RS, Plante M, Kaufman H, *et al.* A phase I trial of pox PSA vaccines (PROSTVAC-VF) with B7-1, ICAM-1, and LFA-3 co-stimulatory molecules (TRICOM) in patients with prostate cancer. *J Transl Med* 2006;4:1.

55 Arlen PM, Skarupa L, Pazdur M, *et al.* Clinical safety of a viral vector based prostate cancer vaccine strategy. *J Urol* 2007;178(4 Pt 1):1515–1520.

56 Kantoff PW, Schuetz TJ, Blumenstein BA, *et al.* Overall survival analysis of a phase II randomized controlled trial of a Poxviral-based PSA-targeted immunotherapy in metastatic castration-resistant prostate cancer. *J Clin Oncol* 2010;28(7):1099–1105.

57 Topalian SL, Hodi FS, Brahmer JR, *et al.* Safety, activity, and immune correlates of anti-PD-1 antibody in cancer. *N Engl J Med* 2012;366(26):2443–2454.

58 Saad F, Olsson C, Schulman CC. Skeletal morbidity in men with prostate cancer: quality-of-life considerations throughout the continuum of care. *Eur Urol* 2004;46(6):731–739; discussion 9–40.

59 Sathiakumar N, Delzell E, Morrisey MA, *et al.* Mortality following bone metastasis and skeletal-related events among men with prostate cancer: a population-based analysis of US Medicare beneficiaries, 1999–2006. *Prostate Cancer Prostatic Dis* 2011;14(2):177–183.

60 Saad F, Gleason DM, Murray R, *et al.* Long-term efficacy of zoledronic acid for the prevention of skeletal complications in patients with metastatic hormone-refractory prostate cancer. *J Natl Cancer Inst* 2004;96(11):879–882.

61  Simonet WS, Lacey DL, Dunstan CR, *et al.* Osteoprotegerin: a novel secreted protein involved in the regulation of bone density. *Cell* 1997;89(2):309–319.

62  Boyle WJ, Simonet WS, Lacey DL. Osteoclast differentiation and activation. *Nature* 2003;423(6937):337–342.

63  Fizazi K, Carducci M, Smith M, *et al.* Denosumab versus zoledronic acid for treatment of bone metastases in men with castration-resistant prostate cancer: a randomised, double-blind study. *Lancet* 2011;377(9768):813–822.

64  Saad F, Smith MR, Shore ND, *et al.* Effect of denosumab on prolonging bone-metastasis free survival (BMFS) in men with nonmetastatic castrate-resistant prostate cancer (CRPC) presenting with aggressive PSA kinetics. *J Clin Oncol* 2012;30:(Suppl;abstr 4510).

65  Lewington VJ, McEwan AJ, Ackery DM, *et al.* A prospective, randomised double-blind crossover study to examine the efficacy of strontium-89 in pain palliation in patients with advanced prostate cancer metastatic to bone. *Eur J Cancer* 1991;27(8):954–958.

66  Serafini AN, Houston SJ, Resche I, *et al.* Palliation of pain associated with metastatic bone cancer using samarium-153 lexidronam: a double-blind placebo-controlled clinical trial. *J Clin Oncol* 1998;16(4):1574–1581.

67  Henriksen G, Breistol K, Bruland OS, *et al.* Significant antitumor effect from bone-seeking, alpha-particle-emitting (223)Ra demonstrated in an experimental skeletal metastases model. *Cancer Res* 2002;62(11):3120–3125.

68  Ritter MA, Cleaver JE, Tobias CA. High-LET radiations induce a large proportion of non-rejoining DNA breaks. *Nature* 1977;266(5603):653–655.

69  Nilsson S, Franzen L, Parker C, *et al.* Bone-targeted radium-223 in symptomatic, hormone-refractory prostate cancer: a randomised, multicentre, placebo-controlled phase II study. *Lancet Oncol* 2007;8(7):587–594.

70  You WK, Sennino B, Williamson CW, *et al.* VEGF and c-Met blockade amplify angiogenesis inhibition in pancreatic islet cancer. *Cancer Res* 2011;71(14):4758–4768.

71  Inaba M, Koyama H, Hino M, *et al.* Regulation of release of hepatocyte growth factor from human promyelocytic leukemia cells, HL-60, by 1,25-dihydroxyvitamin D3, 12-O-tetradecanoylphorbol 13-acetate, and dibutyryl cyclic adenosine monophosphate. *Blood* 1993;82(1):53–59.

72  Ono K, Kamiya S, Akatsu T, *et al.* Involvement of hepatocyte growth factor in the development of bone metastasis of a mouse mammary cancer cell line, BALB/c-MC. *Bone* 2006;39(1):27–34.

73  Hussain M, Smith MR, Sweeney C, *et al.* Cabozantinib (XL184) in metastatic castration-resistant prostate cancer (mCRPC): results from a phase II randomized discontinuation trial. *J Clin Oncol* 2011;29: (Suppl;abstr 4516).

74  Smith MR, Sweeney C, Rathkopf DE, *et al.* Cabozantinib (XL184) in chemotherapy-pretreated metastatic castration resistant prostate cancer (mCRPC): results from a phase II nonrandomized expansion cohort (NRE). *J Clin Oncol* 2012;30:(Suppl;abstr 4513).

75  Buonerba C, Palmieri G, Di Lorenzo G. Docetaxel rechallenge in castration-resistant prostate cancer: scientific legitimacy of common clinical practice. *Eur Urol* 2010;58(4):636–637.

76  Di Lorenzo G, Buonerba C, Faiella A, *et al.* Phase II study of docetaxel re-treatment in docetaxel-pretreated castration-resistant prostate cancer. *BJU Int* 2011;107(2):234–239.

77 Sternberg CN, Petrylak DP, Sartor O, *et al.* Multinational, double-blind, phase III study of prednisone and either satraplatin or placebo in patients with castrate-refractory prostate cancer progressing after prior chemotherapy: the SPARC trial. *J Clin Oncol* 2009;27(32):5431–5438.

78 Mita AC, Denis LJ, Rowinsky EK, *et al.* Phase I and pharmacokinetic study of XRP6258 (RPR 116258A), a novel taxane, administered as a 1-hour infusion every 3 weeks in patients with advanced solid tumors. *Clin Cancer Res* 2009;15(2):723–730.

79 Bissery M-C, Bouchard H, Riou JF, *et al.* Preclinical evaluation of TXD258, a new taxoid. *Proc Am Assoc Cancer Res* 2000;41:214; abstr 1364.

80 Bahl A, Masson S, Malik Z, *et al.* Cabazitaxel for metastatic castration-resistant prostate cancer (mCRPC): interim safety and quality-of-life (QOL) data from the U.K. early access program (NCT01254279). *J Clin Oncol* 2012;30:(Suppl 5;abstr 44).

## CHAPTER 15

# End of Life Care in Prostate Cancer

*John D. Graham*

Beacon Centre, Musgrove Park Hospital, Taunton, Somerset, UK

## Introduction

Despite the many improvements in the management of prostate cancer described in this book and the often quoted statement that more men die with prostate cancer than from it, prostate cancer is the second commonest cause of cancer death in men in North America and Europe [1, 2]. Men with castrate-resistant metastatic prostate cancer (CRPC) are living longer. In the recently published randomized trial of abiraterone prechemotherapy, the survival in the control arm was a median of 27.2 months [3], which compares with a median survival of 10–12 months in the early chemotherapy trials reported in the 1990s [4, 5]. A recent paper showed that the nomograms developed to predict survival of men with metastatic prostate cancer significantly underestimated the survival of a current cohort of chemotherapy-naïve patients from a single institution suggesting that they require updating to reflect improvements in the treatment of men with metastatic prostate cancer [6]. The Halabi nomogram predicted a median overall survival of 21 months and the Smaletz nomogram 18 months when in fact the median survival of the cohort was 30.6 months. To date, none of the new treatments for CRPC cures the disease. Men with metastatic prostate cancer are living longer with better quality of life but the increasing number of treatment options has made the identification and management of end-stage prostate cancer more challenging.

*Prostate Cancer: Diagnosis and Clinical Management*, First Edition.
Edited by Ashutosh K. Tewari, Peter Whelan and John D. Graham.
© 2014 John Wiley & Sons, Ltd. Published 2014 by John Wiley & Sons, Ltd.

# Bone metastases

Almost all men with end-stage prostate cancer have bone metastases. When the disease reaches the point where disease-modifying treatments such as chemotherapy and hormonal therapies are no longer effective, it is often the bone metastases that have the greatest adverse impact on quality of life. There are several issues relating to the management of bone metastases at the end stage of prostate cancer that are different from those covered in Chapter 13. These are bone pain and spinal cord compression.

## Bone pain

Almost half of patients with cancer have their pain undertreated mainly because of health professionals' reluctance to prescribe adequate levels of opiate analgesia [7, 8]. The WHO analgesic ladder provides a simple and practical framework for prescribing pain relief [9]. The National Institute for Health and Clinical Excellence recently published a guideline on the prescribing of strong opioids in palliative care [10]. Radiotherapy is an effective treatment for bone pain with single fractions improving pain in 60% of patients and giving complete pain relief in 30% [11]. The role of single-fraction radiotherapy for neuropathic pain is less clear. There is only one published randomized trial [12]. This showed a higher response rate with fractionated radiotherapy (20 Gy in five fractions) compared with a single 8 Gy, but the difference was not statistically significant. The trial did not mandate three-dimensional imaging of target lesions and the definition of neuropathic pain was not as robust as that advocated in a recent review [13].

The radioactive isotopes strontium-89, samarium-153, and radium-223 have also shown excellent pain-relieving qualities [14–16]. In addition, the latter has also shown improved survival when given to men with metastatic prostate cancer and this will be discussed in more detail below.

Bisphosphonates can also improve bone pain in prostate cancer. In a meta-analysis of studies in prostate cancer, there was an overall pain response rate of 28% but the benefit compared with placebo did not quite reach statistical significance [17]. A large randomized trial of 470 men with prostate cancer comparing the bisphosphonate ibandronate with a single fraction of radiotherapy has been reported [18]. The pain response at 4 weeks was 53% for radiotherapy and 49% for ibandronate. There were more patients with higher pain scores at 4 weeks in the bisphosphonate arm and more patients needed retreatment after ibandronate. Although bisphosphonates can relieve bone pain in men with prostate cancer, the evidence suggests that single-fraction radiotherapy remains the treatment of choice for localized bone pain.

## Spinal cord compression

Spinal cord compression from metastatic prostate cancer is a potentially devastating condition. The rate of onset in prostate cancer is often slower than other cancers and the gradual loss of neurological function may be incorrectly attributed to severe bone pain. Screening studies of asymptomatic men with bone metastases from prostate cancer have shown rates of occult spinal cord compression of up to 44% [19]. A prospective randomized study of MRI screening in prostate cancer patients with bone metastases has recently opened in the United Kingdom.

Once neurological symptoms develop, urgent investigation and treatment are required as pretreatment neurological status is a major factor in determining outcome [20]. Whole-spine MRI is required to make the diagnosis, as multiple levels of cord compression are not unusual. High-dose corticosteroids should be started immediately and treatment with either surgery or radiotherapy considered. Surgical decompression and spinal stabilization have been shown to be superior to radiotherapy resulting in better neurological function. In a meta-analysis, surgical patients were 1.3 times more likely to be ambulatory after treatment and twice as likely to regain ambulatory function [21]. Overall ambulatory success rates for surgery and radiation were 85% and 64%, although the comparison was hampered by significant heterogeneity between the surgical and radiotherapy groups. A Cochrane review of randomized trials comparing surgery plus radiotherapy versus radiotherapy alone recommended surgery for patients who have lost motor function for <48 hours, have localized cord compression, and an estimated life expectancy of >3 months [22]. Non-ambulant patients recovered ambulation after decompressive surgery in 63% of cases versus 19% after radiotherapy alone.

For men with localized spinal cord compression and a reasonable life expectancy, surgical decompression followed by radiotherapy is the treatment of choice.

## Bone-targeted radio-isotopes

Strontium-89 and samarium-153 have been used in clinical practice for many years but a new radio-isotope, radium-223, is due to be licensed in the near future. A recent Cochrane review of randomized trials of strontium-89, samarium-253, and rhenium-186 for the treatment of pain from bone metastases found a moderate effect on pain relief but no evidence of a reduction in analgesic uses and no apparent differences between the three agents [23]. There was no evidence that higher doses of samarium-253 were more effective. All these radioisotopes caused significant hematological toxicity with leucopenia and thrombocytopenia. They have been used predominantly at the end stage of prostate cancer after hormonal therapies and chemotherapy have failed. This may explain the lack of evidence for a significant disease-modifying effect and might also explain the hematological toxicity. There is an unusual trial that showed a significant survival benefit for men given strontium-89 following chemotherapy for metastatic prostate cancer [24] and a similar trial that gave samarium-253 as consolidation following chemotherapy with a docetaxel and estramustine combination [25].

The concept of radio-isotope consolidation with strontium-89 was explored further in the randomized TRAPEZE study following docetaxel chemotherapy [26]. This trial has closed recruitment and results are awaited.

Radium-223 is a new and different radio-isotope that is due to be licensed in 2013 for the treatment of prostate cancer. Unlike strontium-89 and samarium-253, which rely principally on beta-particle emissions for their therapeutic effect, radium-223 is a pure alpha emitter. Each decay produces four alpha particles that deposit large amounts of energy over a much shorter range than beta or gamma particles. This means there is less collateral damage to normal tissues which in the treatment of bone metastases is most importantly the bone marrow. The half-life of radium-223 at 11.4 days is much shorter than the 50.5 days for strontium-89 making it possible to give repeated doses. The preliminary results of the phase III ALSYMPCA study show that radium-223 is potentially disease modifying with an improvement in overall survival of almost 3 months [27]. The trial was in men with CRPC who had two or more symptomatic bone metastases and compared six 4-weekly injections of radium-223 at 50 kBq/kg with best supportive care. The latter could include secondary hormonal therapies but not cytotoxic chemotherapy or radio-isotopes. From June 2008 to February 2011, the trial randomized 541 patients to radium-223 and 268 patients to placebo. Baseline characteristics were well matched and almost 58% had previously received docetaxel chemotherapy. Recruitment was stopped early on the advice of an independent data-monitoring committee because overall survival had crossed a statistically predetermined boundary. Median overall survival was significantly improved at 14.0 months in the radium-223 arm compared with 11.2 months for best supportive care ($p = .00185$; 95% CI $= 0.552$–0.875).

The ALSYMPCA study also showed significant improvements in biochemical endpoints (prostate-specific antigen and alkaline phosphatase) and time to first skeletal-related event (13.6 vs. 8.4 months). Radium-223 even reduced the rate of spinal cord compression from 6% to 3% (HR 0.44; $p = .016$)—the first time this has been demonstrated in a randomized trial in prostate cancer [28]. The response to radium-223 appeared to be greater in men receiving bisphosphonates. It is possible that the inhibition of osteoclast activity by bisphosphonates allows greater binding of radium-223 at the site of bone metastases. Notably there was little toxicity. Even hematological toxicity was low with grade 3 or 4 neutropenia rates of 2% for radium-223 versus 1% for placebo and grade 3 or 4 thrombocytopenia at 4% versus 2%. To date, no pain response or quality of life data from the ALSYMPCA trial has been released.

It is clear that radium-223 offers men with end-stage prostate cancer significant benefits with improved survival, fewer skeletal-related events, and low toxicity even after prior cytotoxic chemotherapy. Its role in earlier stages of the disease and in combination with other disease-modifying treatments remains to be determined.

## Management of end-stage prostate cancer

### Quality of life and coping strategies

Men with metastatic prostate cancer have poorer quality of life and greater health needs than men with localized or locally advanced disease. A recent study from Finland used three quality of life instruments, two generic and one cancer specific, to measure health-related quality of life in 630 men with prostate cancer [29]. Using the generic measure EQ-5D where a score of 1.0 signifies perfect health, men with nonmetastatic disease showed mean scores of 0.87 to 0.90 compared with 0.74 in men with metastatic disease who were receiving active treatment and 0.59 in those receiving palliative care. In metastatic disease, the scores for mobility and vitality were significantly worse than the general population.

In a longitudinal study of over 12 months of men with prostate cancer and their spouses [30], the quality of life of the patients was better than that of the spouses at all stages of disease. Couples' quality of life improved with an increase in social support, open communication, decrease in uncertainty, and improvement in disease symptoms.

Quality-of-life instruments are useful for measuring global changes in populations and have been shown to be predictive of cancer survival [31], but they are less useful at an individual level. This weakness has led to the development of more specific patient-reported outcome measures (PROMs). In prostate cancer, pain response is the most frequently studied PROM but interpretation of the results from different trials is difficult because they often use different tools and different time schedules. Developing and validating PROMs is time-consuming but they offer a potentially valuable means of assessing meaningful outcomes for men with metastatic prostate cancer and deserve to be used more widely [32].

Physical exercise can result in a significant improvement in fatigue experienced by prostate cancer patients. A review [33] found evidence that an exercise program carried out either during or after cancer therapy resulted in a significant reduction of fatigue for patients with prostate and breast cancer.

A meta-analysis of coping strategies in prostate cancer found that men who confront their illness directly obtain psychological and physical benefits [34]. This finding is consistent with the transaction model of stress and coping [35] in which an individual's interpretation of a stressful event determines how they cope with it. Men with prostate cancer and their carers can use either internal or external coping options. Internal options are will power and inner strength which can be enhanced by training such as mindfulness [36]. External options include psychological support from health professionals or via self-help groups.

## Palliative and supportive care

A prospective longitudinal study that included 330 men with prostate cancer found that about 30% of patients had significant unmet needs when assessed with the Supportive Care Needs Survey, a validated 34-item measure that addresses 5 domains: psychological, health system and information, physical and daily activity, patient care and support, and sexuality [37]. Although the majority of the study population had no unmet needs, the findings support the development of care plans and the systematic assessment of patients' needs at various points in the cancer pathway.

Most of the literature on supportive care for prostate cancer patients focuses on the initial diagnosis and treatment. A literature review of patients' and carers' experiences of prostate cancer care found only 1 of 90 studies that dealt with palliative care and no studies that examined end-of-life care [38]. Clearly, there is a need for more research on supportive care for patients and carers dealing with metastatic prostate cancer.

Palliative care is a multiprofessional, holistic approach to managing advanced disease with a limited prognosis. Douglas Macmillan, an English civil servant, founded the Society for the Prevention and Relief of Cancer in 1911 after experiencing the death of his father from cancer. The modern hospice movement was founded by Dame Cicely Saunders in 1967. Palliative care should integrate seamlessly with all cancer treatment services, although historically it has been concentrated in the last few weeks and months of life. An assessment of hospice use by men dying of prostate cancer in the United States found that 53% (7646 of 14 521 men) used a hospice for a median of 24 days [39]. However, <10% of hospice users enrolled with a hospice more than 180 days before death. The men who did not enroll with a hospice underwent more imaging studies and received more high-intensity medical care in the last 6 months of life than those who used hospices. The authors conclude that the numbers of men enrolling for hospice care very close to the end of life remains too high. The association between hospice use and less-intensive medical care warrants further study.

In England, the NHS has promoted an End-of-Life Care program for patients with a terminal diagnosis and a prognosis of <1 year. The Gold Standards Framework has been created by health professionals in primary care to encourage early discussions with patients and their carers about care in the last year of life [40]. It is based on seven key tasks known as the seven C's: communication, coordination, control of symptoms, continuity, continued learning, carer support, and care in the dying phase.

The NHS End-of-Life Care program has also published data on place of death and costs in the last year of life for men with prostate cancer in England [41]. Hospital was the most frequent place of death (Figure 15.1). Table 15.1 shows the number and costs of hospital admissions in the last year of life but does not include costs of community care (outpatient, home, hospice, or nursing home). Patients had an average of 2.4 hospital admissions and the average cost of inpatient care in the final year of life for men with prostate cancer in England was £6931. Emergency admissions were considerably more expensive than elective admissions but the final admission to hospital was the most expensive. The authors of the report recommend better preemptive management to avoid emergency admission.

A small study from the United States of 32 men treated for prostate cancer at 5 military hospitals between 1995 and 1997 found that the mean

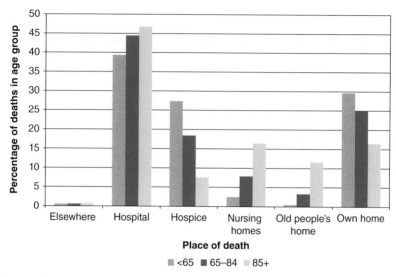

**Figure 15.1** Prostate cancer deaths by age and place of death, percentage of deaths in each age group, England 2001–2010.

total cost of hospitalization, outpatient visits, palliative procedures, and hormonal therapy in the last year of life was $24 660 [42].

It would appear that healthcare resources could be more efficiently used if men with end-stage prostate cancer were offered earlier contact with palliative care and hospice services which might result in fewer emergency admissions to hospital.

**Table 15.1** Admissions, length of stay, and cost in the last year of life, for men dying from prostate cancer in England in 2006–2008

|  | Elective | Emergency | Total |
|---|---|---|---|
| Admissions in the last year of life | 8181 | 41 829 | 50 010 |
| Bed days in the last year of life | 69 482 | 530 288 | 599 770 |
| Average length of stay per admission | 8.5 | 12.7 | 12.0 |
| Average admissions per person | 1.4 | 2.1 | 2.4 |
| Length of stay of final admission | 13.3 | 15.7 | 15.5 |
| **Total Cost (£)** | **15 553 710** | **126 574 654** | **142 128 364** |
| Cost per admission (£) | 1901 | 3026 | 2842 |
| Cost per person (£) | 2691 | 6448 | 6931 |
| Cost of final admission (£) | 2409 | 3323 | 3223 |

*Source: ONS mortality data.*

## Summary

The management of painful bone metastases is a significant issue for men with end-stage prostate cancer. Better use of opioid analgesia is required. The new radio-isotope radium-223 has the potential to improve symptom control after failure of hormonal and chemotherapy treatments.

Earlier involvement of palliative care and hospice services could prevent unnecessary emergency admissions to hospital and might result in more efficient utilization of healthcare resources.

## References

1 Howlader N, Noone AM, Krapcho M (eds). SEER Cancer Statistics Review, 1975–2009 (Vintage 2009 Populations). Bethesda, MD: National Cancer Institute. Available at http://seer.cancer.gov/csr/1975_2009_pops09/, based on November 2011 SEER data submission. Last accessed August 20, 2012 April 2012.

2 Cancer Research UK. UK cancer incidence (2010) and mortality (2010) summary, by Country Summary, April 2013.

3 Ryan CJ, Smith MR, de Bono JS, et al. Abiraterone in metastatic prostate cancer without previous chemotherapy. N Engl J Med 2013;368(2):138–148.

4 Tannock IF, Osoba D, Stockler MR, et al. Chemotherapy with mitoxantrone plus prednisone or prednisone alone for symptomatic hormone-resistant prostate cancer: a Canadian randomised trial with palliative endpoints. J Clin Oncol 1996;14(6):1756–1764.

5 Kantoff PW, Halabi S, Conaway M, et al. Hydrocortisone with or without mitoxantrone in men with hormone-refractory prostate cancer: results of the cancer and leukemia group B 9182 study. J Clin Oncol 1999;17(8):2506–2513.

6 Omlin A, Pezaro C, Mukherji D, et al. Improved survival in a cohort of trial participants with castration-resistant prostate cancer demonstrates the need for updated prognostic nomograms. Eur Urol 2013;64(2):300–306.

7 Deandrea S, Montanari M, Moja L, Apolone G. Prevalence of undertreatment in cancer pain. A review of published literature. Ann Oncol 2008;19(12):1985–1991.

8 Oldenmenger WH, Sillevis Smitt PA, van Dooren S, et al. A systematic review on barriers hindering adequate cancer pain management and interventions to reduce them: a critical appraisal. Eur J Cancer 2009;45(8):1370–1380.

9 WHO: WHO's pain ladder for adults. Available at http://www.who.int/cancer/palliative/painladder/en. Last accessed September 9, 2013.

10 NICE. Opioids in palliative care: safe and effective prescribing of strong opioids for pain in palliative care of adults. Available at http://publications.nice.org.uk/opioids-in-palliative-care-safe-and-effective-prescribing-of-strong-opioids-for-pain-in-palliative-cg140. Last accessed September 9, 2013.

11 Sze W-M, Shelley MD, Held I, et al. Palliation of metastatic bone pain: single fraction versus multifraction radiotherapy – a systemic review of randomised trials. Clin Oncol 2003;15(6):345–352.

12  Roos DE, Turner SL, O'Brien PC, *et al*. Randomised trial of 8 Gy in 1 versus 20 Gy in 5 fractions of radiotherapy for neuropathic pain due to bone metastases (Trans-Tasman Radiation Oncology Group, TROG 96.05). *Radiother Oncol* 2005;75(1): 54–63.

13  Baron R, Binder A, Wasner G. Neuropathic pain: diagnosis, pathophysiological mechanisms, and treatment. *Lancet Neurol* 2010;9(8):807–819.

14  Porter AT, McEwan AJ, Powe JE, *et al*. Results of a randomized phase III trial to evaluate the efficacy of strontium-89 adjuvant to local field external beam irradiation in the management of endocrine resistant metastatic prostate cancer. *Int J Radiat Oncol Biol Phys* 1993;25(5):805–813.

15  Sartor O, Reid RH, Hoskin PJ, *et al*. Quadramet 424Sm10/11 study group. Samarium 153-lexidronam complex for treatment of painful bone metastases in hormone-refractory prostate cancer. *Urology* 2004;63(5):940–945.

16  Nilsson S, Strang P, Aksnes AK, *et al*. A randomised, dose–response, multicenter phase II study of radium-223 chloride for the palliation of painful bone metastases in patients with castration-resistant prostate cancer. *Eur J Cancer* 2012;48(5):678–686.

17  Yuen KK, Shelley M, Sze WM, *et al*. Bisphosphonates for advanced prostate cancer. *Cochrane Database Sys Rev* 2006;(4):CD006250.

18  Hoskin P, Sundar S, Reczko K, *et al* A multicentre randomised trial of ibandronate compared to single dose radiotherapy for localised metastatic bone pain in prostate cancer (RIB). *Eur J Cancer* 2011;47(18) (Suppl 2):6.

19  Bayley A, Milosevic M, Blend R, *et al*. A prospective study of factors predicting clinically occult spinal cord compression in patients with metastatic prostate carcinoma. *Cancer* 2001;92(2):303–310.

20  Loblaw DA, Perry J, Chambers A, Laperriere NJ. Systematic review of the diagnosis and management of malignant extradural spinal cord compression: the Cancer Care Ontario Practice Guidelines Intitiative's Neuro-Oncology Disease Site Specific Group. *J Clin Oncol* 2005;23(9):2028–2037.

21  Klimo P, Thompson CJ, Kestle JRW, Schmidt MH. A meta-analysis of surgery versus conventional radiotherapy of metastatic spinal epidural disease. *Neuro Oncol* 2005;7(1):64–76.

22  George R, Jeba J, Rajkumar G, *et al*. Interventions for the treatment of metastatic extradural spinal cord compression in adults. *Cochrane Database Syst Rev* 2008;(4):CD006716.

23  Roque I, Figuls M, Martinez-Zapata MJ, *et al*. Radioisotopes for metastatic bone pain. *Cochrane Database Syst Rev* 2011;(7):CD003347.

24  Tu SM, Millikan RE, Mengistu B, *et al*. Bone targeted therapy for advanced androgen-independent carcinoma of the prostate: a randomised phase II trial. *Lancet* 2001;357(9253):336–341.

25  Fizazi K, Beuzeboc P, Lumbroso J, *et al*. Phase II trial of consolidation docetaxel and samarium-153 in patients with bone metastases from castration-resistant prostate cancer. *J Clin Oncol* 2009;27(15):2429–2435.

26  A randomised phase III trial of docetaxel plus prednisolone vs docetaxel with prednisolone plus either zoledronic acid, strontium-89 or both agents combined (TRAPEZE). Available at http://www.controlled-trials.com/ISRCTN12808747. Last accessed September 9, 2013.

27  Parker C, Heinrich D, O'Sullivan JM, *et al.* Overall survival benefit and safety profile of radium-223 chloride, a first-in-class alpha-pharmaceutical: results from a phase III randomized trial (ALSYMPCA) in patients with castration-resistant prostate cancer (CRPC) with bone metastases. *J Clin Oncol* 2012;30: (Suppl 5; abstr 8).

28  Sartor AO, Heinrich D, Helle SI, *et al.* Radium-223 chloride impact on skeletal-related events in patients with castration-resistant prostate cancer (CRPC) with bone metastases: a phase III randomized trial (ALSYMPCA). *J Clin Oncol* 2012;30:(Suppl 5; abstr 9).

29  Torvinen S, Farkkila N, Sintonen H, *et al.* Health-related quality of life in prostate cancer. *Acta Oncologica* 2013;52(6):1094–1101. doi:10.3109/0284186X.2012.760848.

30  Song L, Northouse LL, Braun TM, *et al.* Assessing longitudinal quality of life in prostate cancer pateints and their spouses: a multilevel modeling approach. *Qual Life Res* 2011;20(3):371–381.

31  Gotay CC, Kawamoto CT, Bottomley A, Efficace F. The prognostic significance of patient-reported outcomes in cancer clinical trials. *J Clin Oncol* 2008;26(8):1355–1363.

32  Eton DT, Shevrin DH, Beaumont J, *et al.* Constructing a conceptual framework of patient-reported outcomes for metastatic hormone-refractory prostate cancer. *Value Health* 2010;13(5):613–623.

33  Cramp F, Byron-Daniel J. Exercise for the management of cancer-related fatigue in adults. *Cochrane Database Syst Rev* 2012;11:CD006145.

34  Roesch SC, Adams L, Hines A, *et al.* Coping with prostate cancer: a meta-analytic review. *J Behav Med* 2005;28(3):281–293.

35  Lazarus RS, Folkman S. *Stress, Appraisal, and Coping*, New York, NY: Springer Publishing; 1984.

36  Learn mindfulness. Available at http://bemindful.co.uk/learn/about/. Last accessed September 9, 2013.

37  Armes J, Crowe M, Colbourne L, *et al.* Patients' supportive care needs beyond end of cancer treatment: a prospective, longitudinal study. *J Clin Oncol* 2009;27(36):6172–6179.

38  Sinfield P, Baker R, Camosso-Stefinovic J, *et al.* Mens' and carers' experiences of care for prostate cancer: a narrative literature review. *Health Expect* 2009;12(3):301–312.

39  Bergman J, Saigal CS, Lorenz KA, *et al.* Hospice use and high-intensity care in men dying of prostate cancer. *Arch Intern Med* 2011;171(3):204–210.

40  Hansford P, Meehan H. Gold standards framework: improving community care. *End of Life Care* 2007;1:56–61.

41  National End of Life Care Intelligence Network. Deaths from urological cancers in England, 2001–10. Available at http://www.endoflifecare-intelligence.org.uk/view?rid=683. Last accessed October 10, 2012.

42  Piper NY, Kusada L, Lance R, *et al.* Adenocarcinoma of the prostate: an expensive way to die. *Prostate Cancer Prostatic Dis* 2002;5(2):164–166.

## CHAPTER 16

# The Long Perspective: Prostate Cancer as a Chronic Disease

*Peter Whelan*

Pyrah Department of Urology, St. James's University Hospital, Leeds, UK

A great deal of clinical and scientific research into prostate cancer has been carried out over the past 30 years, yet curiously while we have been able to diagnose many more men with the condition and at a much earlier stage, over 90% are localized disease now; our ability to offer definitive prognosis to our patients still relies on nomograms [1] generated by selected patient populations in centers of excellence. Much of what was known in the past seems to have been forgotten. This chapter will review how matters have developed over the last three decades, examine where progress has been made, stress where important lessons have been ignored, and with the use of three case studies, point out where further research needs to be focused and as importantly, where patient education must be improved by physicians. Starting with the knowledge in the prostate-specific antigen (PSA) era, prostate cancer is a disease that will be potentially present for more than 20 years and that therapy next week is the last thing these patients need.

The diagnosis and management of prostate cancer was a relatively straightforward process 30 years ago [2]. Approximately half the patients presented incidentally, most frequently as the result of the histological findings after transurethral resection of the prostate (TURP), whereas the other half presented with advanced disease, with urinary obstruction or the effects of secondary spread such as bone pain or anemia, many of these cases proved fatal. A number of patients were found to have a suspicious prostate and underwent biopsy which itself had complications [3]. What was a reassurance even to the patients found to have metastatic disease was that effective palliative therapy was available, thanks to the work of

*Prostate Cancer: Diagnosis and Clinical Management*, First Edition.
Edited by Ashutosh K. Tewari, Peter Whelan and John D. Graham.
© 2014 John Wiley & Sons, Ltd. Published 2014 by John Wiley & Sons, Ltd.

Huggins [4], by androgen deprivation therapy. In those days, the blunter castration guaranteed most patients, even with substantial metastatic burdens, 2 years of good-quality life, although the hormonal therapy had its side effects. Many patients found with only a small amount of tumor in the chips at TURP, usually taken as less than 5%, were told they had a "small amount of cancer," reassured, and discharged [5]. This was the author's personal practice during this decade with no litigation or clinical problems to make the author regret it. The fact that the histology came from the transitional zone, that the sampling will have been very variable is one matter worthy of review in this period of saturation biopsy.

Although even in 1982 changes were happening with 100 000 cases being diagnosed in the United States with 31 000 deaths, in Europe the figure was that quoted above of approximately half the diagnosed patients dying of the disease. The situation now is that in Europe the ratio is 7.51:1, whereas in the United States it is 8.7:1. This cogently illustrates the level of overdiagnosis as the lifetime risk of death is about 3% not dissimilar to that of the 1980s, even though there has been a fall in mortality of 4% per year during the last 10 years. Part of the problem will have been the failure to always diagnose prostate cancer in the past and in the PSA era the larger number of known prostate cancer patients [6].

The change in the apparent nature of prostate cancer and its management commenced with two unrelated improvements. In 1982, Walsh carried out the first anatomic radical prostatectomy, the product of extensive anatomical research which brought about significant reductions in the troublesome side effects of incontinence and potency [7, 8]. Throughout the 1980s, other major groups such as Catalona [9], Stamey [10], Scardino [11], and the Mayo Clinic [12] produced selected series showing significantly improved, functional results over previous surgical series; what was not appreciated by groups coming after them was the influence of a paper by Jewett, from Johns Hopkins, showing that no patient with a poorly differentiated tumor survived following radical prostatectomy at 15 years [13]. All series from this new era faithfully selected men who did not have high-risk histology. Occasionally, patients were found to have high-grade histology on full pathological examination of the whole specimen, and these were sometimes reported, but they did not do well, as expected.

The second improvement was the finding of PSA and its use as a more effective and reliable substitute for acid phosphatase which had been used hitherto. This was used only in known patients as a monitoring blood test and it proved much more predictable of disease response and disease recurrence. The factor that fused these together was the United States

Food and Drug Administration (FDA) decision to allow PSA to be used as a screening tool [14]. Not surprisingly, large numbers of asymptomatic men were found to have a raised PSA, values of somewhat dubious provenance, as they were drawn from a relatively small group of men, numbered in the hundreds, who were assumed but never confirmed not to have prostate cancer. To hand appeared a certain cure, radical prostatectomy, with good functional results. Out went the practice of no treatment or watchful waiting, although it took several more years before the first randomized trial—the Scandinavian Group-4 study—comparing the two commenced; meaningful results from the trial only began to appear 10 years later [15].

This outcome, although noted by some to be over-zealous at the time [16], was not without its internal sense and coherence, based on concepts at the time. It was assumed that tumors progressed in a stepwise fashion; early disease would worsen and therefore the opportunity to cure was then rather than later. The fact that much of prostate cancer was a very slow growing disease and the use of PSA had moved the time of diagnosis now back to a full decade earlier was ignored in the pursuit of curing those who could be cured. Attempts had been made in the past to pick up patients at an early stage, most notably a German study of the 1970s using rectal examination on an annual basis. This study was repeated well into the PSA era and replicated the poor pick up rate it had demonstrated [17]. Small studies, involving over 800 patients and seemed large at the time, showed opportunistic rectal examination was very unsatisfactory [18]. PSA screening had produced a lot of men with elevated PSA levels and subsequent diagnosis of the disease. The radical prostatectomy rate in the United States and then the rest of the developed world soared and alongside it the complication rate as the procedure was not universally delivered to the same exacting standards of the major centers [19].

An unlooked for but pernicious effect of this rush to therapy, especially a surgical one in which the patient's expectation will have been one of complete cure, was that there was an imperative to treat these patients with "something," if during their follow-up their PSA became measurable, demonstrating that the treatment had failed in its objective; the "something" was hormone therapy. A minor change had come about in the delivery of androgen deprivation therapy, as much by serendipity as anything. Orchidectomy had become the dominant mode of therapy during the 1970s following studies in the late 1960s, showing that high-dose stilboestrol treatment had killed more patients from heart disease than were dying of prostate cancer, although later studies during the 1970s demonstrated that small doses of estrogens had a similar effect to orchidectomy [20]. It also became the clinical practice for some to recommend immediate orchidectomy if there was a large amount of tumor in resected chips or clinically the prostate gland seemed generally abnormal and a needle biopsy was positive. In the early 1980s, a failed contraceptive injection, luteinizing-hormone-releasing hormone (LHRH), was used as a medical substitute for orchidectomy and trials showed equivalent responses [21]. It says a great deal for the skills of marketing, and perhaps financial incentives, that this soon became a billion-dollar-a-year drug. Part of its increased usage was in the growing number of fit men with a rising PSA postsurgery. This led to the greatest failings of this current era in the production of a wholly iatrogenic disease, hormone-resistant nonmetastatic prostate cancer. A known, predictable, effective palliative treatment was sacrificed to try and treat a number, the size and value of which was not known; 2 years of good quality of life when the patient had metastases and needed this therapy was sacrificed to the chimera of effecting a cure with hormones that had never been demonstrated in more than a minority of patients, usually of the order of 10% [22].

As we will see from the three case studies, good can come even from this debacle. These cases seek to show the continuing problems in this disease and to develop the theme that in most men diagnosed contemporarily, time is on their side. They will need to live with the diagnosis for up to a quarter of their lives, much longer than most diabetics. It will seek to show that the focus of research must be on the high-risk groups; and in low-risk ones, a reversal to the former management ethos of earlier times is not only economically vital but in the patient's best interest, and it is our role to educate, as well as give out options mechanistically. In no other disease at present have men the time to determine just what they, individually, want.

The first case concerns a retired doctor aged 68. He sought advice when his brother died from prostate cancer aged 71, especially as his father had died from the disease aged 79. Further enquiry of the family history yielded an uncle, his father's brother, who had been diagnosed with prostate cancer but who had died of a myocardial infarct aged 65. His general physician (GP) recommended a PSA test which came back as 0.1 ng/mL. The GP suggested a further test in a year. He consulted a number of urologists and oncologists but took the advice from a geneticist that he could be at high risk, so recommending a biopsy. With some reluctance he got a radiologist to undertake this and the histology came back as prostate cancer Gleason grade 8 (4+4). He underwent a bone and CT scan and at his request a PET scan, which were all negative and elected to have a robotically assisted radical prostatectomy. He rejected any further PSA tests postoperatively, even hypersensitive assays, but agreed to an annual bone scan which would be done more frequently if he developed symptoms. He indicated that he would probably only accept further therapy if he developed recurrences which became symptomatic. He remains disease-free for 3.5 years on, based on bone scan criteria.

The second case involves a man diagnosed at age 61 years in 1977. This diagnosis followed an episode of urinary retention for which he underwent a TURP. About 22% of the chips were shown to be moderately differentiated prostate cancer (pre-Gleason but probably equivalent to Gleason grade 7) and he was offered immediate orchidectomy. He came under the author's care 10 years or so later when his PSA was >0.05 ng/mL at which level he remained into his early eighties. He was quite fit and thought 20 years long enough to have followed up the disease. A dosimetry bone scan was arranged which showed only age-related changes and no osteoporosis. He was discharged, had no further PSA tests, and died aged 92 of a cerebrovascular accident (CVA).

The third case involves another doctor. He was 57 when he consulted a neurosurgeon friend about a pain in his lower back that had developed 4 weeks previously and had become excruciating over the previous 10 days. An X-ray showed a sclerotic lesion at L3 and a bone scan showed that this was an isolated lesion. Biopsy demonstrated a poorly differentiated prostate cancer Gleason grade 9 (4+5). Subsequent rectal examination demonstrated a hard, malignant feeling gland but this was not biopsied and his PSA was 107 ng/mL. He was seen initially by a radiation oncologist who treated the local lesion with 16 Gy external beam radiotherapy and put him on combined androgen blockade of LHRH injections and an antiandrogen. His PSA rapidly fell in the first 3 months to 0.8 ng/mL and, as his wife was 13 years younger than him, the LHRH was not continued and when at 6 months his PSA had fallen further to 0.4 ng/mL the antiandrogen was also discontinued. He went into a formal program of intermittent therapy with a PSA level of 25 ng/mL as the trigger to recommence the antiandrogen. He achieved more than 2.5 years response to this regime before recommencing the antiandrogen, the PSA kept going up to 31 ng/mL. He was switched to LHRH with the same regime and achieved a further 2 years response before the PSA again rose to over 40 ng/mL and his PSA kept on going up despite the injections. His bone scan throughout this time had shown a fading of the original lesion and no new ones. He achieved a further 18 months response to estrogens, again on an intermittent basis before the PSA rose to over 100 ng/mL and his bone scan showed the presence of new lesions in his ribs and left glenoid.

He had 6 years of symptom-free response, had been off any medication for more than 65% of this time, and had managed to continue working and retired when he wanted to, a few months before the onset of new symptoms. He felt his work defined him and he had wanted to carry on as long as he was well and it was safe to do so. He remained on estrogens, and was offered Taxanes but chose to take just prednisolone, which gave a response of both symptoms and a small fall in his PSA to 87 ng/mL. His left shoulder pain became accentuated 5 months into this treatment but he got symptomatic relief from "spot" radiotherapy to this area. The PSA only rose marginally so when at 10 months he developed generalized bone pain, he opted for strontium-89 which gave symptomatic relief for 4 months. His PSA had now risen to 153 ng/mL and he accepted to go onto Taxetere, although there was some apprehension of marrow problems in view of the relatively recent radioactive isotope treatment. However, he had no such problems and usually had only 1 day in the chemotherapy cycle when he took to his bed, being otherwise very active. There was a decline of the PSA to 98 ng/mL and he remained symptomatically well for a further 8 months. His PSA rose abruptly to 219 ng/mL, he recommended Taxanes but reacted to them badly and declined further treatment. He did accept supportive care, which included several short, localized treatments of radiotherapy for pain and several transfusions. Within the British system, he became part of a hospice system, but slowly as with so many terminal prostate cancer patients, he developed a debilitating weakness but maintained his appetite, bodily functions, and had little pain, and died just about 8 years from the time of diagnosis. From the hormonal studies of the 1980s and early 1990s, one would have predicted that he would have an almost certain 5-year response and he went longer undoubtedly because of other active therapies than hormones.

These three cases illustrate the axiom that an average is one case in a hundred, and that all cases will occur differently and the patients will have different needs. The first case emphasizes the difficulties of the use of PSA. Although in population terms it threw up a great deal of prostate cancer, the majority of the cases are of low risk. We have known since autopsy studies from the 1950s that there is a large amount of indolent cancers in the prostate and that if we live long enough; foci of tumor will be found in most men [23]. A study carried out well into the PSA era showed a three-fold decline in the findings of indolent prostate cancers, unsurprisingly as so many men had had their PSAs measured, been biopsied, and found to have a low-grade tumor, which may or may not have been treated [24]. Thus, proving the obvious that PSA is nondiscriminatory and other factors need to be considered to reduce the overdiagnosis and overtreatment. The first patient would never have been picked up in any PSA screening program, but perhaps investigation of high-risk family groups if carried out under trial conditions may actually lead to a higher pick up rate of significantly at-risk patients. The second problem this patient faced when all current tests showed the disease to be localized was which therapy to have. Few people would have suggested to him active monitoring with no indicators save the presence of metastases to act as markers. On the evidence, the recommendation would have been some form of high-dose radiotherapy [25], primarily because the urological community has done itself no favors in not until now producing a good body of evidence to see whether the findings of Jewett in a small, completely unrepresentative, series is actually true. Extirpative surgery should be able to deliver equivalent outcomes to radiotherapy but perhaps the high doses that can now be delivered does make radiotherapy superior. The serial outcomes of the Scandinavian trial have been salutary. It has shown a modest, about 5–6%, benefit for surgery over watchful waiting, but there has not been the plateauing of the death rate of the treated arm that would be expected once the final cured cohort had been reached [15]. A second, American trial (PIVOT) has also recently reported no difference between their treated arm and the active surveillance arm [26].

Rather than relearning that a lot of prostate cancer is slowly moving the "something must be done" school, with a breathtaking absence of evidence, has continued to promote therapies for low-risk prostate cancer. There has been a major change in the United States in the type of treatment for low- and intermediate-risk disease. This has come about not through any defining trial but exclusively through economics. Brachytherapy, developed in its current state in the 1990s [27], can be delivered as a day case at 60% of the cost of open surgery; the number of treatments of brachytherapy overtook surgical ones in the United States in 2007 and now outnumbers them significantly. Newer treatments with different energy sources are also treating this same group of patients [28]. Not surprisingly, in these economically straitened times a recent paper has made an overwhelming economic case for active surveillance demonstrating a $8 billion saving. There is no clinical, high-grade evidence to gainsay this [29].

In summary for first case, 30 years ago with little knowledge of familial prostate cancer and an aversion to surgery in high-risk patients, assuming it could have been found, although paradoxically, an odd feeling prostate clinically may have led to a biopsy; the likelihood is that this patient would have only presented when he developed symptomatic metastases. There is a chance that at least a prolonged response may have been achieved, but we have no comparative data and know little more than a generation ago, and the patient had to push to get the diagnosis on the advice of a geneticist.

Second case addresses a number of issues. All hormone studies, even in patients with metastases, demonstrate a small 5–10% long-term survival. First, no biochemical abnormality was ever demonstrated in this man so it is possible that the tumor was wholly in the transitional zone and the combination of local surgery and castration may have been curative. We do know that androgen deprivation is not a one-off therapy. Work from 30 years ago showed that if one form of hormone treatment failed either estrogens or orchiectomy [2], using the other often produced a further response and more recent work has shown that several responses can be achieved although the number of responders and duration of responses falls [30]. The important study by Bolla *et al.* [31] showed that radiation therapy plus immediate hormone treatment, in this case for 3 years, produced a significantly better outcome than radiotherapy alone. D'Amico *et al.* [32] demonstrated that the duration of androgen ablation need only 6 months. Some skeptics wondered whether the radiotherapy was actually needed, but an international trial did show a superior outcome to the combination therapy compared with hormones alone [33]. This patient, therefore, in retrospect may have done equally well with radiotherapy which was the standard of care in his day. With the ability to deliver very high radiation doses now to a specific area the need to include hormones is again being debated. When tried in an analogous fashion with radical surgery, they produced no benefit [34] and an arm of a large international antiandrogen trial had to be stopped in low-risk patients who were doing worse than the nontreated arm [35]. Moving hormones upstream, especially if new modes of delivering radiotherapy are good, on their own appears less and less justified.

The last of the cases brings out two very important points that will be examined in some detail. First, the extent and volume of metastatic disease does enable an approximate prognosis in time to be given, whereas never accurate to the month, it does enable a "ballpark figure" of control to be arrived at. Crudely, even the most extensive disease will be unlucky not to get 2 years of good quality of life, and the smaller the burden of disease, the more time can be added; experience rather than pathways may be a better guide. The speed of response to hormones is also a good prognostic indicator and this patient had both. There are genuine hormone nonresponders, but these are small in number. Patients in this situation can, therefore, be given a reasonable time to lead a normal life, as did this man, controlling their own destiny. The other point is that when hormones have failed, the patient becomes a true cancer patient with incurable disease. This man got good responses both from a somewhat eccentric use of steroids but then a confirmed response to Taxanes [36] with little in the way of side effects although he bailed out of a further course as he found the treatment in the oncology ward burdensome as well as reacting badly to a second course, with his whole time being spent as a professional patient. He had the knowledge and insight to opt for some peace and quiet rather than frantically chase down possibilities of treatments that could only offer a few extra weeks.

The point to repeat is that in the hormone-naïve patient a predictable, prolonged response occurs and the profligate use of hormones to treat a biochemical level was and is indefensible. But it is only one of a number of problems that makes a realistic reappraisal difficult in all stages of prostate cancer. Whitmore, a past chief of urology at Memorial Sloan Kettering cancer center stated, "you have to remember that many more people earn their living from prostate cancer than die from it."

In comparison to the massive fall in the death rate from cardiovascular disease that lifestyle changes and active therapy has wrought [37], the modest single-figure percentage reduction in the death rate in one of only two properly randomized trials of active versus palliative therapy in prostate cancer is no advertisement for business as usual. A concern magnified with the move to robotic assisted surgery and its current greater expense is that the increased investment is not justified with the current patient outcomes [38], and the failure to tackle the high-risk cases in a systematic way that can at least be reported and compared with similar groups runs the risk of surgical therapy being considered as a income-generating process for the surgeons but not a good therapeutic option for the patient. Allied to this is the fact that these complex procedures are done by many people, often with low case loads [39], when optimum benefit is least likely to accrue. Radiation therapy offer treatments that are cheaper and delivered as day cases through the high-energy sophisticated equipment that is already tackling large numbers of high-risk patients. The treatment of low- and intermediate-risk cases appears no way inferior, although there are the usual problems of selection bias with no comparative studies. Only a few surgical centers are competing at all with treating the high-risk patient. Looking then at progress over the 30 years, we still seem consciously or unconsciously to be in thrall to Jewett's caution about the bad outcomes of high-risk patients and, however modern robots appear, they are still only performing an extirpative procedure which at present in scientific trials has only shown a marginal benefit for patients over essentially palliative therapy [40]. No robot-assisted randomized trials have yet appeared to show the added value to the patient, although like many things the great value of the robot may be in teaching surgery by means of a simulator so that the trained surgeon minimizes the "learning curve" and ensures better outcomes all round, as radical prostatectomy still seems very dependent on case selection and operator's skill. The best published series are probably those of Myers [41, 42], late of the Mayo Clinic, but procedures that work should not be so capricious, and surgical therapies should be deliverable within fairly narrow limits of outcomes. The robot for its indirect benefits for surgery may be here to stay but possibly not for radical prostatectomy. Analysis from the Scandinavian study suggests that many groups of men such as those with low-risk disease get no benefit at all from the operation and younger groups with more aggressive disease are not benefitting significantly, more data with clear benefit to younger patients urgently need to be generated [40].

Inactive therapy for prostate cancer 30 years ago was much more prevalent and frequently justified because of the known slow growth of many tumors, but also because large numbers of competing morbidities patients had especially cardiovascular ones. Today, the cumulative risks do not appear to be that different. A Swedish cohort study of long-term follow-up of men in a county cancer registry shows that when men are over 70, they are six times more likely to die from co-morbid disease than from their prostate cancer [43]. The second patient was probably overtreated but he fortunately suffered none of the side effects both physically and mentally that can be associated with prolonged androgen deprivation. Overtreatment can inflict needless suffering on patients especially if these agents are used early and the patient can neither see nor derive benefit from them to compensate for these complications.

The third patient, although unable to anticipate a cure of his disease could look forward to a reasonable period of active life and the ability to utilize intermittent hormone therapy which, while not being superior to continuous therapy, appears to be equivalent and certainly enhances retention of potency which was an important issue in this case. The author first gained experience of intermittent hormone therapy from a patient who was on estrogens. He was very compliant during the winter saying that the drugs improved his circulation but come the summer when he was running a park funfair and had a more "active" life (his words), he stayed off the tablets until the funfair shut down, when he then recommenced. He spent approximately 6 months on and 6 months off the drugs and showed no signs of progression until finally removing himself to the coast. The good thing about LHRH and antiandrogens is that all are amenable to intermittent usage without loss of effect [44], and with this, patient-individualized treatment programs can be built around patients' needs and desires.

How can we formulate a rational scheme of dealing with prostate cancer when we rely on a test that fails the first principle of screening in not being able to identify a population that is not at risk? The recent action of the US Preventive Task Force that recommended that screening should not be undertaken is likely to be more than just a straw in the wind [45]. First, we must understand that we have created an environment that needs to be changed. As the disease does not affect individuals in different ways dependent on culture, so treatment advice should not be different. It is counterintuitive for a patient to take a "cancer test" find that it is abnormal, have a biopsy which gives him a diagnosis of prostate cancer, and then be told that we will watch this until it is serious before any treatment will commence: quite reasonably the patient will go off to another doctor who "knows what they are doing." However, the ProtecT study in the United Kingdom has demonstrated that it is quite possible [46], using trained counselors, to convey the appropriate information about not needing to rush a decision and even encourage men to enter a randomized trial. Patient education is our responsibility and patient ignorance is not an excuse to miss this process out.

The default position of all but the most high-risk patient must, given the very long lead time PSA has conferred, be that of active surveillance. Patients must have the benefit of unbiased counseling and the idea reinforced that time for most of these cases is long and not limited [47]. There must be understanding that some patients cannot accept this course of action and some form of active therapy is needed by them psychologically. They must be enabled to have a choice so that the perceived benefits and known side effects are fully understood. Surgical, contemporary series of high-risk patients must be generated or an acceptance made that these patients are not helped by surgery, at the moment we are still influenced by a small selective surgical series from 50 years ago.

The variability of PSA must be emphasized and knowledge that it can rise to 30 ng/mL or more without mishap needs to be reinforced [48].

Evidence of slow progress of the disease even in advanced disease needs to be made known to the patient and efforts need to be made to get them to understand the problems of hormone-resistant nonmetastatic prostate cancer and that they will be trading temporary psychological relief with seeing a falling PSA, for the assurance of effective palliation if the disease progresses. This phase of a rising PSA must be the scene of our most strenuous research efforts. If the prostate is still *in situ* then some form of initial or further local therapy can be used including all the new forms of focused energy but in a properly conducted trial setting in patients showing evidence of activity and therefore, likely to show measurable responses even in this slowly progressive condition [49]. It would also be the ideal phase of the disease to try out novel systemic therapies which have been shown in advanced disease to have some effect, especially those whose mode of action is thought to be through the androgen receptor. But chemotherapy, small molecules, vaccines, etc., need to have the opportunity of having demonstrated an effect in the presence of only small-volume disease. None of the current agents presently being trialed have ever demonstrated the almost magical effect of androgen deprivation therapy on bone and visceral metastases, which so frequently melt away [50]. Such a testing regime would enable us to set out a scheme of sequential therapies for those with active disease which would seek to control it for as long as possible before moving on to the next agent. This would then enable us to reserve androgen deprivation therapy to its rightful place in giving patients a guaranteed period of effective palliation when the disease has progressed and not use up this precious asset in the futile aim of trying to stabilize a biochemical number. It would also demonstrate by analogy to other diseases that we are treating a chronic condition not a rapidly fatal cancer.

This chapter has sought to assert the very long natural history of prostate cancer that now exists, thanks to the widespread use of PSA testing. It has shown that the rush to diagnosis has inevitably led to overtreatment with patients potentially suffering side effects they need not have had. It has shown that this has led to the pernicious misuse of the most consistent active agent in advanced disease, so that whereas 30 years ago they could be assured of at least 2 years of good-quality palliative care, the current very expensive agents give them only a few weeks if they respond.

Prostate cancer causes death but in only a minority of patients diagnosed with the condition. Defining the at-risk patient must be the only worthwhile focus of our research [51]; we have had a decade or more of mass extirpation of the prostate with a very modest reduction in overall mortality of the condition. As stated above, in 1980 31 000 American males died from prostate cancer, in 2013 the predicted death rate is 29 730. In absolute terms, there has been no movement. Relearning some of the lessons of the past will not go amiss especially as we can now add on 10 years to the way we know prostate cancer behaves.

*The old Hollywood scriptwriters always used to ask the film's director whether he wanted the script good or on Tuesday. Over the last couple of decades, we have produced a Tuesday result for our patients, they deserve good.*

## References

1 Kattan MW, Shariat SF, Andrews B, *et al.* The addition of interleukin-6 soluble receptors and transforming growth factor beta improves a preoperative nomogram for predicting biochemical progression in patients with clinically localized prostate cancer. *J Clin Oncol* 2003;21:3573–3579.

2 Whitmore WF. Prostate cancer. Overview: historical and contemporary. *NCI Monogr* 1988;7:7–20

3 Mobley JE, Redman JF, Black RM, *et al.* Hemorrhage from transrectal needle biposy of the prostate. *J Am Med Assoc* 1971;216(11):1868–1867.

4 Huggins C, Stevens RE, Hodges CV. Studies on prostate cancer II. The effects of castration on advanced carcinoma of the prostate gland. *Arch Surg* 1941;43:209–217.

5 Barnes R, Hirst A, Rosenquist R. Early carcinoma of the prostate: comparison of stages A and B. *J Urol* 1976;115:404–409.

6 Schroeder FH, Roobol MJ. Prostate cancer epidemic in sight? *Eur Urol* 2012;61(6): 1079–1092.

7 Walsh PC, Lepor H, Eggleston JC. Radical prostatectomy with preservation of sexual function, anatomical and pathological associations. *Prostate* 1983;4:473–485.

8 Walsh PC, Quinlan D, Morton RA, *et al.* Radical retropubic prostatectomy. Improved anastomosis and urinary continence. *Urol Clin North Am* 1990;17:679–684.

9 Catalona WJ, Bigg SW. Nerve sparing radical prostatectomy. Evaluation of results after 250 patients. *J Urol* 1990;143:538–543.

10 Stamey TA, McNeal JE, Freiha FS, *et al.* Morphological and clinical studies on 68 consecutive radical prostatectomies. *J Urol* 1988;139:1235–1244.

11 Eastham J, Scardino P. Radical prostatectomy for clinical stages T1 and T2 prostate cancer. In: *Comprehensive Textbok of Genito – Urinary Oncology* (eds N Vogelzang, P Scardino, W Shipley, *et al.*). Philadelphia, PA: Lippincott Williams & Wilkins; 1999. pp 727–738.

12 Lerner SG, Blute ML, Lieber MM, *et al.* Morbidity of contemporary radical retropubic prostatectomy for localized prostate cancer. *Oncology* 1995;9(5):328–335.

13 Jewett HJ. The present status of radical prostatectomy for stages A and B prostate cancer. *Urol Clin North Am* 1975;2:105–112.

14 United States Department of Health & Human Services. *U.S. Food and Drug Administration Approves Test for Prostate Cancer* (Press Release). Silver Spring, MD: FDA; 1994.

15 Bil-Axelsson A, Holmberg L, Filen F, *et al.* Radical prostatectomy versus watchful waiting in localized prostate cancer: the Scandinavian prostate cancer trial group-4 randomised trial. *N Eng J Med* 2011;364(18):1708–1712.

16  Whelan P. Are we promoting stress and anxiety? *BMJ* 1997;315:1549.

17  Lubbolt HJ, Bex A, Swoboda A, *et al.* Early detection of prostate cancer in Germany, study using digital rectal examination and 4.0ng/ml prostate specific antigen. *Eur Urol* 2001;39(2):131–137.

18  Chodak GW, Schoenberg HW. Early detection of prostate cancer by routine screening. *J Am Med Assoc* 1984;252(23):3261–3264.

19  Fowler FJ, Barry MJ, Lu-Yao G, *et al.* Patient-reported complications and follow-up treatment after radical prostatectomy. The National Medicare Experience: 1988–1990 (updated June 1993). *Urology* 1993;42:622–629.

20  Byar DP. The Veterans Administration Cooperative Urological Research Group's studies of cancer of the prostate. *Cancer* 1973;32:1126–1135.

21  Vogelzang NJ, Chodak GW, Soloway MS, *et al.* Goserelin versus orchidectomy in the treatment of advanced prostate cancer. Final results of a randomized trial. Zoladex Prostate Study Group. *Urology* 1995;46:220–226.

22  Schroeder FH, Crawford DP, Axcrona K, *et al.* Androgen deprivation therapy; past, present, and future. *BJU Int* 2012;109(Suppl. 6):1–12.

23  Edwards CN, Steinthorsson E, Nicholson D. An autopsy study of latent prostate cancer. *Cancer* 1953;6(3):531–554.

24  Konety BR, Bird VY, Deorah S, *et al.* Comparison of incidence of latent prostate cancer delineated at autopsy before and after prostate specific antigen. *J Urol* 2005;174(5):1785–1788.

25  Prada PJ, Gonzalez H, Fernandez J, *et al.* Biochemical outcome after high dose rate intensity modulated brachytherapy with external beam radiotherapy: 12 years of experience. *BJU Int* 2011;109:1787–1793.

26  Wilt T. Prostate intervention versus observation trust (PIVOT). Initial results. *NCI Cancer Bull* 2011;8(11):12.

27  Blasko JC, Ragde H, Grimm PD. Transperineal ultrasound guided implantation of the prostate, morbidity and complications. *Scand J Urol Nephrol* 1991;137:113–118.

28  Ahmed HU, Zackarakis E, Dudderidge T, *et al.* High intensity focused therapy for localized prostate cancer, the first UK series. *Br J Cancer* 2009;101:19–26.

29  Keegan KA, Dall'era MA, Durbin-Johnson B, *et al.* Active surveillance for prostate cancer compared with immediate treatment – an economic analysis. *Cancer* 2012; 118:3512–3518.

30  Kotwal S, Whelan P. Does failure of single hormone therapy delineate hormone refractoriness for prostate cancer? *Scand J Urol Nephrol* 2008;42(2):116–120.

31  Bolla M, Collette L, Blank L, *et al.* Long term results from immediate androgen suppression and external radiation in patients with locally advanced prostate cancer(an EORTC study): a phase III randomized trial. *Lancet* 2002;360:103–106.

32  D'Amico AV, Chen MH, Renshaw AA, *et al.* Androgen suppression and radiation versus radiation alone for prostate cancer, a randomized trial. *J Am Med Assoc* 2008;299:289–295.

33  Warde P, Mason M, Ding K, *et al.* Combined androgen deprivation therapy and radiation therapy for locally advanced prostate cancer: a randomized, phase 3 trial. *Lancet* 2011;378(9809):2104–2111.

34  Soloway MS, Sharifi R, Waisman Z, *et al.* Prospective trial comparing radical prostatectomy alone versus radical prostatectomy preceded by androgen blockade in clinical B2 (T2bNxMO) prostate cancer. *J Urol* 1995;154920:424–428.

35 Casodex Summary of Product Characteristics, April 2009 Electronic Medicines Compendium Website. Available at www.medicines.org.uk/guides/casodex. Last accessed July, 2012.

36 Tannock IF, de Wit R, Berry WR, *et al.* Docetaxol plus prednisone or mitoxantrone for advanced prostate cancer. *N Eng J Med* 2004;351:1502–1512.

37 Peeters A, Nusselder WJ, Stereton C, *et al.* The reduction of cardiovascular deaths in last 15 years. *Eur J Epidemiol* 2012;26(5):364–373.

38 Barbash GL, Giled SA. New technology and health care costs. *N Eng J Med* 2010;363:701–704.

39 Savage CC, Vickers AJ. Low annual caseloads in US systems including radical prostatectomy. *J Urol* 2009;182(6):2677–2679.

40 Vickers A, Bennette C, Steineck G, *et al.* Individualised estimation of the benefit of radical prostatectomy from the Scandinavian Prostate Cancer Group randomized trial. *Eur Urol* 2012;62:204–209.

41 Myers RP. Localised prostate cancer. Important points of conduct for radical retropubic prostatectomy. *Eur Urol Suppl* 2002;1(1):15–19.

42 Hubanks JM, Umbreit EC, Karnes RJ, Myers RP. Open radical retropubic prostatectomy using high anterior release of the levator fascia and constant haptic feedback in bilateral neurovascular bundle preservation plus early postoperative phosphodiesterase type 5 inhibition: a contemporary series. *Eur Urol* 2012;61:878–884.

43 Stattin P, Holmberg F, Johansson JE, *et al.* Outcomes in localized prostate cancer: National Prostate Cancer Register of Sweden follow-up study. *J Natl Cancer Inst* 2010;102(13):950–958.

44 Calais da Silva FM, Bono AV, Whelan P, *et al.* Intermittent androgen deprivation for locally advanced and metastatic prostate cancer: results from phase3 study of South European Uro-oncology group. *Eur Urol* 2009;55:1269–1277.

45 Chou R, Croswell JM, Dana T, *et al.* Screening for prostate cancer: a review of evidence for the US Preventive Services Task Force. *Ann Intern Med* 2011;155(11):762–771; quoted Albertsen P. *Eur Urol* 2012;62:201–203.

46 Donovan J, Hamdy F, Neal DF, *et al.* Prostate testing for cancer and treatment (ProtecT) feasibility study. *Health Technol Assess* 2003;7(14).

47 Studer U, Collette L, Whelan P, *et al.* Using PSA to guide timing of androgen deprivation in patients with T0–T4 prostate cancer not suitable for local curative treatment (EORTC 30891). *Eur Urol* 2008;53:941–949.

48 Studer U, Whelan P, Albrecht W, *et al.* Immediate or deferred androgen deprivation in patients with T0–T4 N0-2 M0 prostate cancer not suitable for local curative treatment: EORTC trial 30891. *J Clin Oncol* 2006;24:1868–1876.

49 Ripert T, Azemar AM, Menard J, *et al.* Six years experience with high intensity focused ultrasonography for prostate cancer: oncological outcomes using the new 'Stuttgart' definition for biochemical failure. *Eur Urol* 2010;57:1899–1905.

50 Shore N, Mason M, de Reijke TM. New developments in castrate-resistant prostate cancer. *BJU Int* 2012;109(Suppl. 6):22–32.

51 McGuire BB, Helfand BT, Kundu S, *et al.* Association with prostate cancer risk alleles with unfavourable pathological features in potential candidates for active surveillance. *BJU Int* 2012;110:338–343.

## CHAPTER 17

# The Future: What's in the Toolkit for Prostate Cancer Diagnosis and Treatment?

*Norman J. Maitland*

Department of Biology, YCR Cancer Research Unit, University of York, Heslington, York, UK

## Introduction

As a basic scientist it is often difficult to convince my scientific colleagues of the need to consider the clinical consequences of their research. The phrase "translational research" was often interpreted to mean "soft" science. Collaboration with the pharma industry, on whom we are increasingly reliant for the budgets to bring a new treatment to reality, was viewed as worse that Faust selling his soul to the devil.

Translational medical research only emerges from a hard understanding of how things *work*, just like an engineering or architectural project is based on sound mathematics and physics. Experimental design should always, for medical researchers, encompass the clinical situation. In the prostate cancer literature, on an internet search reveals almost half a million references which link prostate cancer treatment to the LNCaP cell line. How many of these are actually in the clinic? The gap between the lab and the clinic shows every sign of widening, as the depth of our understanding of the scientific basis of cancer increases. This is in spite of governmental and charity directives to include an impact or translational statement (in a format understandable by the educated common man) in all applications for funding.

I hope to illustrate some of the opportunities, which may become available to clinicians as a result of basic science. However, it is important for *both* professions to bridge the "gulf of translation." Perhaps we need to

---

re-examine how clinicians treat prostate cancer in the light of new scientific developments, rather than the scientists designing new agents to fit established treatment regimes.

## The future of diagnosis

Accurate diagnosis is probably one of the greatest challenges extant in the prostate cancer field. We have had a test in routine practice, for prostate-specific antigen (PSA), for more than 20 years [1]. It has been refined, but it is still registering sensitivity and selectivity scores, which do not satisfy both patients and clinicians. The same is true for histopathological diagnosis. The Gleason system has been in use since 1987 (although most of the hard work was done in the 1960s) [2]. It has now been further improved, but still excludes the influence of gene expression [3]. Some time ago, state-of-the-art gene expression array technology showed that there was a distinction between the Gleason patterns 3 and 4 [4]. New markers, for example, genes such as AMACR or p63 can refine this diagnosis, but much is still dependent on the skill and discrimination of the histopathologist [5].

There is also the enduring problem of: (i) the requirement for multiple biopsies, (ii) the limitations in the biopsy procedure (anterior sites are difficult to access), and most of all (iii) the "snapshot" nature of the procedure. A histopathologist can only read the section placed on the microscope stage, and there is a frequent upgrading of tumors after radical prostatectomy. What is required is a means of imaging the entire prostate (and the local lymph nodes) in a non-invasive manner, which can define the extent of the tumor and its grade, extension within and locally outside the prostate.

This can be addressed on two levels. The first level involves monitoring for overt signs of metastases, and the physical ability to spread via the vascular/lymphatic systems, by monitoring serum-borne markers. The second means is to devise real-time imaging which can distinguish a potentially malignant mass from an organ-confined non-malignant mass of the same size. This can be achieved either by direct monitoring of genes, or of processes associated with malignant change. Sophisticated contrasting agents for ionic content/charge, pH, and various metabolites such as the predominant polyamines in prostate combined with improved-resolution NMR, PET, and combined imaging such as infrared spectroscopy could resolve these differences and are in clinical trial.

Direct exploitation of the altered state of invasive tumor cells, based on previously determined gene expression signatures, could be combined with imaging, in a more sophisticated form of the prostatscint assay, which detected the elevated expression of prostate-specific membrane antigen (PSMA) [6]. Unexpectedly, PSMA was also found on tumor (and other) neovasculature, which increased the noise in the assay, but enhanced the signal in a highly vascularized tumor. For an improved-resolution assay to work, we require both an accessible tumor and an antibody/peptide reagent which is both specific for malignancy and preferentially localized to the external surface of the tumor cells. Accessibility of an intravenously applied imaging agent can be restricted both by the size and charge of the reagent. Improvements in antibody technology such as high-affinity single-chain "exotic" antibodies, like those from camelids (e.g., llamas); dual-specificity reagents; aptamers; and high-affinity modified peptides are all available in experimental systems: but will they pass the clinical tests?

## A soluble problem: serum biomarkers

If we accept that all interventions in cancer patients are likely to alter the natural history of the disease, then non-invasive, remote monitoring is most desirable. However, what is the best source of biomarkers? Do we exploit molecules secreted into the blood, urine, or indeed seminal fluid? All three sources can provide different information about the status of clinical disease (Table 17.1). A full discussion of all biomarkers is out with this review but can be found elsewhere [7]. However, the ideal marker should be (i) stable (to enable clinical sampling without a need for expensive shipping and storage), (ii) be expressed at levels with a sufficient dynamic range to permit the stratification of patients, (iii) be amenable to a practical noncomplex assay (to eliminate laboratory errors), but perhaps most importantly, (iv) must reflect the natural history of the tumor, and not just prostate *disease*. Ideally, one would want a stable molecule whose level increased with the severity of disease, and was able to distinguish non-malignant from malignant disease, and not just the degree of vascularization (for example) of a lesion in the prostate.

**1. Secreted proteins:** The classical secreted marker protein for prostate cancer remains PSA, which replaced prostatic acid phosphatase some 20 years ago. Although considerable clinical information can be gained from PSA measurements, particularly when the bound:free ratio and ultrasensitive assays are performed [8], there is an urgent need for new markers, to augment PSA (as a combination) or indeed to replace it.

**Table 17.1** Advanced diagnostic tools for the early detection of metastatic prostate cancer

| Diagnostic tool | Biological material | Source of clinical material | Comments |
| --- | --- | --- | --- |
| ELISA | Protein | B, U, PS/SF, C | Established and highly sensitive method, capable of detecting <1 ng protein in routine setting, e.g., PSA |
| Autoantibodies | Protein | B | Antibodies from patient serum directed against random peptides which can distinguish (used as a panel of multiple targets) malignant tumors |
| MicroRNA | RNA | B, U(?), C | Small highly stable RNA involved in gene control; expression is changed in cancers; can be identified in blood |
| Fragmented RNA | RNA | B, U(?), C | Like miRNA, fragmented RNA can be readily isolated from venous blood |
| Exosomes | Small vesicles | B, U, PS/SF(?) | Endosome-derived vesicles (40–100 nm diameter), secreted by many cell types; they contain many protein and miRNA biomarkers to distinguish cancer from normal patients, and can influence the immune response against tumors |
| Oncosomes | Large vesicles | B, U(?), PS/SF (?) | Large (1–10-$\mu$m diameter) vesicles, derived from bulky cellular protrusions in metastasizing cancer cells, which contain enzymes and RNA; they have a biological effect on endothelial cells, and fibroblasts as well as other tumor cells |
| Imaging | Intact cells | B, tissue, whole body | The ability to locate small tumors by MRI, NMR, and advanced fluorescence techniques will provide an essential addendum to previous TNM staging; development of enhancers to distinguish cancer cells essential |
| Circulating tumor cells | Intact cells | B | CTCs are cells sloughed off from tumors after the cancer has spread or has access to the bloodstream through angiogenesis; most CTCs are nonviable although there may be a small percent of CSCs |

B, blood sample; U, urinary sediment; PS/SF, prostate secretion (after massage)/seminal fluid; C, cells or tissues.

For example, the expression of proteins normally restricted to primitive undifferentiated cells such as *engrailed* has recently been proposed [9]. A more unusual marker, microseminoprotein B (MSMB)—whose presence in urine is "off" in cancer, and whose expression may be linked to genetic susceptibility, is also in trials [10]. It will be some time yet before these markers emerge from the testing stage.

**2. Secreted vesicular vehicles:** Exosomes [11] and their larger relatives oncosomes [12] have been known for some time, but their role as a depositary of genetic information and proteins has only recently been fully realized in prostate cancers. They are membrane vesicles of varying diameters, which are shed from many cell types, including cancers, leaving an imprint in body fluids such as the bloodstream (and urine) of protein microRNA, and messenger RNA from the cells in which they originated. They are more commonly secreted from rapidly turning over cancer cells. Only a rigorous examination of clinically collected fluids (in contrast to laboratory models) will prove their utility.

**3. Micro and messenger RNA:** Despite its apparent ability in a laboratory setting, it is clear that RNA can persist in the bloodstream, and that the presence of a tumor results in a unique pattern of expression. Cancer-specific signatures for microRNAs, which control the expression of whole sets of genes, have been found in cancer [13]. Perhaps more surprising is the regular isolation of cellular messenger RNA from a variety of genes, which has led to the development of diagnostic "signatures," also able to distinguish malignant disease. However, completely different gene sets were presented in these two recently published studies [14,15]. Unless there is a subtle difference in isolation technique that biases against some genes, how can two similar studies result in two very different mRNA profiles? If these issues can be resolved, and the natural reluctance of clinical laboratories to embrace nucleic acid technology, such as the PCA3 [16] which is the closest-to-clinic RNA-based diagnostic test (discovered in 1998, but only licensed 12 years later), then nucleic acid detection can make a real impact diagnostically.

**4. Circulating tumor cells:** Of all the material secreted into the bloodstream (and urinary deposits in the case of bladder cancer), cells sloughed off from primary tumors, metastatic deposits, and relapsing tumors after therapy failure seem to offer the most immediate diagnostic tool. In prostate, these cells have been selected on the basis of known tumor markers. For example, using the Veridex Cellsearch system, after purging of the more prevalent hematopoietic cells, epithelial antigens such as EPCAM, low-molecular-weight cytokeratins (CK18), and androgen receptor are used to positively identify CTCs, further confirmed by the presence of a TMPRSS2–ERG fusion detected by fluorescence *in situ* hybridization [17]. At sensitivity levels of 5 CTCs/mL of venous blood, Scher *et al.* showed that it was possible to discriminate patients with frankly metastatic disease at a significance of $p<.0001$ [18]. If such assays could detect micrometastases, in the "difficult" classes of patients with small Gleason pattern 4 or border-line Gleason 3 tumors, then the real value of CTCs would be realized.

Given the relative rarity of CTCs, and the potential for contamination with cells from other sources, the cancer origins sometimes remain in doubt. Detection of the cancer-specific TMPRSS2–ERG fusion gene is one approach, but a combination with oncolytic viruses which selectively repli-cate in tumor cells could result in a traffic light system wherein the CTCs are labeled with a fluorescent marker, relative to normal and hematopoi-etic cells from blood (R. Rodriguez, Johns Hopkins, USA, personal com-munication, 2011). Should such labeling occur before (by intravenous inoculation of a tracker virus) or after biopsy/blood sample? In terms of sensitivity, the intravenous inoculation would be best, but for safety pur-poses the latter will prevail. The same technique has already been used in solid tumors as an indicator of tumor extent by injection of a labeling virus prior to surgery [19].

Equally, the precise nature of the CTCs is open to discussion. The prostate phenotype selected is equivalent to luminally differentiated fast-growing tumor cells, and not the more primitive phenotype of tumor (and metastasis)-inducing cells. We have termed these rare cells: tumor-inducing cells (TICs) or cancer stem cells (CSCs) [20]. A recent study of CTCs in breast cancer detected this more primitive CSC phenotype in single-cell whole-genome expression profiling. Perhaps significantly, the expression profiles were totally different from the most commonly used cell line models for breast cancer therapeutic development [21].

## Genetic markers of familial and sporadic prostate cancers

Prediction of at-risk patients, who may have a familial susceptibility (between 5% and 25%) to develop prostate cancer [22] has been the aim of linkage studies for almost two decades. In general, familial cancer pre-disposes to early-onset (probably below age of 60 years) prostate cancer, and the same disease in one or more first-degree male relatives. A decreas-ing age of onset in successive generations is also significant. The first simple family trees have now been replaced by analysis of progressively more precise milestones on the human genome, starting with microsatellites, and culminating now in total genome sequencing. As the total human genome sequence can be determined for $1000, the large international consortia of multiple families can now reach statistical significance for risk factors, bringing new precision to Genome Wide Association Studies (GWAS) [23]. More recently, the existence of common, frequent prostate cancer risk genes (or alleles) has probably been disproved, unlike the BRCA genes in breast cancer, and the most recent studies are designed to identify rarer susceptibility loci [24]. If a truly applicable panel of markers is derived, then it provides the opportunity to screen early in life. With this ability to determine (a risk factor) comes an ethical responsibility. Insurance companies can already refuse cover to an older man with low Gleason grade cancer—for which the prognosis is good. If a young man inherits a panel of susceptibility loci, would he then become uninsurable too? "Genetic ethics" have failed to keep pace with the explosion in genetic technology.

## Chemoprevention

It is very appealing to think that, with our current understanding, we can prevent prostate cancer; especially as the tumor is normally considered to be a late-initiating tumor, that is, in older men. Our current thinking exploiting mathematical models and other biological techniques, including the accumulation of the necessary mutations, suggests that this may well be a false assumption, and that prostate cancer may start as early as puberty, when the large tissue expansion within the prostate occurs. The exceptional longitudinal study, based on stored serum from Sweden, also implies that elevated PSA levels, perhaps diagnostic of the very earliest stages of prostate cancer development, can be detected in men in their thirties rather than the more substantial increases in PSA seen in men in their fifties and sixties [25]. Therefore, any application of a chemoprevention may well be too late if applied at the age of 40, as some studies have recommended [26]. The early development and pre-tumor progression are indicated in Figure 17.1.

Chemical intervention such as androgen blockade may even, according to the results of the two American trials where the effects of 5-alpha-reductase inhibitors was reported, do more harm than good in some patients. Although the REDUCE and PCPT trials achieved their overall aim of reducing the prostate cancer incidence, there was an increase in both the

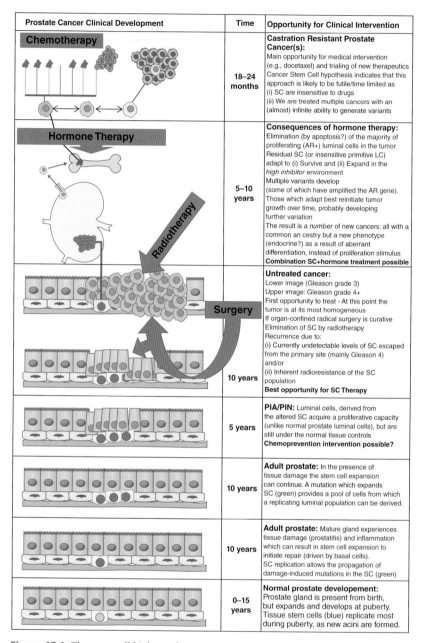

**Figure 17.1** The stem cell biology of prostate cancer treatment. We propose that the outcome of prostate cancer treatments is modified by the existence of a rare population of tissue and cancer stem cells (indicated by small cells with contrasting nuclei).

malignancy and the death rate from high-grade cancers which adopted a less differentiated high Gleason grade "morphology" [27,28]. Based on the existence of malignancy-initiating CSCs, which are impervious to androgen blockade, the latter treatment would result in an amplification of the undifferentiated cells within a cancer equivalent to the observed pathology, in more than 2000 fatal cases observed from the 25 000 men in the REDUCE/PCPT trials. The United States Food and Drug Administration (FDA) took the decision not to support finasteride and dutasteride as chemopreventives. However, we do know that these drugs are given for the medical control of benign prostatic hyperplasia. Perhaps greater care should be taken to diagnose any underlying cancers when used for this purpose.

## Heterogeneity and prostate cancer treatments

Prostate cancer treatment has altered little in strategy since the 1960s when Huggins showed that castration was an effective treatment. After this, the concept of androgen and total androgen blockage became an important part of the urologist's armory. However, it is clear that such medical treatments are almost inevitably time-limited and once relapsed, prostate cancer has a very different (neuroendocrine) nature to that which entered the treatment in the first place [29]. The same limitations probably apply to the application of standard chemotherapeutics such as cisplatin/docetaxel. Although the former shows a spectacular response in other male tumors such as germ cell tumors, in prostate cancer the responses have in general been disappointing, with the initial regression followed by an aggressive and malignant relapse.

There can be no doubt that the outcome of prostate cancer, in both treatment-naïve and advanced castration-resistant prostate cancer (CRPC) is influenced by androgens. As a result, a tremendous effort has been placed into understanding androgen signaling and in the design of novel inhibitors based on this paradigm. Among the more recent innovations, Abiraterone [30] strikes at the heart of the supply of raw materials for androgen synthesis, and is complemented by the next-generation blockade of androgen receptor activity by agents such as MDV3100 for the treatment of advanced prostate cancers [31].

However, even these sophisticated therapies only rarely offer more than a few extra months of life to the patient. There are two explanations for this: either the cells very rapidly develop a resistance to the drugs, or (based on the kinetics of response) there is a preexisting resistant CSC fraction, which can change and adapt to the post-therapy environment, as the tumor mass is being eliminated [20]. Although prostate cancer models in the laboratory are adaptable, primary human tumors are sufficiently heterogeneous to contain resistant cells, and according to our hypothesis, have a primitive-therapy-resistant phenotype similar to tissue stem cells. Whichever hypothesis is adopted, we do persist in treating prostate cancers as a monoclonal, homogeneous mass of cells. Even when proposing combination therapies, the proposal is frequently to target the same pathway in the cancer cells simultaneously or sequentially at two different points (e.g., Abiraterone and MDV3100).

Rather than deal with each individual type of prostate cancer, begining with early-stage organ-confined tumors of low Gleason grade, compared with high Gleason grade and progressing through to the highly malignant castration-resistant forms, I propose that we should adopt an overall strategy to match the genetic heterogeneity and biology of the tumor to the therapies which are applied. It makes absolute sense in biological and genetic terms to treat *early* prostate cancers with medical therapies, if such therapies were available and effective.

Current surgical treatments are effective if cancers are caught at an early stage—but at a price [32]. Radiotherapy can be extremely effective if applied to a primary lesion, but in those difficult cases where there is local capsular penetration or perhaps localized spread to lymph nodes, our success rates with the latter two strategies, although improving, still leave much to be desired. In those extreme cases where the patient presents with high-grade locally advanced disease with spread to the lymph nodes, it appears as if there is little we can do except to prolong life. Some of the current new medicines in the clinic, together with their rather modest survival advantages, are listed in Table 17.2. How then can genetics and biology help promote a new generation of prostate cancer treatments?

## Should biology drive treatment strategies rather than vice versa?

Our laboratory has pioneered a new approach to the heterogeneity of responses seen in the treatment of prostate cancers. The hypothesis derives from the existence of cells within many tumor types which have unique properties (see Table 17.3), the most notable of which is an enhanced

**Table 17.2** Some new treatments for prostate cancer

| Treatment | Disease stage | Median/mean survival (months) | Placebo/*SOC* comparator | Therapeutic advantage (months) |
|---|---|---|---|---|
| Docetaxel (2004) | CRPC (TAX327) | 18.9 | *16.4* | 2.5 |
| Abiraterone (2008–2011) | CRPC (COU-AA-301) | 14.8 | 11.2 months | 3.6 |
| Provenge (2010) | CRPC (SELECT) | 25.8 | 21.7 months | 4.1 |
| MDV3100 (2011) | CRPC (AFFIRM) | 18.4 | 13.6 months | 4.8 |
| Radium-223 chloride (2011) | CRPC (Bone) (ALSYMPCA) | 14 | 11 months | 3 |

Note: Survival with placebo shown in standard type while survival with SOC shown in italics.
SOC, standard of care.

**Table 17.3** Properties of cancer stem cells

| Cancer stem cell property | Stem cell characteristics | Cancer characteristics |
|---|---|---|
| Can reconstitute the original tumor at another site in the patient, by surviving outside the prostate | ✓ | ✓ |
| Shows relative resistance to chemo- and radiotherapies | ✓ | ✓ |
| Is responsible for tumor regeneration after injury | ✓ | ✓ |
| Can divide for the lifetime of the tumor/host organism | ✓ | ✓ |
| Divides asymmetrically to produce another SC and a progenitor which replenishes the tumor mass | ✓ | ✗ |
| Constitutes a small fraction of the tissue/tumor cells | ✓ | ✓ |
| Quiescent (silent and static) or slowly proliferating | ✓ | ✗ |
| Displays properties and appearance quite different from the rest of the cells in a tumor | ✓ | ✗ |
| Can differentiate to produce a lineage of other differentiated cell types: including those we currently recognize as "prostate cancer" | ✓ | ✗ |
| Can maintain its population independently of input from other cell populations | ✓ | ✓ |
| Can invade and penetrate the prostate capsule/blood vessels and lymphatics: resulting in metastasis | ✗ | ✓ |

ability to initiate new tumors compared with the rest of the cells, which constitute the majority of the cells in a tumor. Since our identification of these cells *in vitro* and *in vivo*, we now know much more about the genes which they express and can begin to formulate ideas about how to treat them. The development of *stem cell therapies* has been covered elsewhere [33], but assuming that they can be developed, how could this hypothesis influence our treatment decisions for prostate cancer?

As outlined diagrammatically in Figure 17.1, we can divide tumor (and prostate) development into a series of somewhat artificial stages. Using stem cell, or even the historical stochastic models of tumor resistance development, it is clear that by the time we are most actively treating the cancer by means other than surgery, we are dealing with a cancer which has developed into a number of variants, still rooted in the original cancer, but with multiple genetic variants [34], *selected* by the treatments applied. Since cells have multiple means to develop drug resistance, and many pathways to achieve excessive growth and inhibition of cell death, a drug-resistant tumor could be derived by activating one of these mechanisms. As the stem cells in cancer are quiescent [35], and do not express many of the proliferative and differentiation-associated antigens present in prostate cancers, they can act as a reservoir for selection of new resistant tumor clones. New "resistance" mutations (which require a round of cell division to become established in a population) may even be promoted by the temporary release of quiescence, induced by the therapies, in a similar manner to the expansion of tissue stem cells in normal skin as a response to wounding, that is, the chemotherapy- and radiotherapy-induced damage to the bulk tumor cells.

If we assume that CRPC (top box in Figure 17.1) is indeed a multiplicity of cancers, then it is indeed surprising that our therapies have any effect at all, let alone the ability to achieve a cure. We can still achieve tumor shrinkage, but variants emerge all too rapidly. Surgically, if every man had his prostate removed by the age of 30, then we could probably eliminate the tumor: an overtreatment, but elective surgical mastectomies are carried out in women with high breast cancer risk. In our experiments, we have shown that the CSC population in prostate (like some other tumors) is remarkably resistant to radiotherapy, but that high doses of radiation are just as cytotoxic to the CSCs as to the bulk tumor. The approach here must be to better visualize and target the tumor, assuming that there has been no early spread from the primary tumor. Our increasing knowledge of the type of mutations found in real tumors (compared with cancer cell lines, which contain multiple cell-culture-induced changes) suggests that genetic changes predisposing to metastatic spread may be present at a very early stage, and certainly that relatively few "good" (i.e., low grade) prostate cancers develop into metastatic disease, as suggested by the colon cancer paradigm more than 20 years ago [36]. The key transition is from pre-malignancy (prostatic inflammatory atrophy (PIA) or prostatic intraepithelial neoplasia (PIN)) to cancer.

Next, if we are to treat the tumor medically, then either a combination of agents to eliminate both the bulk tumor (a replicating luminal-like cell mass) *and* the underlying (undifferentiated) cancer stem cell population must be used, or agents to block different signaling pathways should be used. Will the proposed combinations of androgen response inhibitors be successful? In the short term they may enhance PSA responses, but will probably suffer the same fate as previous total androgen blockades in the longer term, that is relapse and emergence of an altered tumor type.

The timing of application of such combinations is also critical (Figure 17.2, Plate 17.2). A cytoreductive agent, which results in the stimulation of an SC response, could be applied in advance of the anti-CSC agent. The primary application of an anti-CSC drug is unlikely to have any effect at all on either tumor mass or PSA responses (and would be treated as a failure), although it may restrict the establishment of new tumors by removing circulating CSCs. Therefore, small molecules with tumor-penetrating properties would be needed, but a combination of agents to disrupt tumor structure followed by, for example, a cytotoxic antibody or similar reagent to target the stem cells within the tumor could be equally effective.

Another prospect which we have recently raised is the application of nontoxic (or at least the use at nontoxic doses) of differentiating agents such as retinoic acid which acts to push stem cells toward a more treatable cell type, which can then be killed with our current agents [37]. These lower doses of a "fate-modifying" drug would have precisely the opposite effect to a normal anticancer agent, when the PSA response is measured. As we are *increasing* the number of PSA-secreting luminal cells, by differentiating the precursors, then the initial PSA levels would *rise*, but a more prolonged nadir after secondary treatment is predicted: together with a longer-lasting tumor response. In the past, agents such as retinoic acid have been used over a vast concentration range in small trials, as toxins, and were also classed as failures.

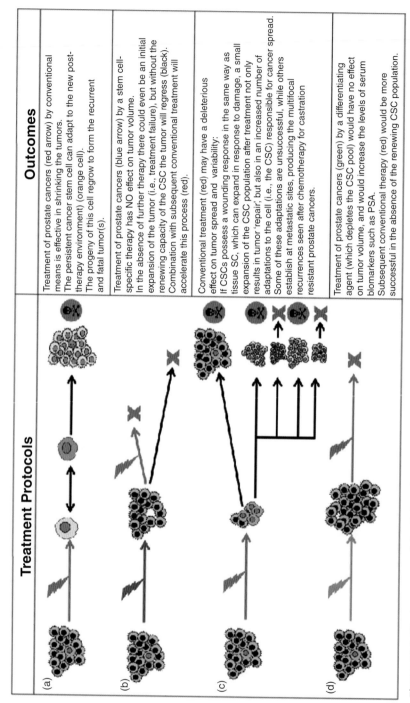

**Figure 17.2** The importance of the timing of treatments to account for the existence of cancer stem cells. (See also Plate 17.2.)

## Treatment Protocols

## Outcomes

(a) Treatment of prostate cancers (red arrow) by conventional means is effective in shrinking the tumors.
The persistent cancer stem cell can adapt to the new post-therapy environment (orange cell).
The progeny of this cell regrow to form the recurrent and fatal tumor(s).

(b) Treatment of prostate cancers (blue arrow) by a stem cell-specific therapy has NO effect on tumor volume.
In the absence of further therapy there could even be an initial expansion of the tumor (i.e., treatment failure), but without the renewing capacity of the CSC the tumor will regress (black).
Combination with subsequent conventional treatment will accelerate this process (red).

(c) Conventional treatment (red) may have a deleterious effect on tumor spread and variability:
If CSCs possess a wounding response in the same way as tissue SC, which can expand in response to damage, a small expansion of the CSC population after treatment not only results in tumor 'repair', but also in an increased number of adaptations to the cell (i.e., the CSC) responsible for cancer spread. Some of these adaptations are unsuccessful, while others establish at metastatic sites, producing the multifocal recurrences seen after chemotherapy for castration resistant prostate cancers.

(d) Treatment of prostate cancers (green) by a differentiating agent (which depletes the CSC pool) would have no effect on tumor volume, and would increase the levels of serum biomarkers such as PSA.
Subsequent conventional therapy (red) would be more successful in the absence of the renewing CSC population.

# Conclusions: how soon will the future come?

To a biologist, the ability to put ideas and experimental results into clinical practice remains surprisingly difficult, and the time to the clinic for any new therapy is frustratingly (in the light of the European Clinical Trial Directive) lengthy. Many cancer treatments, developed in the few prostate cancer cell lines available to the pharmaceutical industry, perform poorly in man. Is this the result of a poor agent, or a poor preclinical testing system?

I would argue that our best testing system is in man, and that biology is failing the efforts of the drug design chemists in this regard. However, an unwavering persistence with cell replication inhibition (tumor shrinkage) and serum PSA decrease as preferred endpoints is equally short-sighted. Given the discussion in the previous section, and the information in Figure 17.2, short-term tumor shrinkage could occur at the expense of the derivation of new CSC derivatives, which are both malignant and resistant to chemotherapies. Thus, a deeper knowledge of the biology is required. We have an immediate opportunity to take the first steps in this by looking carefully at trial design, which only rarely involves nonclinical academics. We now know from DNA sequencing studies that each patient's tumor is somehow different at the genome level, but has solved its primary biological tasks, that is, an ability to survive and grow in spite of physiological/immunological control, in an individual way. This implies that every patient requires his own medicine—or combination of medicines! The natural evolution of this is the current moves to develop biologically/genetically stratified trials, where patient susceptibility is assessed prior to entry, giving the best opportunity for success [38]. A further advance might be to conduct parallel trials in the laboratory on harvested tumor material from patients under treatment: could this approach predict outcome more rapidly and allow tailoring of treatments more precisely?

Finally, as implied in Figure 17.2, there is a serious restriction on the use of new agents in patients for whom there is an established treatment. The application of monotherapy drug treatments (beyond phase I for toxicity) in CRPC patients is genetically flawed, as we would be treating multiple cancers and not one at this point. The overall survival figures (not the changes in survival) almost certainly reflect this. We can only advance treatments by expanding the patient pool back down the progression chart to the point where the initiating cell pool is more homogeneous.

The need for such new approaches has never been greater, as our ability to diagnose prostate cancers in an ageing population continues to increase.

## Acknowledgments

I thank all the members of the YCR Cancer Research Unit, in York, and Yorkshire Cancer Research for their continuing support for my biological research on prostate cancer.

## References

1 Vickers AJ, Roobol MJ, Lilja H. Screening for prostate cancer: early detection or overdetection? *Ann Rev Med* 2012;63:161–170.
2 Gleason DF. Histologic grading of prostate cancer: a perspective. *Hum Pathol* 1992;23(3):273–279.
3 Epstein JI. An update of the Gleason grading system. *J Urol* 2010;183(2):433–440.
4 True L, Coleman I, Hawley S, *et al.* A molecular correlate to the Gleason grading system for prostate adenocarcinoma. *Proc Natl Acad Sci U S A* 2006;103(29):10991–10996.
5 Browne TJ, Hirsch MS, Brodsky G, *et al.* Prospective evaluation of AMACR (P504S) and basal cell markers in the assessment of routine prostate needle biopsy specimens. *Hum Pathol* 2004;35(12):1462–1468.
6 Pan MH, Gao DW, Feng J, *et al.* Biodistributions of 177Lu- and 111In-labeled 7E11 antibodies to prostate-specific membrane antigen in xenograft model of prostate cancer and potential use of 111In-7E11 as a pre-therapeutic agent for 177Lu-7E11 radioimmunotherapy. *Mol Imaging Biol* 2009;11(3):159–166.
7 You J, Cozzi P, Walsh B, *et al.* Innovative biomarkers for prostate cancer early diagnosis and progression. *Crit Rev Oncol Hematol* 2010;73(1):10–22.
8 Peltola MT, Niemela P, Alanen K, *et al.* Immunoassay for the discrimination of free prostate-specific antigen (fPSA) forms with internal cleavages at Lys((1)(4)(5)) or Lys((1)(4)(6)) from fPSA without internal cleavages at Lys((1)(4)(5)) or Lys((1)(4)(6)). *J Immunol Methods* 2011;369(1–2):74–80.
9 Pandha H, Sorensen KD, Orntoft TF, *et al.* Urinary engrailed-2 (EN2) levels predict tumour volume in men undergoing radical prostatectomy for prostate cancer. *BJU Int* 2012;110(6 Pt B):E287–E292.
10 Whitaker HC, Kote-Jarai Z, Ross-Adams H, *et al.* The rs10993994 risk allele for prostate cancer results in clinically relevant changes in microseminoprotein-beta expression in tissue and urine. *PLoS ONE* 2010;5(10):e13363.
11 Mitchell PJ, Welton J, Staffurth J, *et al.* Can urinary exosomes act as treatment response markers in prostate cancer? *J Transl Med* 2009;7:4.
12 Di Vizio D, Kim J, Hager MH, *et al.* Oncosome formation in prostate cancer: association with a region of frequent chromosomal deletion in metastatic disease. *Cancer Res.* 2009;69(13):5601–5609.

13  Selth LA, Tilley WD, Butler LM. Circulating microRNAs: macro-utility as markers of prostate cancer? *Endocr Relat Cancer* 2012;19(4):R99–R113.

14  Olmos D, Brewer D, Clark J, *et al.* Prognostic value of blood mRNA expression signatures in castration-resistant prostate cancer: a prospective, two-stage study. *Lancet Oncol* 2012;13(11):1114–1124.

15  Ross RW, Galsky MD, Scher HI, *et al.* A whole-blood RNA transcript-based prognostic model in men with castration-resistant prostate cancer: a prospective study. *Lancet Oncol* 2012;13(11):1105–1113.

16  Aubin SM, Reid J, Sarno MJ, *et al.* Prostate cancer gene 3 score predicts prostate biopsy outcome in men receiving dutasteride for prevention of prostate cancer: results from the REDUCE trial. *Urology* 2011;78(2):380–385.

17  Attard G, Swennenhuis JF, Olmos D, *et al.* Characterization of ERG, AR and PTEN gene status in circulating tumor cells from patients with castration-resistant prostate cancer. *Cancer Res* 2009;69(7):2912–2918.

18  Scher HI, Jia X, de Bono JS, *et al.* Circulating tumour cells as prognostic markers in progressive, castration-resistant prostate cancer: a reanalysis of IMMC38 trial data. *Lancet Oncol* 2009;10(3):233–239.

19  Adusumilli PS, Stiles BM, Chan MK, *et al.* Real-time diagnostic imaging of tumors and metastases by use of a replication-competent herpes vector to facilitate minimally invasive oncological surgery. *FASEB J* 2006;20(6):726–728.

20  Maitland NJ, Collins AT. Prostate cancer stem cells: a new target for therapy. *J Clin Oncol* 2008;26(17):2862–2870.

21  Navin N, Kendall J, Troge J, *et al.* Tumour evolution inferred by single-cell sequencing. *Nature* 2011;472(7341):90–94.

22  Goh CL, Schumacher FR, Easton D, *et al.* Genetic variants associated with predisposition to prostate cancer and potential clinical implications. *J Intern Med* 2012;271(4):353–365.

23  Jin G, Lu L, Cooney KA, *et al.* Validation of prostate cancer risk-related loci identified from genome-wide association studies using family-based association analysis: evidence from the International Consortium for Prostate Cancer Genetics (ICPCG). *Hum Genet* 2012;131(7):1095–1103.

24  Kote-Jarai Z, Olama AA, Giles GG, *et al.* Seven prostate cancer susceptibility loci identified by a multi-stage genome-wide association study. *Nat Genet* 2011;43(8):785–791.

25  Vickers AJ, Cronin AM, Bjork T, *et al.* Prostate specific antigen concentration at age 60 and death or metastasis from prostate cancer: case-control study. *BMJ* 2010;341:c4521.

26  Lilja H, Cronin AM, Dahlin A, *et al.* Prediction of significant prostate cancer diagnosed 20 to 30 years later with a single measure of prostate-specific antigen at or before age 50. *Cancer* 2011;117(6):1210–1219.

27  Crawford ED, Andriole GL, Marberger M, Rittmaster RS. Reduction in the risk of prostate cancer: future directions after the Prostate Cancer Prevention Trial. *Urology* 2010;75(3):502–509.

28  Andriole GL, Bostwick DG, Brawley OW, *et al.* Effect of dutasteride on the risk of prostate cancer. *N Engl J Med* 2010;362(13):1192–1202.

29  Abrahamsson PA. Neuroendocrine cells in tumour growth of the prostate. *Endocr Relat Cancer* 1999;6(4):503–519.

30  de Bono JS, Logothetis CJ, Molina A, *et al.* Abiraterone and increased survival in metastatic prostate cancer. *N Engl J Med* 2011;364(21):1995–2005.

31  Scher HI, Beer TM, Higano CS, *et al.* Antitumour activity of MDV3100 in castration-resistant prostate cancer: a phase 1-2 study. *Lancet* 2010;375(9724):1437–1446.

32  Schroder FH, Hugosson J, Roobol MJ, *et al.* Prostate-cancer mortality at 11 years of follow-up. *N Engl J Med* 2012;366(11):981–990.

33  Maitland NJ, Collins AT. Cancer stem cells – a therapeutic target? *Curr Opin Mol Ther* 2010;12(6):662–673.

34  Baca SC, Prandi D, Lawrence MS, *et al.* Punctated evolution of prostate cancer genomes. *Cell* 2013;153(3):666–677.

35  Moore N, Lyle S. Quiescent, slow-cycling stem cell populations in cancer: a review of the evidence and discussion of significance. *J Oncol* 2011;2011.

36  Fearon ER, Vogelstein B. A genetic model for colorectal tumorigenesis. *Cell* 1990;61(5):759–767.

37  Rane J, Pellacani D, Maitland NJ. Advanced prostate cancer: a case for adjuvant differentiation therapy. *Nat Rev Urol* 2012;9(10):595–602.

38  Trusheim MR, Burgess B, Hu SX, *et al.* Quantifying factors for the success of stratified medicine. *Nat Rev Drug Discov* 2011;10(11):817–833.

# Index

Note: Page number followed by f and t denotes figure and table respectively.

*Prostate Cancer: Diagnosis and Clinical Management*, First Edition.
Edited by Ashutosh K. Tewari, Peter Whelan and John D. Graham.
© 2014 John Wiley & Sons, Ltd. Published 2014 by John Wiley & Sons, Ltd.